Pocketbook
Seventh Edition

From the publishers of the *Tarascon Pocket Pharmacopoeia*

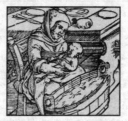

Prashant Mahajan, MD, MPH, MBA
Professor of Emergency Medicine and Pediatrics
Vice-Chair, Department of Emergency Medicine
Section Chief, Pediatric Emergency Medicine
University of Michigan
C. S. Mott Children's Hospital of Michigan

JONES & BARTLETT
LEARNING

World Headquarters
Jones & Bartlett Learning
5 Wall Street
Burlington, MA 01803
978-443-5000
info@jblearning.com
www.jblearning.com

Jones & Bartlett Learning books and products are available through most bookstores and online booksellers. To contact Jones & Bartlett Learning directly, call 800-832-0034, fax 978-443-8000, or visit our website, www.jblearning.com.

Substantial discounts on bulk quantities of Jones & Bartlett Learning publications are available to corporations, professional associations, and other qualified organizations. For details and specific discount information, contact the special sales department at Jones & Bartlett Learning via the above contact information or send an email to specialsales@jblearning.com.

19396-1

Production Credits
VP, Product Management: Amanda Martin
Director of Product Management: Matthew Kane
Product Manager: Joanna Gallant
Product Assistant: Melina Leon, Emmy Boes
Project Specialist: Jennifer Risden
Digital Project Specialist: Angela Dooley
Sr. Marketing Manager: Lindsay White
Product Fulfillment Manager: Wendy Kilborn
Composition: S4Carlisle Publishing Services
Project Management: S4Carlisle Publishing Services
Cover Design: Michael O'Donnell
Media Development Editor: Troy Liston
Rights & Media Specialist: John Rusk
Cover Image (Title Page): Courtesy of the U.S. National Library of Medicine
Printing and Binding: Cenveo

Library of Congress Cataloging-in-Publication Data

Names: Mahajan, Prashant (Professor of pediatric emergency medicine),
    author. I Rothrock, Steven G. Tarascon pediatric emergency pocketbook.
Title: Tarascon pediatric emergency pocketbook / Prashant Mahajan.
Other titles: Pediatric emergency pocketbook
Description: Seventh edition. I Burlington, MA : Jones & Bartlett Learning,
    [2021] I Preceded by Tarascon pediatric emergency pocketbook / by Steven
    G. Rothrock. 6th ed. c2011. I Includes bibliographical references and index. I
Identifiers: LCCN 2019043386 I ISBN 9781284193961 (paperback)
Subjects: MESH: Emergency Treatment--methods I Pediatric Emergency
    Medicine--methods I Handbook
Classification: LCC RJ370 I NLM WS 39 I DDC 618.92/0025--dc23
LC record available at https://lccn.loc.gov/2019043386

6048

Printed in the United States of America
24 23 22 21 20   10 9 8 7 6 5 4 3 2 1

CONTENTS

Contents

Jason Miller, MD, Fellow, Department of Pediatrics, Division of Pediatric Emergency Medicine, Children's Hospital of Michigan, Detroit, MI

Aditi Mitra, MD, Fellow, Department of Emergency Medicine, Division of Pediatric Emergency Medicine, University of Michigan, Ann Arbor, MI

Jennifer Noble, MD, Assistant Professor, Department of Pediatrics, Division of Pediatric Emergency Medicine, Children's Hospital of Michigan, Detroit, MI

Nehal Patel, MD, Fellow, Department of Pediatrics, Division of Pediatric Emergency Medicine, Children's Hospital of Michigan, Detroit, MI

Yagnaram Ravichandran, MD, Attending Physician, Pediatric Emergency Medicine, Dayton Children's Hospital, Dayton, OH

Natalie Schellpfeffer, MD, Assistant Professor, Department of Emergency Medicine, Division of Pediatric Emergency Medicine, University of Michigan, Ann Arbor, MI

Melissa Skaugset, MD, Director of Quality & Safety, Department of Emergency Medicine, Mary Bridge Children's Hospital, Tacoma, WA

Emily Supenia, PharmD, BCPS, Clinical Pharmacist—Emergency Medicine, Department of Pharmacy, University of Michigan, Ann Arbor, MI

Karen Szczepanski, MD, Clinical Staff Physician, Department of Pediatrics, Division of Pediatric Emergency Medicine, Cincinnati Children's Hospital Medical Center, Cincinnati, OH

Sarah Tomlinson, MD, Assistant Professor, Department of Emergency Medicine, Division of Pediatric Emergency Medicine, University of Michigan, Ann Arbor, MI

Elizabeth VanWert, PharmD, BCPS, Clinical Pharmacist—Emergency Medicine, Department of Pharmacy, University of Michigan, Ann Arbor, MI

Margaret Wolff, MD, MHPE, Associate Professor, Department of Emergency Medicine, Division of Pediatric Emergency Medicine, University of Michigan, Ann Arbor, MI

Angela Zamarripa, MD, Assistant Professor, Department of Emergency Medicine, Spectrum Health, Michigan State University, Grand Rapids, MI

ABBREVIATIONS

bid	twice per day	**IV**	intravenous
BP	blood pressure	**J**	joules
cm	centimeters	**kg**	kilogram
CNS	central nervous system	**m²**	square meter
CSF	cerebrospinal fluid	**mcg**	micrograms
dl	deciliter	**mEq**	milliequivalent
D₅W	5% dextrose in H₂O (D₁₀W, 10% dextrose; D₂₅W, 25% dextrose; D₅₀W, 50% dextrose)	**ml**	milliliters
		mm	millimeters
		ms	milliseconds
		NS	normal saline
ET	endotracheal	**O₂**	oxygen
F	French	**PO**	by mouth
g	grams	**PMN**	neutrophil
Hb	hemoglobin	**PR**	by rectum
HR	heart rate	**prn**	as needed
ICP	intracranial pressure	**RR**	respiratory rate
Ig	immunoglobulin	**SC**	subcutaneous
IM	intramuscular		

1 ■ ABUSE (NONACCIDENTAL TRAUMA)

ABUSE (NONACCIDENTAL TRAUMA)

SUSPECT IF:

1. **History:** Delay in seeking care, inconsistent stories, inappropriate affect of caregivers, pattern of injury does not match history.
2. **Pattern of Injury:**
   - **Bruising:**
     - If present on any region in infants <4 months of age or in a child that is not mobile
     - If located on neck, ear, torso, genitalia, buttocks in a child <4 years of age
     - If shape of causative agent is maintained, typically hand/finger markings, buckle, belt, looped cord, spatula, cigarette or car cigarette lighter, hanger, kitchen utensil or teeth[1]
   - **Burns:**
     - If there are clear demarcation lines; these are seen in immersion injuries
     - If the splash-burn injury is not consistent with the developmental age of the child
     - If the scald is of uniform depth, has sharply delineated borders, if flexures are spared, if there is involvement of buttocks, perineum and lower limbs, if there is a glove or stocking distribution, or if there is symmetrical distribution
   - **Cold injuries:** If the child presents with signs of cold injuries or hypothermia with no obvious medical explanation
3. **Fractures:** Long bone fractures especially in a child that is not walking
     - Fractures in children <18 months
     - Multiple fractures at one time and/or at different stages of healing
     - Rib fracture in the absence of major injury, birth trauma, or underlying bone disease
     - Scapula, skull, and sternum fractures
     - Avulsion fracture of clavicle or acromion
     - Metaphyseal corner fractures, bucket handle fractures
     - Spinal fractures
     - Fractures on either side of the spine and close to the sternum (shaken baby)
4. **Intracranial injuries:** If multiple hemorrhages over convexity of brain or, in interhemispheric fissures or, if hypoxic ischemic injury or, if associated with retinal hemorrhages

5. **Visceral injuries:** In the absence of major accidental trauma or unsuit-
   able explanation
6. **Oral injury:** Frenular tear highly suspicious

Because the history is unreliable and physical examination findings are not
sensitive, abusive head trauma (AHT) is notoriously difficult to diagnose and
the consequences of missing AHT can be devastating. The neurological examination is tremendously limited in children <1-year-old, and AHT is more
common than anyone likes to think. The Pittsburg Infant Brain Injury Score is
a clinical predictor rule developed to help clinicians consider AHT as a cause
of an infant's presenting symptoms. This should be considered in infants who
present with a brief, resolved, unexplained event (BRUE), emesis (>4 episodes) without diarrhea, seizures, scalp swelling, bruising, lethargy, or other
neurologic symptoms. The 5-point clinical prediction rule includes: abnormal
skin exam (2 points); age≥3 months (1 point); head circumference >85th
percentile (1 point); and serum hemoglobin <11.2 g/dl (1 point). Using a
prediction rule cut-off score of 2 points yielded sensitivity of 93%, specificity of 53%, and positive predictive value of 39% for abnormal neuroimaging.
Clinicians should also measure hemoglobin and obtain a head circumference
to help make their decision. Head CT or MRI should be routinely used in these
children who meet the above criteria.[2,3]

Suspect sexual abuse: If a girl or boy has genital/anal lesion without any
explanation or if there is associated genital symptoms with behavioral or emo-
tional changes. If there is anal fissure or gaping anus with no medical explanation. If there are one or more foreign bodies in vagina or anus.

Consider sexual abuse: If a child younger than 13 years has Hepatitis B or
anogenital warts or sexually transmitted infections like gonorrhea, chlamydia,
syphilis, genital herpes, hepatitis C, HIV, or trichomonas infection and there is
no evidence of mother to child transmission during birth or nonsexual transmission from a member of the household. Consider sexual abuse if the above
mentioned symptoms are seen in older children from nonconsensual sexual
activity, or if the relationship is incestuous, or is with a person in a position of
trust, or if there is clear difference in mental capacity between the young person
and their sexual partner.

Table 1-1 Appearances of Bruises Over Time

- Bruises of any color (red, blue, purple, yellow, green, gray) can occur at any time.
- Evidence for accurately dating bruises is lacking.
- Abuse should be suspected if injuries occur over nonbony prominences such as
  ears, neck, face, hands, back, buttocks, forearm, foot, and abdomen, especially in
  children <4 years, or if the mechanism does not fit the injury pattern.

Modified from Maguire S, Mann M. Systematic reviews of bruising in relation to child abuse—what have we
learnt: an overview of review updates. *Evid Based Child Health.* 2013;8(2):255-263.

Table 1-2 Bony Injuries Associated with Child Abuse

Fractures associated with a high or moderate specificity for abuse	• Rib fractures (especially posteromedial have highest probability of abuse), scapular fractures, sternal fractures • Metaphyseal-epiphyseal fractures [e.g., corner fractures (bucket-handle fractures), metaphyseal lucency] • Spinous process, vertebral body fractures, and subluxations • Fractures in different stages of healing or delayed presentation • Fractures inconsistent with history or developmental age • Skull fractures—if multiple, bilateral, or cross suture lines • Pelvic fractures (rare) or spine fractures without significant force • Femur fractures in nonambulatory patients • Midshaft humeral fractures ≤1–2 years old
Fractures associated with a low specificity for abuse	• Clavicle fractures due to birth (infants <22 days or infants <30 days with a healing fracture) • Distal tibia spiral fractures (toddler's fracture), unless nonambulatory • Supracondylar fractures, fractures of the hands or feet (except digital fractures in nonambulatory infants or multiple fractures) • Torus fractures of long bones

Modified from Kemp A, Dunstan F, Harrison S, et al. Patterns of skeletal fractures in child abuse: systematic review. *BMJ.* 2008;337:a1518; Borg K, Hodes D. Guidelines for skeletal survey in young children with fractures. *Arch Dis Child Educ Pract Ed.* 2015;100:253-256; Flaherty EG, Perez-Rossello JM, Levine MA, et al. Evaluating children with fractures for child physical abuse. *Pediatrics.* 2014;133:e477-e489.

Table 1-3 Appearances of Fractures Over Time

Age of fracture	Fracture appearance
4–10 days	Resolution of soft-tissue swelling
10–14 days	New periosteal bone
14–21 days	Fracture line definition lost and soft callus present
21–42 days	Hard callous present
2–24 months	Remodeling of fracture

Table 1-4 Head Injury Associated with Abuse

- Subdural hematoma
- Extra-axial hemorrhages (esp. interhemispheric, multiple bleeds, or in posterior fossa)
- Parenchymal brain injury (e.g., contusion, axonal injury, laceration)
- Retinal hemorrhage (usually bilateral)

Modified from Kemp AM. Abusive head trauma: recognition and the essential investigation. *Arch Dis Child Educ Pract Ed.* 2011;96(6):202-208; Choudhary AK, Servaes S, Slovis TL, et al. Consensus statement on abusive head trauma in infants and young children. *Pediatr Radiol.* 2018;48(8):1048-1065.

REFERENCES

1. Pierce MC, Kaczor K, Aldridge S, O'Flynn J, Lorenz DJ. Bruising characteristics discriminating physical child abuse from accidental trauma. *Pediatrics.* 2010;125(1):67-74.
2. Berger RP, Fromkin J, Herman B, et al. Validation of the Pittsburgh infant brain injury score for abusive head trauma. *Pediatrics.* 2016;138(1). doi:10.1542/peds.2015-3756.
3. Hymel KP, Armijo-Garcia V, Foster R, et al. Validation of a clinical prediction rule for pediatric abusive head trauma. *Pediatrics.* 2014;134(6):e1537-e1544.

2 ■ ADVANCED LIFE SUPPORT

VITALS AND RESUSCITATION EQUIPMENT

Table 2-1 Age-Based Estimates for Vital Signs and Weight

Age	Weight (kg)	Heart rate[1] BPM*	Respiratory rate/minute	Systolic BP[2] mm Hg	Diastolic BP[2] mm Hg
Premature	1	145	~ 40	42 ± 10	21 ± 8
Premature	1–2	145	~ 40	40 ± 10	28 ± 8
Newborn	2–3	125	~ 40	60 ± 10	37 ± 8
1 month	4	120	24–35	80 ± 10	46 ± 16
6 months	7	130	24–35	89 ± 29	60 ± 10
1 year	10	120	20–30	96 ± 30	66 ± 25
2–3 years	12–14	115	20–30	99 ± 25	64 ± 25
4–5 years	16–18	100	20–30	99 ± 20	65 ± 20
6–8 years	20–26	100	12–25	100 ± 15	60 ± 10
10–12 years	32–42	75	12–25	110 ± 17	60 ± 10
>14 years	>50	70	12–18	118 ± 20	60 ± 10

*BPM—beats per minute.
[1]Heart rate rises 10–14 beats/minute for each 1°C rise in temperature. [2]BP—mean ± 2 standard deviations.
Modified from Thompson, M., Harnden, A., Perera, R., Mayon-White, R., Smith, L., McLeod, D., & Mant, D.
Deriving temperature and age appropriate heart rate centiles for children with acute infections. *Archives of Disease in Childhood*, 2009;94(5):361-365. doi:10.1136/adc.2008.145011

Table 2-2 Resuscitation Equipment: First Drug Dose Based on Length, Weight, or Age[1]

Age	3 months	6 months	1 year	2 years	3 years	5 years	10 years
Length (cm)	50–58	58–70	70–85	85–95	95–107	107–124	138
Weight (kg)	5–6	7–8	9–11	12–14	15–17	18–24	32
Bag mask	Infant	Infant	Child	Child	Child	Child	Adult
Oral airway	Infant	Infant	Child	Child	Child	Child	Sm[2] adult
LMA	1	1	2	2	2	2.5	3
O₂ mask	Newborn	Newborn	Peds	Peds	Peds	Adult	Adult
ET tube[3]	3–3.5	3.5–4	3.5–4	4–4.5	4.5	5	6–6.5
Laryngoscope	1 Miller	1 Miller	1 Miller	2 Miller	2[4]	2[4]	2–3[4]
Suction catheter	8F	8F	8–10F	10F	10F	10F	10F
NG tube	5–8F	5–8F	8–10F	10F	10–12F	12–14F	16–18F
Urine catheter	5–8F	5–8F	8–10F	10F	10–12F	10–12F	12–14F

(Continued)

Table 2-2 Resuscitation Equipment: First Drug Dose Based on Length, Weight, or Age[1] (*Continued*)

Age	3 months	6 months	1 year	2 years	3 years	5 years	10 years
Length (cm)	50–58	58–70	70–85	85–95	95–107	107–124	138
Weight (kg)	5–6	7–8	9–11	12–14	15–17	18–24	32
Chest tube	10–12F	12–14F	16–20F	20–24F	20–24F	24–32F	28–32F
Amiodarone	25–30	35–40	45–55	60–70	75–85	90–120	160
Ampicillin	250–300	350–400	450–550	600–700	750–850	900–1,200	1,600
Atropine	0.1–0.12	0.14–0.16	0.18–0.22	0.24–0.28	0.3–0.34	0.36–0.48	0.6
Bicarb (mEq)	5–6	7–8	9–11	12–14	15–17	18–24	32
Ceftriaxone	250–300	350–400	450–550	600–700	750–850	900–1,200	1,600
Cefotaxime	250–300	350–400	450–550	600–700	750–850	900–1,200	1,600
Defibrillator (J)	10–12	14–16	18–22	24–28	30–34	36–48	64
Dextrose (g)	5–6	7–8	9–11	12–14	15–17	18–24	32
Epinephrine	0.05–0.06	0.07–0.08	0.09–0.11	0.12–0.14	0.15–0.17	0.18–0.24	0.32
Lidocaine	5–6	7–8	9–11	12–14	15–17	18–24	32
Lorazepam	0.5–0.6	0.7–0.8	0.9–1.1	1.2–1.4	1.5–1.7	1.8–2.4	3.2
Normal saline[5]	100–120	140–160	180–220	240–280	300–340	360–480	640
Succinylcholine	10–12	14–16	14–16	18–21	15–17	18–24	32

[1]All drugs are in mg unless otherwise specified. [2]Sm—small. [3]Uncuffed (if cuffed ET tube used in child, subtract 1). [4]Miller or Macintosh. [5]Bolus in ml for hypovolemia.

CPR, NEWLY BORN

Table 2-3 CPR Maneuvers and Techniques in Newborns, Infants, and Children

Maneuver	Newly born/neonate	Infant (<1 year)	Child (1–8 years)
Open Airway	Head tilt, chin lift (jaw lift without head tilt if trauma), all ages		
Breathing Initial	May require 30–40 cm H_2O pressure	Two breaths to make chest rise	Two breaths to make chest rise
Subsequent (if no CPR)	30–60 breaths/minute	12–20 breaths/minute	12–20 breaths/minute
Subsequent (during CPR)	30–60 breaths/minute	8–10 breaths/minute	8–10 breaths/minute
Circulation[1] Check pulse	Umbilical/brachial	Brachial or femoral	Carotid
Compress at	Lower 1/3 sternum	Lower 1/3 sternum	Lower 1/3 sternum
Compress with	Two thumbs encircle chest with hands	Two thumbs encircle chest with hands	Heel of one hand

Table 2-3 CPR Maneuvers and Techniques in Newborns, Infants, and Children (*Continued*)

Maneuver	Newly born/neonate	Infant (<1 year)	Child (1–8 years)
Depth	*One-third depth of chest for all listed ages*		
Rate[2]	120/minute	100–120/minute	100–120/minute
Ratio[3,4]	3:1—interpose breaths	15:2	15:2
Foreign Body Airway Obstruction[5]	Back blows Chest thrusts	Back blows Chest thrusts	Chest thrust, back blows, or abdominal thrusts

[1]Also check for normal breathing, movement, or coughing. Gasping is not considered as breathing normally. Laypeople do not check pulse. [2]Total number of events: compressions plus breaths per minute. [3]Ratio of 3:1 in neonates with 90 compressions and 30 breaths per minute. Rescuers may consider higher ratios of 15:2 if cardiac etiology is suspected for the arrest. Coordinated CPR should be continued until HR is ≥60/minute. [4]Ratios are for two-person CPR only. [5]Only if obstruction is severe and victim is unable to make a sound. Older than age 1 year, chest thrusts transmit higher airway pressures and induce less trauma than abdominal thrusts.

Visit the following website for current recommendations: https://www.ilcor.org/consensus-2015/costr-2015-documents/

Modified from Gateway to ILCOR 2010. www.americanheart.org/ILCOR

Table 2-4 Newly Born Resuscitation

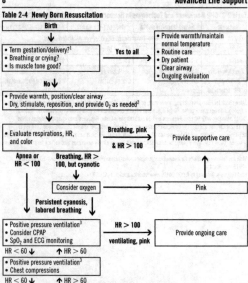

¹Meconium management: *Intrapartum*—Do not deep suction mouth, pharynx, and nose after delivery of the head. *Following delivery*—Place on mother and suction with bulb syringe and gentle cutaneous stimulation while drying recommended if vigorous infant. Immediate positive pressure ONLY if (1) depressed respirations, (2) absent or diminished muscle tone, or (3) HR < 100 beats/minute. Suctioning of the trachea before initiating positive pressure ventilation (positive pressure) is NOT recommended. ²Begin positive pressure/resuscitation with 21% FiO₂ and titrate up as required (≤ 35 weeks 25–30% FiO₂). ³Consider endotracheal (ET) intubation (ETI) if positive pressure ventilation is ineffective at this step. ETI also indicated if ineffective bag mask ventilation, chest compressions, ET medication administration, congenital diaphragmatic hernia, or birth weight < 1,000 g.

Modified from American Heart Association and American Academy of Pediatrics. 2005 American Heart Association (AHA) guidelines for cardiopulmonary resuscitation (CPR) and emergency cardiovascular care (ECC) of pediatric and neonatal patients: neonatal resuscitation guidelines. *Pediatrics.* 2006;117(5):e1029–e1038.

Table 2-5 Newly Born Resuscitation—Withholding or Discontinuing

Withhold resuscitation (Do not begin)	• Death is certain based on weight (<400 g), age < 22 weeks, or congenital anomaly incompatible with life (e.g., anencephaly, trisomy 13 or 18) • If condition with uncertain prognosis (22–24 weeks), survival borderline, high morbidity, and anticipated burden to child are high, then follow parent's wishes • Resuscitation is nearly ALWAYS indicated if high survival and acceptable morbidity (e.g., ≥ 24 weeks and most congenital malformations)
Discontinue (stop) resuscitation	• If no signs of life (no heart rate or respirations) after 10 minutes of continuous and adequate resuscitation

Modified from American Heart Association Recommendations. Visit the following website for final 2018 recommendations: Retrieved from https://eccguidelines.heart.org/circulation/cpr-ecc-guidelines/

Table 2-6 Size of Endotracheal Tube/Laryngoscope Blade for Newly Born

Gestational age	Birth weight (g)	Size of ET tube[1,2]	Blade size[3]
<28 weeks	< 1,000	2.5	Number 0 straight
28–34 weeks	1,000–2,000	2.5–3.0	Number 0 straight
34–38 weeks	2,000–3,000	3.0–3.5	Number 0 straight
>38 weeks	Term (>3,000)	3.5	Number 0–1 straight

[1] Internal diameter in millimeters. [2] Depth at gum line = Infant's nasal-tragus length (NTL) + 1 cm.
[3] Wide/fat straight blades (e.g., Wis-Hipple, Flagg) may be superior to thin (Miller) blades for manipulating normally large neonatal/infant tongues.

Table 2-7 Normal Blood Pressure for Different Birth Weights

Weight	<1 kg	1–2 kg	2–3 kg	> 3 kg
Systolic BP	40–60	50–60	50–70	50–80
Diastolic BP	15–35	20–40	25–45	30–50

Table 2-8 Apgar Scoring[1]

Sign	0	1	2
Heart rate	Absent	<100	>100
Respiratory effort	Absent	Slow/irregular	Good, cry
Muscle tone	Flaccid	Some extremity flexion	Active motion
Reflex irritability	No response	Grimace	Vigorous cry
Color	Pale	Cyanotic	Completely pink

[1] Apgar is checked at 1 and 5 minutes postdelivery. A score of 0–3 requires intense resuscitation, a score of 4–7 requires some intervention, and a score of 7–10 is normal.

GLUCOSE AND HYPOGLYCEMIA

Hypoglycemia = a blood glucose <40–45 mg/dl in neonates (<35–40 if premature). Due to inaccuracy of bedside glucose, give glucose to all neonates with bedside glucose <50 mg/dl. *Dose:* 5 to 10 ml/kg of D_{10}.

Table 2-9 Normal Arterial Blood/Hematocrit (Hct) Values in Full-Term Newly Born[1]

Age	PaO_2	$PaCO_2$	pH	Base excess	Hct (vol.%)
1 hour	63 mm Hg	36 mm Hg	7.33	−6.0 mEq/L	53
24 hours	73 mm Hg	33 mm Hg	7.37	−5.0 mEq/L	55

[1]Healthy newborns take >10 minutes to achieve a pre-ductal O_2 saturation > 95%, and up to 1 hour post-ductal.

■ Drug Therapy

IO route can be used for therapy if IV or umbilical vein unavailable.

Epinephrine—Indicated if HR < 60 after 30 seconds of effective ventilation and high-quality CPR. Dose at 0.01–0.03 mg/kg IV/IO/umbilical vein (0.1–0.3 ml/kg of 1:10,000; higher for endotracheal 0.05–0.1 mg/kg every 3–5 minutes) (0.1–0.3 ml/kg of 0.1 mg/ml) every 3–5 minutes prn. ET dose 0.05–0.1 mg/kg, 0.5–1 ml/kg; of 1 mg/ml.

Dopamine—Use if unresponsive hypotension. See Table A-2 for infusion.

Glucose—Hypoglycemia is most common in premature or small-for-gestational-age infants following a prolonged and difficult labor, mothers on ritodrine or terbutaline, and infants of mothers with diabetes. Hypoxia, hypothermia, hyperthermia, and sepsis deplete glucose stores. Treat with 5–10 ml/kg of $D_{10}W$ IV push, then infuse 6–8 ml/kg/minute.

Naloxone—0.01–0.1 mg/kg IV/ET/umbilical vein/IM/SC if severe respiratory depression and maternal narcotic administration in prior 4 hours. Caution: Naloxone may precipitate seizures if mother used narcotics chronically.

Sodium bicarbonate—Do not use unless specific circumstances or severe and refractory acidosis. 1–2 mEq/kg IV/umbilical vein of 0.5 mEq/ml solution over ≥ 2 minutes. IV push may cause venous irritation/CNS bleed.

Volume—NS or O neg blood at *10 ml/kg IV/umbilical over 5–10 minutes.* Do not use LR for fluid resuscitation.

UMBILICAL ARTERY/VEIN CATHETERIZATION

The umbilical vein is a single thin-walled vessel that is the preferred access site during newly born resuscitation. Prep abdomen/cord in a sterile manner. Loosely tie umbilical tape to cord base for anchoring/hemostasis. Cut cord with scalpel 2 cm from abdominal wall.

Umbilical vein—Remove visible clot, flush catheter with heparin. Use 3.5–4F catheter if <2 kg and 5–8F for >2 kg neonates. Advance umbilical catheter (5–8F) through vein until blood return or 4–5 cm. Lateral clavicle to umbilicus length in cm × 0.6 places catheter tip above diaphragm. Tighten umbilical tape to secure catheter and withdraw after resuscitation.

Umbilical artery—After dilating with iris forceps, insert tip of catheter to lumen. (1) Use nomogram with total body length to estimate depth; **OR** (2) for thoracic umbilical artery catheter, estimate shoulder to umbilicus (S-U) distance. If (S-U) < 13 cm, insert S-U distance + 1 cm. If S-U > 13 cm, insert to depth of S-U distance + 2 cm; **OR** (3) if birth weight < 1.5 kg insertional length = [4 × weight (kg) + 7] cm. Correct position verified by catheter position between T6 and T10 on radiography.

Modified from Wright, I. M. R., Owers, M., & Wagner, M. The umbilical arterial catheter: A formula for improved positioning in the very low birth weight infant. *Pediatric Critical Care Medicine*, 2008.9(5):498-501.

INTRAOSSEOUS (IO)

May be placed more quickly than umbilical line in critically ill, term neonates. Place IO in proximal tibia (1–2 cm distal + medial to tuberosity), distal tibia (medial malleolus; tibial shaft junction), or distal femur (as condyle tapers into shaft). After site is sterilized, puncture skin, direct needle slightly away from growth plate. Push and rotate gently until "pop" and advance 0.5–1 cm. Confirm by (1) aspiration of marrow OR (2) easy infusion of 3 ml NS with aspiration of injected fluid that returns with pink tinge. Aspirate for labs (hemoglobin, type and cross-match, electrolytes, BUN, creatinine, blood count) and infuse medications/fluid/blood with large syringe. Pressure infusion required for infusion. Any advanced life support drug or blood can be given IO. Watch for extravasation. Remove as soon as alternate access site is obtained.
See specific scenarios next.

Table 2-10 Management of the Critically Ill Neonate (≤ 28 days old)

Perform Initial Resuscitation
• Check O_2 saturation, administer 100% O_2, ventilate or intubate if needed.
• Apply cardiac monitor; assess heart rate, rhythm, perfusion, blood pressure; and examine.
• Obtain IV/IO access and administer NS (10 ml/kg in newborn, 20 ml/kg if older) if hypoperfusion (e.g., low blood pressure, altered mentation, poor skin signs) *UNLESS* congestive heart failure present (see Congestive Heart Failure, which follows).
• Check glucose, administer D_{10} (5–10 ml/kg) if <30–40 mg/dl newborn, <50 mg/dl in infant
• Labs (cultures, CBC, electrolytes, UA), ECG, CXR, and other tests (e.g., ultrasound, CT) as indicated.

Figure 2-1 Management considerations for the critically ill neonate (≤ 28 days old)

Address Following Scenarios If Present	
Scenario	**Management Considerations**
HR > 220 beats/minute →	• Cardioversion (synchronized) at 0.5–1 J/kg if shock, extreme dyspnea, or otherwise unstable • Adenosine or amiodarone (see pages 48, 336)
Congestive Heart Failure →	• Lasix 1 mg/kg IV, ± dobutamine or dopamine • See pages 52–53, 336 • See unresponsive hypoxia, which follows
Cyanosis—unresponsive *(pO₂ < 50 after 100% O₂ administration X 10 minutes)* →	• *No congestive heart failure present:* "Tet spell": knee-chest position, saline IV (if no congestive heart failure), NaHCO₃, phenylephrine, and prostaglandin E1 (see page 337) • *Congestive heart failure present:* e.g., transposition of great arteries; treat congestive heart failure (see previous), and prostaglandin E1
Acute Stridor *(intubate if needed)* →	• Consider laryngomalacia, tracheomalacia, or brainstem lesion (bilateral vocal cord paralysis)
Bilious Vomiting →	• IV fluids, NG tube, ± IV antibiotics • Surgical consult (± upper GI series after consult) • See pages 284–285
Lethargy with Recurring Hypoglycemia, or Acidosis, High Ammonia →	• IV fluids, replace glucose • Management differs with metabolic error • See pages 197–198, metabolic errors
Hypoglycemia, Low Sodium, High Potassium, ± Ambiguous Genitalia →	• IV fluids, treat hypoglycemia • Hydrocortisone 25 mg IV (draw extra blood) • See pages 69–70, adrenal crisis
Inconsistent Story (Trauma or Altered Sensorium) →	• CT head (abdomen/pelvis), skeletal survey • Manage trauma, pages 315–329 • Report to police, child protective services
Other Cases →	• Consider sepsis and administer fluids, antibiotics, vasopressors, and blood as needed

Table 2-11 Pulseless Cardiac Arrest

Provide CRP, attach monitor and defibrillator, estimate weight
using Broselow-Luten tape, and assess rhythm

VF/Pulseless VT[1]	PEA[2] or Asystole
Defibrillation[3] • Shock once at 2 J/kg or • Use AED > 1 year • **Resume CPR for 5 cycles (2 minutes)**	• **Resume CPR** • Give epi[4] IV or IO at 0.01 mg/kg (0.1 ml/kg) • Repeat every 3–5 minutes

During CPR—15 compressions and 2 breaths
for two-person CPR, secure airway and confirm
placement with waveform capnography. After
intubation perform CPR without pausing for breaths
(8–10 breaths/minute) via ET tube

Search for and treat causes of cardiac arrest:
hypovolemia, hypoxia, hydrogen ion (acidosis),
hypo/hyperkalemia, hypoglycemia, hypothermia,
toxins, tamponade, tension pneumothorax, trauma,
thrombosis (coronary or pulmonary)

If VF/pulseless VT persist after 2 minutes CPR • Shock at 4 J/kg or use AED > 1 year • Resume CPR • Give epinephrine IV/IO or ET tube	**Resume CPR** For 5 cycles (2 minutes) • If pulseless VT or VF, see VT/VF algorithm to left
After 5 cycles of CPR, recheck rhythm; if VF/pulseless VT persist: Shock once at 4–10 J/kg or use AED > 1 year **Consider one of the following:** (1) **Amiodarone** 5 mg/kg IV/IO (max 300 mg, repeat second dose if necessary) (2) **Lidocaine** 1 mg/kg IV/IO (3) **Magnesium** sulfate 25–50 mg/kg IV/IO (max 2 g) if Torsades de pointes	After meds, continue CPR for 5 cycles (2 minutes) and recheck rhythm: **If VF/pulseless VT,** resume CPR, recheck rhythm 2 minutes followed by shock and epi every 3–5 minutes and antiarrhythmics **If Asystole/PEA,** treat per PEA/asystole

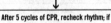

[1]VF—ventricular fibrillation; VT—ventricular tachycardia. [2]PEA—pulseless electrical activity. [3]Biphasic defibrillation is superior to monophasic. Limited evidence suggests 2 J/kg is too low a dose. May give 2–10 J/kg, not to exceed adult dose. [4]Give epinephrine (epi) every 3–5 minutes.

VASCULAR ACCESS

See pages 10–11 for techniques of umbilical vein/artery and intraosseous access, and pages 97–99 for subcutaneous fluid options (not for use during acute resuscitation).

Table 2-12 Central Venous Catheter Diameter Based on Age and Site (int. diameter-French)

Age (years)	Weight (kg)	Internal jugular vein	Subclavian vein	Femoral vein
0–0.5	3–7	3F	3F	3F
0.5–2	7–15	3F	3F	3–4F
3–6	15–25	4F	4F	4–5F
7–12	25–60	4–5F	4–5F	5–8F

Table 2-13 Right Internal Jugular and Right Subclavian (SC) Central Venous Catheter Depth (cm)[1,2]

Initial catheter insertion based on patient height/length	Height < 100 cm	Height ≥ 100 cm
	Initial Catheter Depth = Height (cm)/10 − 1 cm	Initial Catheter Depth = Height (cm)/10 − 2 cm

	Approx. age	Weight (kg)	Length/Depth (cm)
Initial catheter insertion based on patient weight (Note: Chart and formula are based on patient's weight when known, and age is only approximated based on patient's weight)	0–2 months	3.0–4.9	5
	> 2–5 months	5.0–6.9	6
	6–11 months	7.0–9.9	7
	1–2 years	10.0–12.9	8
	> 2–6 years	13.0–19.9	9
	> 6–9 years	20.0–29.9	10
	> 9–12 years	30.0–39.9	11
	> 12–14 years	40–50	12

[1]If <100 cm, puncture skin for SC vein 1 cm lateral to mid clavicle, 2 cm lateral if ≥100 cm. [2]Formulas will place 97–98% of catheters above right atrium.
Modified from Dean B. Andropoulos, The Optimal Length of Insertion of Central Venous Catheters for Pediatric Patients, *Anesthesia & Analgesia.* 2001;93(4):883-886.

Table 2-14 Femoral Vein Catheter Mean Length/Insertion Depth

Age	Weight (kg)	Height (cm)	Length (cm)	Age	Weight (kg)	Height (cm)	Length (cm)
1 month	4.2	55	15.7	2 years	12.8	88	24.2
3 months	5.8	61	17.3	4 years	16.5	103	28.1
6 months	7.8	68	19.1	6 years	20.5	116	31.4
9 months	9.2	72	20.1	8 years	26	127	34.2
1 year	10.2	76	21.1	10 years	31	137	36.8
1.5 years	11.5	83	22.9	12 years	39	149	39.9

3 ■ AIRWAY AND ANESTHESIA

AIRWAY MANAGEMENT

Table 3-1 Endotracheal Tube (ET Tube) Size and Depth, and Laryngoscope Size

Age	Laryngoscope[1]	Weight (kg)	ET tube size	ET tube depth[2]
Premature	Straight 0	1.5	2.5–3.0	8
Term	Straight 0–1	3.0	3.0–3.5	9
3 months	Straight 1	5–6	3.5	9–10
6 months	Straight 1	7–8	3.5–4.0	10
1 year	Straight 1	10	4.0–4.5	11
2 years	Straight 1	12	4.0–4.5	12–13
3 years	Miller/Macintosh 2	14	5.0	15
4 years	Miller/Macintosh 2	16	5.5	16.5
5 years	Miller/Macintosh 2	18	5.5	16.5
6–7 years	Miller/Macintosh 2	20–22	6.0	18
8–10 years	Miller/Macintosh 2	25–30	6.0–6.5	18–18.5
10–12 years	Miller/Macintosh 2	30–35	6.5	18.5
12–14 years	Miller/Macintosh 3	35–40	7.0	21

[1]Wide/fat straight blades (Wis-Hipple, Flagg) may be superior to thin (Miller) blades for manipulating normally large tongues in infants younger than 1 to 2 years old.
[2]The calculation (internal diameter × 3 cm) can be used to estimate ET tube depth (at incisors or gum line) if older than 2 years old. If younger than 2 years old, this calculation slightly overestimates ET tube depth.

ET TUBE SELECTION

- Uncuffed tube internal diameter estimate (mm) = (age in years ÷ 4) + 4.
- Cuffed tube internal diameter estimate (mm) = (age in years ÷ 4) + 3.
- Note in previous table, these formulas may overestimate tube size if younger than 2 years old.
- Use uncuffed ET tubes or low-pressure/high-volume cuffed tubes for those younger than 8 years old. If cuffed tube is used, keep inflation pressure less than 20 cm H_2O.
- See pages 5-6, and previously for age, length/weight-based estimate for ET tube size.

GLIDESCOPE (VIDEO-ASSISTED) DIFFICULT AIRWAY OPTION

A curved plastic laryngoscope blade with 60° upward angulation and video incorporated into the undersurface of its curved side allows for a better larynx view.

Technique—(1) Insert the blade down *midline* of the tongue until the glottis/vocal cords are seen; (2) insert ET tube stylet in front of the camera; (3) advance disengaged ET tube (without advancing stylet) through the glottis, into the trachea.

Table 3-2 GlideScope Video Laryngoscope (GVL) Sizes

	Age (approximate)	Weight	GVL size[1,2]
GlideScope video laryngoscope (GVL) sizes www.verathon.com	Premature–neonate	< 3.6 kg	GVL 1
	Newborn–1 year	1.8–10 kg	GVL 2
	1–18 years	10 kg to adult	GVL 3
	12 years to adult	40 kg to obese	GVL 4
	12 years to adult	40 kg to obese	GVL 5

[1]Video baton 1–2 used with GVL 1 and 2, video baton 3–4 used with GVL 3 and 4. [2]A rigid stylet (GlideRite) can be used with the GVL 3, 4, and 5 with ET tubes that have ≥6 mm internal diameter.

Table 3-3 Steps for Rapid Sequence Intubation (RSI)

Equipment
• Ready two wall-suction devices with Yankauer tips; check laryngoscope lights.
• Appropriate-size ET tube and backup 0.5 to 1 size smaller; consider stylet.
• Check integrity of cuff, if present (use no cuff or low-pressure cuff for those younger than 8 years).

Patient Preparation and Medications
• Raise bed (e.g., patient's nose at intubator's xiphoid), prepare alternate airway: jet ventilation, cricothyrotomy (older than 8 years), estimate weight (e.g., Broselow-Luten tape).
• Confirm working pulse oximeter, cardiac monitor, end-tidal CO_2 detector.
• Specify person for (1) cricoid pressure (uncertain benefit, may obstruct airway), (2) neck immobilization, (3) handling ET tube, (4) watching O_2 saturation and cardiac monitors, and (5) medications.
• Position head appropriately (sniffing position if no trauma).
• Draw up all drugs in syringes and ensure secure IV access is available.
• Preoxygenate with 100% oxygen for at least 3–4 minutes (if time permits).
• Consider lidocaine 1–1.5 mg/kg (max 100 mg) IV if head injury (however, no clear evidence that in acute traumatic injury pretreatment with lidocaine before RSI reduces ICP).
• **Atropine** 0.01 mg/kg IV (no minimum dose but max dose is 0.5 mg), use if neonate, preexisting bradycardia, or in those who receive a second dose of succinylcholine (current PALS recommendations do not include routine use and do not require a minimum dose).
• Most experts do not routinely use atropine as a defasciculating agent.
• Administer *sedating* and then *paralyzing* agent IV; apply Sellick maneuver.

Modified from de Caen AR, Berg MD, Chameides L, et al. Part 12: Pediatric advanced life support: 2015 American Heart Association guidelines update for cardiopulmonary resuscitation and emergency cardiovascular care. *Circulation.* 2015;132(18 Suppl 2):S526–S542.

Table 3-4 Drugs for Rapid Sequence Intubation

Agent	Dose IV (mg/kg)	Onset (minutes)	Key properties
Defasciculating drug—for use if using succinylcholine as paralytic			Not recommended in children by most experts (esp. younger than 5 years)
Rocuronium	0.06–0.1	2–3	
Vecuronium	0.01	3	Minimal tachycardia
Sedating drug			
Etomidate	0.3–0.4	<1	Minimal blood pressure effect
Fentanyl	2–6 mcg/kg	1–2	↑ ICP, chest wall rigidity
Ketamine	1–2	<1	↑ BP, ↑ ICP, ↑ GI, and eye pressure
Midazolam	0.1–0.2	1–3	Hypotension
Thiopental	3–5	<1	Hypotension, bronchospasm
Paralyzing drug			
Rocuronium[1,2]	0.6–1.2	0.5–1.5	*Esmeron*, rapid onset, lasts 25–60 minutes
Succinylcholine[3]	1–2	<1	Fasciculation ↑ BP, ICP, GI, eye pressures, malignant hyperthermia, hyperkalemia
Vecuronium[2]	0.1–0.2	1–4	Prolonged action
Reversal drug (if nondepolarizing agent used)			
Sugammadex* (*Bridion*)	16 mg/kg for neuromuscular blockade due to a single dose of rocuronium 2–4 mg/kg (routine reversal dose)	3 minutes	Only for use in older than 2 years; can cause anaphylaxis, bradycardia

[1]Caution: Hyperkalemic cardiac arrest may occur if muscular dystrophy (especially if undiagnosed). [2]Use initial priming dose (1/10 of paralyzing dose) 3 minutes prior to paralyzing dose of rocuronium or vecuronium to speed time to paralysis. [3]Use 2–3 mg/kg if younger than 1 year, 1.5–2 mg/kg at 1–5 years, and 1–1.5 mg/kg for older than 5 years.

Pongrácz A, Szatmári S, Nemes R, Fülesdi B, Tassonyi E. Reversal of neuromuscular blockade with sugammadex at the reappearance of four twitches to train-of-four stimulation. *Anesthesiology.* 2013;119(1):36-42.

Modified from Walls RM, Murphy MF. *Manual of Emergency Airway Management.* 3rd ed. Philadelphia, PA: Lippincott Williams & Wilkins; 2008, 432 pp.

Table 3-5 Checklist After Performing Intubation

- Check tube placement (CO_2 detector/capnography preferred).*
- Inflate cuff (if present) then release cricoid pressure.
- Measure and record tube depth (see below).
- Reassess clinical status, $\downarrow$ HR = esophageal intubation.
- Obtain CXR to verify correct placement depth.
- Consider longer-acting sedative and paralytics.

*Use DOPE mnemonic to check when poor oxygenation or ventilation occur: Displacement, Obstruction, Pneumothorax, Equipment failure.

Table 3-6 Formulae for Estimating Depth of ET Tube After Intubation

- Distance in cm from mid-trachea to incisors/gum line = $3 \times$ (ET tube ID*)
- Distance in cm from mid-trachea to incisors/gum line = 12 + (age in years)/2
- Distance in cm from mid-trachea to incisors/gum line = (height in cm)/10 + 5
- Distance in cm from mid-trachea to nares (for nasotracheal) = 12 + (age in years)/2

*ID—internal diameter (in mm).

Table 3-7 Laryngeal Mask Airway (LMA) Sizes

Mask size	Patient weight (kg)	Maximum cuff volume (ml)	Maximum ET tube* size (mm) uncuffed
1	<5	≤4	3.5
1.5	5–10	≤7	4
2	10–20	≤10	4.5
2.5	20–30	≤14	5
3	30–50	≤20	6
4	50–70	≤30	6
5	70–100	≤40	7
6	>100	≤50	7

*Maximum ET tube size that can be placed through an *LMA Classic* if it is used as a conduit during tracheal intubation. If *LMA Fastrach* is used, an 8.0 mm cuffed ET tube can be placed through a 3, 4, or 5 LMA. *LMA Supreme* allows drainage of gas and fluids away from the airway; *LMA CTrach* aids in difficult intubations.

Table 3-8 Tracheostomy Tube Replacement Sizes

Age	Size	Inner diameter (mm)	Outer diameter (mm)	Suction catheter size (French)*
Premature	00	3.1	4.5	6
Newborn–3 months	0	3.4	5.0	6, 8
3–10 months	1	3.7	5.5	6, 8

Table 3-8 Tracheostomy Tube Replacement Sizes (*Continued*)

Age	Size	Inner diameter (mm)	Outer diameter (mm)	Suction catheter size (French)*
10–12 months	2	4.1	6.0	6, 8
13–24 months	3	4.8	7.0	8, 10
2–9 years	4	5.0	8.5	8, 10
10–11 years	6	7.0	10.0	12, 14
≥ 12 years	6	7.0	10.0	12, 14
	8	8.5	12.0	14, 16
	10	9.0	13.0	16, 18

*Size of catheter for suctioning tracheostomy tube.
Data from J. Byron Mullins, Airway resistance and work of breathing in tracheostomy tubes, *Laryngoscope.* 1993;103:1367.

RESCUE PROCEDURE FOR TRANSTRACHEAL JET VENTILATION

Place a 14-gauge IV catheter attached to a 5 ml syringe through a cricothyroid membrane. Remove the needle, leaving the catheter, and confirm placement by aspirating air. Attach a 3.0 mm ET tube adapter to the IV catheter, or attach a 3 ml locking syringe (without plunger) to a 3 mm ET tube adapter. Attach a 10–50 pounds per square inch (psi) 100% O_2 source (15 l/minute) and deliver O_2 at 20 bursts/minute with an inspiratory to expiratory ratio of 1:3.

Table 3-9 Parameters for Transtracheal Jet Ventilation

Age (years)	Initial PSI	Tidal volume (ml)
< 5	5	100
5–8	5–10	240–340
8–12	10–25	340–625
> 12	30–50	700–1,000

Table 3-10 Initial Ventilator Settings for Volume Limited Ventilators

Age (years)	Tidal volume (ml/kg)	Rate[1]	Inspiratory time[2]	PEEP[3]
0–1	8–10	20	0.8	3–5
1–3	10	16	0.9	3–5
4–10	8	12	1	3–5
≥ 11–12	6–8	10	1	3–5

[1]Breaths/minute. [2]Seconds. [3]Positive End-Expiratory Pressure, cm H_2O.

Table 3-11 Guidelines for Mechanical Ventilation

Item	Neonates and young infants (younger than 1 year)[1]	Older children
Ventilator	Pressure-limited if weight < 10 kg	Volume limited
Resp rate	30–40 per minute	Normal for age (12–20)
I:E ratio[2]	1:2	1:2
PEEP[3]	Start at 3–5 cm H_2O	Start at 3–5 cm H_2O
PSV	Initial pressure support ventilation (PSV) 10 cm H_2O, may ↑ to 35 cm	
FiO_2	5–10% above preintubation FiO_2, adjust to oxygen saturation	
Setting	Begin peak inspiratory pressure at 16 mm Hg, ↑ 2 mm Hg until adequate excursion	Tidal volume 5–8

[1]Pressure-limited ventilators may also be used in disorders causing low lung compliance (e.g., acute respiratory distress syndrome) since mean airway pressure is more easily manipulated. See pages 273-274 for *noninvasive ventilation*. [2]Inspiratory/expiratory ratio: During ventilation of lungs with normal compliance and diffusion characteristics I:E is typically 0.5 (1:2). In poorly compliant lungs with impaired diffusion, inspiration may be prolonged (or inverted > 1) to an I:E of 2 or 3:1. Prolonged inspiration can ↑ mean airway pressure and ↓ cardiac output. Shortened exhalation may lead to overdistention and gas trapping. [3]Positive end expiratory pressure is used to recruit lungs and restore functional residual capacity (FRC) preventing atelectasis.

ANALGESIA

Table 3-12 Maximum Dose of Local Anesthetics Without (*and With*) Epinephrine

Bupivacaine (*Marcaine, Sensorcaine*)[1]	2.5 mg/kg (*3 mg/kg*)
Lidocaine (*Xylocaine*)[2]	5 mg/kg (*7 mg/kg*)
Mepivacaine (*Carbocaine*)	4 mg/kg (*7 mg/kg*)
Prilocaine (never use for younger than 6 months old)	5.5 mg/kg (*8.5 mg/kg*)

[1]Due to cardiac toxicity, never use for IV regional anesthesia or hematoma block.
[2]For IV regional anesthesia (Bier blocks) max lidocaine dose is 3 mg/kg with even less for mini-Bier block. Use preservative-free lidocaine without epinephrine for Bier or hematoma blocks.

Table 3-13 Oral Analgesic Agents (Liquid Preparations)

Agent	Dose (mg/kg)	Frequency	Concentration and comments
Acetaminophen	15	Every 4 hours	80 mg/0.8 ml (dropper) or 160 mg per 5 ml
Acetaminophen with codeine	0.5 to 1	Every 4–6 hours	Acetaminophen 120 mg + codeine 12 mg per 5 ml (dose in mg/kg based on codeine)

Table 3-13 Oral Analgesic Agents (Liquid Preparations) (*Continued*)

Agent	Dose (mg/kg)	Frequency	Concentration and comments
Aspirin	10–15	Every 4 hours	No elixir available
Hydrocodone*	0.1–0.2	Every 4–6 hours	*Hycet elixir* (2.5 mg hydrocodone/108 mg Tylenol/5 ml also contains 7% alcohol) *Lortab elixir* (2.5 mg hydrocodone/167 mg Tylenol/5 ml also contains 7% alcohol)
Ibuprofen (suspension)	5–10	Every 6–8 hours	*Children's Motrin* or *Advil:* 100 mg per 5 ml
Oxycodone*	0.05 to 0.2	Every 4–6 hours	5 mg/5 ml (solution) and 20 mg/ml (concentrate)—exercise *caution* because the presence of two preparations and a high concentration increases dosing error risk. Max dose 10 mg
Naproxen suspension*	5–7	Every 8–12 hours	125 mg per 5 ml

*Only approved for select ages/indications; consult manufacturer's product labeling.

Table 3-14 Topical Analgesia*

Use	Agent	Onset (minutes)
Un-intact skin	• LET (lidocaine 4%, epinephrine 0.1%, tetracaine 0.5%)—apply with cotton ball, not gauze. Use 1–3 ml (1 ml per cm to maximum 3 ml). 90–95% effective on face/scalp, 50% on limbs/torso.	20–30
	• EMLA (2.5% prilocaine, 2.5% lidocaine) may be used on un-intact skin if LET unavailable (less effective on un-intact skin). Use ≤ 1 g per 10 cm^2.	45–60
Intact skin	• EMLA (See un-intact skin above)	45–60
	• LMX4 or 5 (4–5% liposomal lidocaine formerly ELA-Max)—use ≤ 1 g per 10 cm^2	30
	• Synera–(lido/tetracaine) apply patch to vascular access site or needle stick (only if older than 3 years)	20–30
	• Topicaine (4–5% lidocaine gel)–apply < 0.3–0.4 g per 10 cm^2	30–60

(*Continued*)

Table 3-14 Topical Analgesia* (*Continued*)

Use	Agent	Onset (minutes)
Needle-free injection (pre-IV)	• *J-tip:* Buffered lidocaine (0.25 ml of 1% buffered lidocaine or alternate dosing) via compressed CO_2	3
	• Zingo: 0.5 mg lidocaine delivered via helium-powered device	3
Iontophoresis	• 1 ml of lidocaine 2% with 1:100,000 epinephrine added to drug electrode. Apply 1 milliampere (mA) to site and slowly increase until tingling sensation gone to a total dose of 30 mA. Place ground electrode onto major muscle of child or parent.	10–15

*Healthcare workers are advised to review package inserts, mixture components, side effects, contraindications, indications, and dosing (especially maximum total dose per age/size) prior to using these agents.

Table 3-15 Analgesia and Sedation

Agent Trade name	Dose	Route	Onset (minutes)	Duration (hours)	Comments and select properties*
Diazepam *Valium*	**Sedative:** Younger than 6 months: not recommended 6 months–6 years: < 0.5 mg/kg Older than 12 years: 0.12–0.8 mg/kg OR 0.04–0.20 mg/kg **Status epilepticus:** 0.2–0.5 mg/kg OR 6 months–5 years: 0.2–0.5 mg/kg Older than 5 years: 1 mg	PO IV/IM PR IV	< 1	1–2	↓ Respirations, ↓ BP
Etomidate *Amidate*	0.1–0.4 mg/kg	IV	< 1	< 0.25	Administer over 1 minute, causes myoclonus, vomiting
Fentanyl *Sublimaze*	1–3 mcg/kg 1–1.5 mcg/kg	IV Intranasal (use with atomizer)	2–3	0.5	↓ Respirations, ↓ BP, bradycardia, rare chest wall rigidity (due to rapid administration)

Table 3-15 Analgesia and Sedation (*Continued*)

Agent *Trade name*	Dose	Route	Onset (minutes)	Duration (hours)	Comments and select properties*
Flumazenil *Romazicon*	0.01 mg/kg (maximum dose of 0.05 mg/kg up to max of 1 mg)	IV	< 1	1	Reverses benzodiazepines (e.g., lorazepam, midazolam, diazepam)
Ketamine *Ketalar*	1–2 mg/kg 4 mg/kg 5–10 mg/kg	IV IM PO	< 1 5 30	0.25 0.5–1 1–2	Elevated BP, ↑ intracranial/ocular pressure, rare laryngospasm
Methohexital	20 mg	PR	15	0.5	↓ Respirations, ↓ BP
Midazolam *Versed*	0.10 mg/kg 0.10–0.15 mg/kg 0.2–0.3 mg/kg 0.5 mg/kg	IV IM Intranasal PO/PR	2 10–15 10–15 15–30	0.5 0.75 1 1–1.5	↓ Respirations, ↓ BP Start IV dose at 0.05–0.10 mg/kg with slow titration to max of 0.4–0.5 mg/kg
Morphine	0.1 mg/kg	IV	< 5	3–4	↓ Respirations, ↓ BP
Naloxone *Narcan*	0.01–0.1 mg/kg	IV, IM, SC	< 1	< 1	Reverses narcotics, erratic absorption SC, use low dose first
Nitrous oxide	30%	Inhaled	1–2	< 0.1	Patient holds mask to self-titrate
Propofol *Diprivan*	1–2 mg/kg (Max 1st dose 40 mg)	IV	< 1	< 0.25	Pain on IV site, respiratory depression, apnea, hypotension; don't use if allergy to egg yolk, lecithin, soybean oil, glycerol, EDTA (infuse 0.1–0.3 mg/kg/minute); not recommended for younger than 3 years old

(*Continued*)

Table 3-15 Analgesia and Sedation (*Continued*)

Agent *Trade name*	Dose	Route	Onset (minutes)	Duration (hours)	Comments and select properties*
Thiopental *Pentothal*	3–5 mg/kg 25	IV PR	< 1 5	0.1–0.5 0.5–1.0	Slow IV at 1 mg/kg every 1–2 minutes; causes histamine release, ↓ respi- ration, ↓ BP
Dexmedeto- midine *Precedex*	Loading 0.5–1.0 mcg/kg Maintenance 0.3–2.0 mcg/ kg/hour	IV	< 5	2–3	Hypotension, bradycardia, and cardiac arrest

*Only those thoroughly familiar with pediatric airway management, appropriate monitoring, and medication action and side effects should administer these agents.

4 ■ ANAPHYLAXIS

Table 4-1 Management of Anaphylaxis

Airway	Assess and support the airway. Administer 100% oxygen. Consider early intubation if airway edema is suspected.		
Cardiac	Apply cardiac monitor and pulse oximeter; assess vitals frequently. Initiate chest compressions if cardiovascular arrest occurs.		
Skin	Remove the inciting allergen, if possible. Apply ice to bite, sting sites.		
Drugs	**Dose**	**Route**	**Indications and Detail**
Epinephrine	0.01 mg/kg (max of 0.5 mg) (Conc. 1:1,000) Immediately and then every 5–15 minutes as necessary	IM	First line of treatment. Inject IM into anterolateral thigh, NOT subcutaneously.
	0.1–1 mcg/kg/minute (to a maximum of 10 mcg/minute)	IV*	IV epinephrine infusion if persistent shock exists despite IM epinephrine and fluid resuscitation See IV drip, Table A-2
Other vasopressors	Consider norepinephrine or vasopressin if IV fluids and epinephrine drip fail to resolve hypotension.		
Normal saline	20 ml/kg Give as quickly as possible	IV Intraosseous access if IV access is not readily available.	Hypotension (repeat as needed)
Methylprednisolone (Solumedrol) or Dexamethasone	1–2 mg/kg (max 120 mg) 0.6 mg/kg (max 10 mg)	IV IV/PO	Second-line agent**
Diphenhydramine (Benadryl) or Cetirizine	1 mg/kg (max 50 mg) 2.5–10 mg	PO/IV/IM PO	Second-line agent** Relieve the cutaneous symptoms Onset of action is faster for cetirizine than Benadryl

(*Continued*)

Table 4-1 Management of Anaphylaxis (*Continued*)

Famotidine or Ranitidine	0.5 mg/kg (max 20 mg) 1 mg/kg (max 50 mg)	IV IV	H2 blocker Second-line agent** Combined effect of H1 and H2 antagonist is superior to H1 alone in treating cutaneous manifestations
Glucagon	20–30 mcg/kg bolus* (max 1 mg), followed by continuous infusion at 5–15 mcg/minute	IV *Administer bolus slowly over 5 minutes as rapid administration can induce vomiting	Consider for patients on β blockers when anaphylaxis is refractory to IV epinephrine and fluid
Albuterol	2.5–5 mg every 15 minutes	Nebulized/ Metered-dose inhaler (2–6 inhalations)	Bronchospasm refractory to epinephrine
Racemic epinephrine	Currently not recommended. Anecdotal evidence that it may decrease oropharyngeal edema and make airway management less difficult in anaphylaxis		
Patient positioning	Place adults and adolescents in recumbent position; place young children in position of comfort; place pregnant patient on left side.		
Observation	Per expert opinion observe all for 4–8 hours. Consider longer observation/admission if severe or refractory symptoms or with a history of asthma or risk factors for severe anaphylaxis.		
Follow-up	Prescribe epinephrine auto-injector [e.g., Twinject (0.15 mg) if 15 to < 30 kg, or Twinject (0.3 mg) if ≥ 30 kg, each device has two doses OR EpiPen (0.3 mg) if ≥ 30 kg or EpiPen Jr (0.15 mg) if 15 to <30 kg, each as single dose or 2-Pak to all with serious symptoms]. Educate patient, patient provider, and family on the use of auto-injector Provide anaphylaxis action plan Outpatient allergy-immunology referral		

*Monitor closely, as life-threatening complications (e.g., ischemia, arrhythmias) can occur.
**Efficacy of the second-line agents has not been proven.
Modified from Lieberman P, Nicklas RA, Randolph C, et al. Anaphylaxis—a practice parameter update 2015. *Ann Allergy Asthma Immunol.* 2015;115(5):341-384; Campbell RL, Li JTC, Nicklas RA, et al. Emergency department diagnosis and treatment of anaphylaxis: a practice parameter. *Ann Allergy Asthma Immunol.* 2014;113:599-608.

HEREDITARY ANGIOEDEMA

Table 4-2 Hereditary Angioedema

A rare genetic condition with autosomal dominant inheritance. Affected individuals have either a reduced level (type I) or functional deficiency (type II) of C1 esterase inhibitor (C1-INH) or excessive bradykinin due to an increased factor XII activity (type III). It causes recurrent painful episodes of swelling, typically in the face, hands, feet, or genitals. May also occur in the airways and intestinal tract. Manifestations include abdominal pain, nausea, vomiting, diarrhea, and possible life-threatening airway obstruction. Trauma, stress, infections, surgery, and drugs (e.g., estrogens) are typical precipitants.

Acute management: (1) If (there is) isolated extremity (or) truncal edema, a wait and see approach is appropriate. Alternatively, increase Danazol by 2.5–5 mg/kg/day in those already taking this agent to abort an attack. Tranexamic acid (not FDA approved) is another prophylactic agent. (2) First-line agent for severe attacks is C1-INH concentrate (Cinryze), 10–20 units/kg IV (if <50 kg), 1,000 units (if 50–100 kg), or 1,500 units IV (if >100 kg). (This agent is not FDA approved in children.) Recombinant C1 inhibitor (Ruconest) and bradykinin B2-receptor antagonist (Icatibant) are other available options. Ecallantide (Kalbitor)—30 mg (3 doses of 10 mg each)—given at three separate sites subcutaneously is approved in children > 12 years. Discuss appropriate use and dosing of these drugs in children with pediatric allergist or hematologist. If previously mentioned medicines are unavailable or contraindicated, consider fresh frozen plasma (FFP) (may worsen attacks). Consider intubation if progressive laryngeal edema; epinephrine (dosing mentioned previously) administered IM (or IV if life-threatening) may or may not be effective. However, steroids and antihistamines are ineffective for hereditary angioedema.

Modified from Cicardi M, Aberer W, Banerji A, et al. Classification, diagnosis, and approach to treatment for angioedema: consensus report from the Hereditary Angioedema International Working Group. *Allergy.* 2014;69: 602-616.

5 ■ BRIEF RESOLVED UNEXPLAINED EVENT (BRUE)

This term [formerly *apparent life-threatening event (ALTE)*] describes a sudden, brief (<1 minute in duration), unexplained but now resolved event in infants younger than 1 year with a normal physical examination.[1]

DIAGNOSIS OF BRUE

Includes one or more of the following criteria that lasted for less than 1 minute in an infant with no other explanation for the event and whose physical examination is reassuring:

1. Cyanosis or pallor
2. Absent, decreased, or irregular breathing
3. Marked change in tone (hyper- or hypotonia)
4. Altered level of responsiveness

- If the criteria are met, obtain an appropriate history and physical exam.
- Diagnosis of BRUE can only be made when there is no explanation for a qualifying event after a complete history and physical.

BRUE RISK CLASSIFICATION

Infants are categorized into two groups:

LOW-RISK PATIENTS

1. Age > 60 days
2. Gestational age > 32 weeks and postconception age > 45 weeks
3. Occurrence of only 1 BRUE (no prior BRUE ever and not occurring in clusters)
4. Duration of BRUE < 1 minute
5. No cardiopulmonary resuscitation by a trained medical provider
6. No concerning historical features
7. No concerning physical examination findings

HIGH-RISK PATIENTS

1. Patients who do not meet criteria as low risk by default are considered high risk.
2. History and physical examination suggest the need for further investigation, monitoring, and/or treatment.[1]

MANAGEMENT RECOMMENDATIONS

LOW-RISK PATIENTS

- **Should** educate caregivers about BRUE and ensure timely follow-up.
- **Should not**:
  - Obtain laboratory studies, CBC, comprehensive metabolic panel, CSF, blood cultures, ammonia, blood gases, urine organic acids, plasma amino acids, or acylcarnitines.
  - Obtain chest X-ray, echocardiogram, or EEG.
  - Obtain viral respiratory test, urinalysis, blood glucose, serum bicarbonate, serum lactic acid, or neuroimaging; admit the patient to the hospital solely for cardiorespiratory monitoring.
  - Initiate home cardiorespiratory monitoring.
  - Prescribe acid suppression therapy or antiepileptic medications.
- **May consider** obtaining pertussis testing and 12-lead ECG; monitoring the patient with continuous pulse oximetry and serial observations (1–4 hours)

HIGH-RISK PATIENTS

- Common etiologies in these infants include gastroesophageal reflux, seizures, child abuse, bronchiolitis, and pertussis.
- Less common etiologies are inborn errors of metabolism, arrhythmias, increased intracranial pressure, toxic ingestions, and craniofacial anomalies and syndromes.
- Evaluate the patient accordingly.
- Admit for further evaluation and management; however, no guidelines exist for management of high-risk infants.

REFERENCES

1. Tieder JS, Bonkowsky JL, Etzel RA, et al. Brief resolved unexplained events (formerly apparent life-threatening events) and evaluation of lower-risk infants: executive summary. *Pediatrics.* 2016;137.
2. Kondamudi N, Virji M. *Brief Resolved Unexplained Event (BRUE).* Treasure Island: StatPearls; 2019.
3. Colombo M, Katz ES, Bosco A, Melzi ML, Nosetti L. Brief resolved unexplained events: retrospective validation of diagnostic criteria and risk stratification. *Pediatr Pulmonol.* 2019;54(1):61-65.

6 ■ BIOLOGIC, CHEMICAL, AND RADIATION EXPOSURES

Visit www.cdc.gov for updates/information regarding biologic/chemical exposures. Visit https://orise.orau.gov/reacts/ or call (865) 576-1005 regarding radiation exposure. Contact the Centers for Disease Control and Prevention (CDC) for further information regarding biologic, chemical, and radiation exposures. CDC Bioterrorism Preparedness and Response Center: (770) 488-7100.

   General rules—Gown, gloves, and high-efficiency particulate air (HEPA) filter masks protect against most biologic agents, soap/water removes most biologic agents from skin, and hypochlorite (0.1%) bleach removes most contaminants from objects.

BIOLOGIC

Exposure to biologic agents can be due to various dispersal techniques, such as contaminated water and aerosol sprays. Symptoms can appear from days to weeks after exposure. There are three categories based on ease of dissemination, morbidity and mortality, panic potential, and level of public health requirements.

CATEGORY A (HIGHEST PRIORITY)

- *Bacillus anthracis* **(Anthrax):** It is a spore-forming organism found in soil normally transmitted by handling contaminated animals or animal products. Symptoms begin 1 to 60 days after exposure. Cutaneous signs include pruritic macule or papule, edema, painless ulceration, and eschar. Lymphangitis or painful lymphadenopathy can occur. Gastrointestinal symptoms and signs include abdominal pain, vomiting, hematemesis, or bowel perforation. Inhalation signs include cough, chest pain, fever, chills, hemorrhagic mediastinitis, pleural effusions, respiratory failure, or shock. Diagnosis may include PCR testing of skin lesions or serum for anthrax lethal factor toxin. Gram-positive rods in a typical "jointed bamboo rods appearance" in culture or short chains of two to four cells in direct clinical samples (unspun peripheral blood smear, CSF, or vesicular fluid) are highly suggestive of anthrax. Postexposure chemoprophylaxis for penicillin-resistant strains or prior to susceptibility results is for 60 days after exposure with one of the following:

Medication	Dose	Maximum dose	Interval
In penicillin-resistant strains or before susceptibility results:			
Ciprofloxacin	30 mg/kg/day	500 mg/dose	Divided every 12 hours
Doxycycline			
<45 kg	4.4 mg/kg/day	100 mg/dose	Divided every 12 hours
>45 kg	100 mg/dose		Divided every 12 hours
Clindamycin	30 mg/kg/day	900 mg/dose	Divided every 8 hours
Levofloxacin			
<50 kg	16 mg/kg/day	250 mg/dose	Divided every 12 hours
>50 kg	500 mg/day		Every 24 hours
In penicillin-susceptible strains:			
Amoxicillin	75 mg/kg/day	1,000 mg/day	Divided every 8 hours
Pen VK	50–75 mg/kg/day		Divided every 6–8 hours

A three-dose anthrax vaccine adsorbed (AVA) BioThrax is recommended for an adult post exposure but it is currently not FDA approved for children younger than 18 years. However, it will be available to children older than 6 weeks as an investigational vaccine through an expedited process at the time of an event and should be given at 0, 2, and 4 weeks in addition to the chemoprophylaxis. In children younger than 6 weeks, chemoprophylaxis should be provided, but the vaccine should be delayed until the infant is older than 6 weeks of age.

Treatment of confirmed cases of cutaneous anthrax without systemic signs includes a single oral antimicrobial agent (same antimicrobials and doses as given in the previous table) for 7 to 10 days in a naturally acquired infection, and for 60 days if following bioterrorism. Treat inhalational, gastrointestinal, or other systemic involvement without meningitis with two parenteral antimicrobials as follows:

Treatment of Anthrax (Systemic Without Meningitis)

Medication	Dose	Maximum dose	Interval	Route
Bactericidal agent (one of the following):				
Ciprofloxacin	30 mg/kg/day	400 mg/dose	Divided every 8 hours	IV
Meropenem	60 mg/kg/day	2,000 mg/dose	Divided every 8 hours	IV

(Continued)

Treatment of Anthrax (Systemic Without Meningitis) (*Continued*)

Levofloxacin		250 mg/dose		
<50 kg	20 mg/kg/day		Divided every 12 hours	IV
>50 kg	500 mg/day		Every 24 hours	IV
Imipenem/ Cilastatin	100 mg/kg/day	1,000 mg/dose	Divided every 6 hours	IV
Vancomycin	60 mg/kg/day		Divided every 8 hours	IV
OR for penicillin-susceptible strains:				
Ampicillin	200 mg/kg/day	3,000 mg/dose	Divided every 6 hours	IV
Penicillin G	400,000 units/ kg/day	4 mU/dose	Divided every 4 hours	IV
PLUS one of the following protein synthesis inhibitors:				
Clindamycin	40 mg/kg/day	900 mg/dose	Divided every 8 hours	IV
Linezolid	30 mg/kg/day	600 mg/dose	Divided every 8 hours (<12 years) Divided every 12 hours (>12 years)	IV
Rifampin	20 mg/kg/day	300 mg/dose	Divided every 12 hours	IV

Data from Bradley JS, Peacock G, Krug SE, et al. Pediatric anthrax clinical management. *Pediatrics.* 2014;133(5):e1411-e1436. doi:10.1542/peds.2014-0563.

Treat children who have systemic anthrax with meningoencephalitis with a bactericidal fluoroquinolone (e.g., ciprofloxacin or levofloxacin) PLUS a beta lactam (e.g., meropenem) PLUS a protein synthesis inhibitor (e.g., linezolid, clindamycin). Antitoxin (AIG or raxibacumab) is recommended for all systemic diseases. Consider steroids for all cases with cerebral edema or meningoencephalitis.

- **Clostridium botulinum (Botulism):** A neurotoxin that causes neuroparalysis with three main presentations, which include infant, foodborne, and wound botulism. Symptoms can begin from 6 hours up to 10 days following exposure. Signs for infants and children include constipation, diminished gag reflex, weak neck muscles, or respiratory failure. Adults have weak jaw clench, difficulty speaking and swallowing, drooping eyelids, diplopia, descending proximal to distal muscle weakness, or respiratory failure. Botulism differs from other flaccid paralysis in the following ways: (a) symmetry, (b) first manifests with cranial nerve palsies, (c) descending paralysis, and (d) absence of sensory nerve dysfunction. Laboratory confirmation is done by demonstrating the presence of botulinum toxin in serum, stool, or food, or by microbiologic culture. However, it is not advised to wait for laboratory results but rather to treat based on clinical findings. Treatment includes supportive care. There is an antitoxin (botulinum antitoxin or BabyBIG) that can be given to halt the paralysis and reduce the risk of complications from botulism, but it does not reverse paralysis.

- *Yersinia pestis* (Plague): The plague is transmitted to humans by a rat flea bite, and there are three types: bubonic, pneumonic, and septicemic with pneumonic being the most severe and the only one with human-to-human transmission. Symptoms begin from 1 to 10 days following exposure. Signs include tender and enlarged lymph nodes called buboes, fever, chills, myalgia, pulmonary edema, abdominal pain, sepsis, or pneumonia. Diagnosis includes PCR testing, formalin-fixed tissues by hematoxylin and eosin stain (H&E, gram), or silver impregnation and Giemsa stains. Treatment in children includes streptomycin 15 mg/kg two times per day IM (max 2 g/day), gentamycin 2.5 mg/kg/dose every 8 hours IV/IM, levofloxacin 8 mg/kg/dose every 12 hours (max 250 mg/dose) IV or PO, ciprofloxacin 20 mg/kg two times per day (max 500 mg/dose) PO, or doxycycline 200 mg everyday (> 45 kg) or 2.2 mg/kg two times per day (max of 100 mg every day) for < 45 kg IV or PO. Post-exposure chemoprophylaxis in children for 7 days with ciprofloxacin 20 mg/kg two times per day (max 1 g) PO, or doxycycline PO 200 mg everyday or 2.2 mg/kg two times per day (max of 200 mg) if < 45 kg.
- *Variola major* (Smallpox): Symptoms begin from 7 to 19 days after exposure. Signs include fever, myalgia, or lesions that progress from macules and papules all the same stage on face and extremities to vesicles and umbilicated pustules. Diagnosis includes samples from vesicle fluid or skin samples by PCR of variola DNA or by electron microscopy. Treatment is supportive care with antibiotics reserved only for secondary bacterial infection. There is a vaccine that may be effective if given within 3 days to help decrease the incidence of disease and decrease the incidence of death. The FDA has approved three antivirals (tecovirimat, cidofovir, and brincidofovir) but they have not been tested on people with smallpox.
- *Francisella tularensis* (Tularemia): This bacterium can be spread by ticks, deerflies, or contact with an infected animal, as well as by breathing in contaminated dust or drinking contaminated water. Symptoms begin from 2 to 14 days. Signs include fever, sepsis, pneumonia, necrotizing lymphadenitis, skin ulcer with corresponding lymph node involvement, or conjunctivitis with ulcers. Diagnosis includes direct examination of secretions, exudates, or biopsy specimens using gram stain, direct fluorescent antibody, or immunohistochemical stains. Treatment with antibiotics for 10 to 21 days with streptomycin 15 mg/kg IM two times per day (max of 2 g/day), or gentamicin 2.5 mg/kg IM/IV every 8 hours everyday or

doxycycline 2.2 mg/kg two times per day (maximum of 100 mg/dose) or ciprofloxacin 15 mg/kg two times per day (maximum of 400 mg/dose). Ciprofloxacin, however, is not currently approved by the FDA for treatment of human beings for tularemia.

- **Viral Hemorrhagic Fever (Marburg, Ebola, Lassa Virus):** Caused by families of the RNA virus, all of these viruses can show signs of fever, bleeding, facial and chest flushing, petechiae, edema, hypotension, vomiting, and headache, leading to multiple organ failures and hypovolemic shock due to bleeding diathesis or circulatory compromise.
  - Symptoms begin for Lassa in 1 to 3 weeks after exposure and can be detected by enzyme-linked immunosorbent assay (ELISA) testing for Lassa antigen, IgM and IgG, or PCR testing. Treatment with ribavirin seems to be effective if given early on in clinical illness. Symptoms for Marburg begin 2 to 10 days after exposure and can be detected by ELISA testing or PCR. There is no treatment except supportive care. Ebola symptoms begin 2 to 21 days after exposure and can be detected by ELISA or PCR. There is no cure, and treatment includes supportive care.

CATEGORY B (SECOND-HIGHEST PRIORITY)

- **Brucella (Brucellosis):** This can be contracted by consumption of undercooked meat or unpasteurized milk. Symptoms begin 5 days to 6 months after exposure. Signs include fever, foul-smelling sweat (described as similar to wet hay), arthralgia, night sweat, vomiting, diarrhea, abdominal pain, enlarged liver, liver abscess, enlarged spleen, arthritis, optic neuritis, or endocarditis. Diagnosis can be done by PCR or microagglutination. Treatment includes antibiotics for 6 weeks with doxycycline 100 mg two times per day or if children are younger than 8 years of age then trimethoprim 5 mg/kg, sulfamethoxazole 25 mg/kg (TMP-SMZ) two times per day.
- **Clostridium perfringens Epsilon Toxin:** Toxin types B and D bind to endothelial cells of the brain capillary vessels and pass though the blood-brain barrier. Symptoms begin 6 to 24 hours after exposure. It causes devastating neurological signs and there is no cure.
- **Coxiella burnetii (Q Fever):** Can be contracted via inhalations from spore-like variants, contact with animal-infected secretions, and can also be tick-borne. Symptoms begin 2 to 3 weeks after exposure. Signs include flu-like symptoms, upper respiratory infection, cough, confusion, vomiting, or diarrhea. It can progress to atypical pneumonia with respiratory distress. It can also cause granulomatous hepatitis as well as retinal vasculitis. Diagnosis includes PCR testing or indirect immunofluorescence antibody using *burnetii* antigens. Treatment is most effective if started within the first 3 days of symptoms. Antibiotics include doxycycline 100 mg bid for 14 days or if younger than 8 years of age then TMP-SMZ 8–12 mg/kg/day (max 320 mg/day trimethoprim).
- **Ricin:** This is a toxin from the castor oil plant and found in the beans. A dose as small as the size of a few grains of table salt can kill a human.

Symptoms begin 4 to 10 hours after ingestion, 4 to 8 hours after inhalation, and within 12 hours following injection. Signs include abdominal pain, vomiting, diarrhea, fever, necrotizing pneumonia, pulmonary edema, or shock. Diagnosis by ELISA. Treatment includes charcoal lavage and supportive care.

- **Staphylococcus aureus Enterotoxin B:** This is a toxin that can be administered by food or water or inhaled as an aerosol. Symptoms from 4 to 10 hours after exposure. Signs include fever, headache, pulmonary edema, vomiting, diarrhea, intestinal cramping, or toxic shock syndrome with high fever, hypotension, rash, and peeling of skin. Diagnosis includes ELISA or PCR testing. Treatment includes supportive care because there is no cure.
- **Alpha Viruses (Viral Encephalitis—Venezuelan, Eastern, and Western Equine):** These are mosquito-borne viral pathogens that cause progressive central nervous system disorders. Venezuelan equine presents with symptoms 1 to 6 days after exposure as compared to Eastern and Western equine, which are between 5 and 14 days. Signs include flu-like symptoms, fever, headache, vomiting, confusion, seizures, or focal neurological deficits. Diagnosis includes serology testing with specific IgM antibodies in serum or CSF. Treatment includes supportive care because there is no cure. About 33% of Eastern equine is fatal compared to 15% of Western equine.

CATEGORY C (THIRD-HIGHEST PRIORITY)

- **Flavivirus (Yellow Fever):** This is a mosquito-borne disease. Symptoms begin 3 to 6 days after exposure. Signs include fever, headache, dizziness, jaundice, hemorrhage, or shock. Diagnosis is done by ELISA. Treatment includes supportive care because there is no cure.

CHEMICAL WEAPONS

- **Blistering Agents**
  - **Mustard Gas/Lewisite:** Can cause skin erythema or vesicles, eye inflammation, or respiratory inflammation with delayed blistering up to 12 hours later. Decontaminate with soap and water for skin contamination, but if eye contact with the gas, then irrigate with water immediately for most effectiveness. Treatment for mustard gas is supportive care. Treatment for lewisite includes supportive care as well as dimercaprol 3–4 mg/kg IM every 4–6 hours for systemic effects in severe cases.
- **Blood Agents**
  - **Cyanide:** a colorless gas with a faint, bitter almond smell. It inhibits cytochrome oxidase causing cellular anoxia and lactic acidosis. Symptoms can begin 1 to 20 minutes after exposure. Signs include convulsions, cyanosis, fatigue, headache, hypotension, loss of consciousness, metabolic acidosis, palpitations, vomiting, or death.

Treatment includes 100% oxygen and hydroxocobalamin 70 mg/kg IV (max 5 g) or cyanide antidote kit. The cyanide antidote kit includes amyl nitrite, which is inhaled for 30 seconds per minute for 3 minutes, sodium nitrate 10 ml (300 mg) IV, and sodium thiosulfate 1.65 mg/kg (max 12.5 g or 50 ml).

- **Nerve Agents:**
  - **Cyclosarin (GF), Sarin, Soman, Tabun, VX:** Organic chemicals (organophosphates) that disrupt nerve transfer messages to organs, are easily vaporized, can enter though the respiratory system, and can be absorbed through the skin. Most are colorless and tasteless with a slight fruity odor, except for VX, which has a faint fishy odor. Symptoms begin within minutes. Signs include bronchial constriction, cramps, diarrhea, increased secretions, miosis, respiratory arrest, tremors, sweating, paralysis, or loss of consciousness. Decontaminate by removing clothes, irrigating skin with soapy water, and irrigating eyes and wounds with sterile water. Treatment includes atropine 0.05 mg/kg IV/IM (max 2 mg) every 2 to 5 minutes to control bronchial secretions or bronchospasms. Give pralidoxime 25 mg/kg IV/IM (max 1 g IV or 2 g IM) with or after atropine, can repeat within 30 to 60 minutes up to a total of 45 mg/kg, and then every 12 hours up to two doses. If seizures, then give benzodiazepines. There is a nerve agent antidote kit called DuoDote, which is 2 mg atropine and 500 mg pralidoxime per auto injector, convulsive antidote nerve agent (CANA) with diazepam 10 mg auto injector.

RADIATION

Decontamination should be done as soon as possible with removal of clothing, irrigation of wounds with normal saline, irrigation of eyes with sterile water, and irrigation of skin with warm water and soap.

Cutaneous radiation syndrome occurs when exposed to high radiation with symptoms 12 to 20 days after irradiation. Symptoms include blistering, erythema, desquamation, and ulceration. Treat the area as if it was a thermal burn.

Acute radiation syndrome can occur after whole-body exposure from a minimum dose of 1 gray (Gy) to a fatal dose of greater than 10 Gy. There are four states of acute radiation. The first phase is called prodrome, which occurs within minutes to days following exposure with symptoms that include nausea, vomiting, diarrhea, anorexia, abdominal cramping, and dehydration. The next stage is the latent stage in which the patient feels healthy for a few hours to weeks. The manifest illness stage is the third stage and can last from hours to months. There are also three syndromes. In the hematopoietic syndrome, the person develops pancytopenia, infections, and hemorrhage. In the gastrointestinal syndrome, the person develops pancytopenia, but the GI tract cells are drying thus leading to infection, dehydration, and electrolyte imbalance. The cardiovascular/central nervous system syndrome symptoms include confusion, vomiting, diarrhea, and loss of consciousness. The last stage ranges from recovery to death. Often death occurs a few months after hematopoietic syndrome, within 2 weeks of gastrointestinal syndrome, and within 3 days of cardiovascular/central nervous system syndrome.

Treatment includes contact precautions, isolation, antibiotics, platelet transfusion, growth factors transfusion, hydration, and parenteral nutrition.

Potassium iodide (KI) should be administered within 6 hours after exposure to radioactive iodine. The use of KI reduces the risk of thyroid cancer after the release of radioactive iodine only.

Daily Potassium Iodide (KI) Dose for Radiation Exposure

Population	Predicted thyroid exposure (rad)	Daily KI dose
Adults > 40 years	> 500	130 mg
Adults > 18 to 40 years	≥ 10	130 mg
Pregnancy or lactating	≥ 5	130 mg
> 12 to 18 years (if ≥70 kg, treat as adult)	≥ 5	65 mg
> 3 to 12 years	≥ 5	65 mg
> 1 month to 3 years (dilute in milk, formula, H_2O)	≥ 5	32 mg
< 1 month	≥ 5	16 mg

Data from www.fda.gov/Drugs/EmergencyPreparedness/BioterrorismandDrugPreparedness and www.cdc.gov

7 ■ BURNS

Table 7-1 Fluid Resuscitation in Burn Victims

• Intravenous fluid resuscitation required if ≥ 10% total BSA burns.	
• Partial- and full-thickness (not erythema) are used to calculate the total BSA.	

Pediatric burn fluid resuscitation formula	
Parkland formula	• LR* 4 ml/kg/% BSA** burn in first 24 hours (from time of burn) + maintenance fluid, with 1/2 over first 8 hours, and 1/2 over subsequent 16 hours
Cincinnati (young children)	• 4 ml/kg/%TBSA*** burn +1,500 ml/m² total BSA of LR. 1/2 over first 8 hours, and 1/2 over next 16 hours • First 8 hours add 50 mEq/l of sodium bicarbonate. Second 8 hours only LR. Third 8 hours of first 24 hours only, add 12.5 g of 25 albumin/l of crystalloid • D₅W as needed
Cincinnati (older children)	• 4 ml/kg/%TBSA burn + 1,500 ml/m² total BSA of LR. 1/2 over first 8 hours, and 1/2 over next 16 hours; no albumin • D₅W as needed
Galveston	• 5,000 ml/m² BSA burn + 2,000 ml/m² total BSA of LR. 12.5 g of 25% albumin/l of crystalloid. • D₅W as needed • 1/2 over first 8 hours, and 1/2 over next 16 hours.

Use 5% dextrose in maintenance fluids in children < 30 kg _(See Table 13.18 for maintenance rate)_	

Adult (teenager) burn fluid resuscitation formula	
Parkland formula	• 4 ml/kg/%TBSA burn of LR 1/2 over first 8 hours, and 1/2 over next 16 hours • No colloid or glucose
Modified Brooke	• 3 ml/kg/%TBSA burn of LR. 1/2 over first 8 hours, and 1/2 over next 16 hours • No colloid or glucose

*LR—Ringer's lactate solution. **BSA—body surface area. ***%TBSA—Percent total body surface area.

Table 7-2 Estimation of Burns in Children as a Percentage of Body Surface Area (BSA)*

Age in years	<1	1	5	10	15
Head (%)	19	17	13	11	9
Neck (%)	2	2	2	2	2
Trunk (anterior or posterior) (%)	13	13	13	13	13
One buttock (%)	2.5	2.5	2.5	2.5	2.5
Genitalia and perineum (%)	1	1	1	1	1
One forearm (3) or upper arm (4) (%)	3–4	3–4	3–4	3–4	3–4
One hand (2.5) or foot (3.5) (%)	2.5–3.5	2.5–3.5	2.5–3.5	2.5–3.5	2.5–3.5
One thigh (%)	5.5	6.5	8	8.5	9
One leg (below knee) (%)	5	5	5.5	6	6.5

* Entire palm of the individual, regardless of age, can be used to estimate 1% of the BSA.

Burns Admission Criteria
5–10% TBSA partial thickness burns
2–5% full thickness burn
Circumferential burn
Inhalation burn
High-voltage injury
Associated medical conditions or suspected abuse

Burn Center Referral Criteria
Partial-thickness burns ≥ 10% BSA
≥ 2% full thickness burns in any age group
Burns to face, hands, feet, genitalia, perineum, or major joints
Chemical burns
High-voltage burn
Inhalational injury
Concomitant major trauma
Preexisting medical disorders that could complicate management, prolong recovery, or affect mortality
Inadequate support or suspected abuse

Asymptomatic children with exposure to common household current (120–240 V) require no treatment and no observation if there are no burns and no symptoms upon ED arrival.

Modified from American College of Surgeons. Chapter 14: Guidelines for trauma centers caring for burn patients. In: Resources for optimal care of the injured patient, 2014, chapter 14; 100-106 Jamshidi R, Sato TT. Pediatrics in Review Vol.34 No.9 September 2013, https://doi.org/10.1053/j.sempsurg.2019.01.013., Mary K. Arbuthnot DO , Alejandro V. Garcia MD , Early Resuscitation and Management of Severe Pediatric Burns, Seminars in Pediatric Surgery (2019), doi: https://doi.org/10.1053/j.sempsurg.2019.01.013

8 ■ CARDIOVASCULAR DISORDERS

ENDOCARDITIS PROPHYLAXIS

Table 8-1 Cardiac Conditions Requiring Infective Endocarditis (IE Prophylaxis)[1–3]

- Prior infectious endocarditis or any prosthetic cardiac valve
- Congenital heart disease (CHD)—only CHD categories below require prophylaxis:
  - Unrepaired CHD including those who have had shunts for palliation
  - Repaired CHD with residual defects at or adjacent to prosthetic patch or device
  - First 6-month post-op: Completely repaired CHD defects with prosthetic graft or device
- Post-cardiac transplantation with valve regurgitation

[1]Prophylaxis only required before dental procedures or if invasive respiratory tract procedure with incision or biopsy of respiratory mucosa. [2]Prophylaxis is no longer recommended prior to GU or GI procedures. [3]See Table 18-1 for antibiotic regimens. Modified from Wilson W, Taubert KA, Gewitz M, et.al. Prevention of infective endocarditis: guidelines from the American Heart Association: a guideline from the American Heart Association Rheumatic Fever, Endocarditis, and Kawasaki Disease Committee, Council on Cardiovascular Disease in the Young, and the Council on Clinical Cardiology, Council on Cardiovascular Surgery and Anesthesia, and the Quality of Care and Outcomes Research Interdisciplinary Working Group. *Circulation.* 2007;116(15):1736-1754; Nishimura RA, Otto CM, Bonow RO, et al. 2017 AHA/ACC focused update of the 2014 AHA/ACC guideline for the management of patients with valvular heart disease: a report of the American College of Cardiology/American Heart Association task force on clinical practice guidelines. *Circulation.* 2017;135(25):e1159-e1195.

ECG EVALUATION

Table 8-2 Normal ECG Values

Age	P-R interval[1]	QRS interval[1]	QRS axis (mean)	QTc[2]
0–7 days	0.08–0.12	0.04–0.08	80–160 (125)	0.34–0.54
1–4 weeks	0.08–0.12	0.04–0.07	60–160 (110)	0.30–0.50
1–3 months	0.08–0.12	0.04–0.08	40–120 (80)	0.32–0.47
3–6 months	0.08–0.12	0.04–0.08	20–80 (65)	0.35–0.46
6–12 months	0.09–0.13	0.04–0.08	20–100 (65)	0.31–0.49
1–3 years	0.10–0.14	0.04–0.08	20–100 (55)	0.34–0.49
3–8 years	0.11–0.16	0.05–0.09	40–80 (60)	< 0.45
8–16 years	0.12–0.17	0.05–0.09	20–80 (65)	< 0.45

[1]Seconds. [2]QTc = QT interval/(square root of RR interval).

Table 8-3 ECG Diagnosis of Chamber Enlargement (Hypertrophy)

Right ventricular hypertrophy (RVH)	Biventricular hypertrophy
• R in V1 > 20 mm (> 25 mm < 1 month) • S in V6 > 6 mm (> 12 mm < 1 month) • Upright T in V3R, R in V1 after 5 days • QR pattern in V3R, V1	• RVH and (S in V1 or R in V6) exceeding mean for age • LVH and (R in V1 or S in V6) exceeding mean for age
Left ventricular hypertrophy (LVH)	**Right atrial enlargement**
• R in V6 > 25 mm (> 21 mm < 1 year) • S in V1 > 30 mm (> 20 mm < 1 year) • R in V6 + S in V1 > 60 mm (use V5 if R in V5 > R in V6) • Abnormal R/S ratio • S in V1 > 2 × R in V5	• Peak P value > 3 mm (< 6 months), > 2.5 mm (≥ 6 months) **Left atrial enlargement** • P in II > 0.09 seconds • P in V1 with late negative deflection > 0.04 seconds and > 1 mm deep

Table 8-4 ECG Features of Disorders Associated with or Mistaken for Disease States[1]

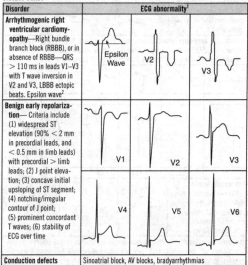

Disorder	ECG abnormality[1]
Arrhythmogenic right ventricular cardiomyopathy—Right bundle branch block (RBBB), or in absence of RBBB—QRS > 110 ms in leads V1–V3 with T wave inversion in V2 and V3, LBBB ectopic beats. Epsilon wave[2]	Epsilon Wave / V2 / V3
Benign early repolarization— Criteria include (1) widespread ST elevation (90% < 2 mm in precordial leads, and < 0.5 mm in limb leads) with precordial > limb leads; (2) J point elevation; (3) concave initial upsloping of ST segment; (4) notching/irregular contour of J point; (5) prominent concordant T waves; (6) stability of ECG over time	V1 / V2 / V3 V4 / V5 / V6
Conduction defects	Sinoatrial block, AV blocks, bradyarrhythmias

(Continued)

Table 8-4 ECG Features of Disorders Associated with or Mistaken for Disease States[1] (Continued)

Disorder	ECG abnormality[1]		
Drugs and toxins	See specific drug or toxin in the "Toxicology" section.		
Hyperkalemia—*Early* narrow or peaked T waves, short QT interval, *later* widened QRS with ↓ P wave height, then loss of P waves, AV block, sine wave pattern, asystole	$K^+ > 6$ mEq/l tall T wave	$K^+ > 7.5$ mEq ↑ PR, ↑ QRS	$K^+ > 9$ mEq/l, no P, sinusoidal
Hypocalcemia—Prolonged QT (see pages 44 (prolonged QT syndrome) and 47)	Prolongs QT by lengthening ST segment, also ↓ T wave voltage, flat T waves, terminal T wave inversion, or deeply inverted T waves (if severe), rare ST elevation		
Hypokalemia—ST depression, flat T waves, and prominent U wave (arrow); prolonged QT			
Hypertrophic cardiomyopathy (idiopathic subaortic stenosis): Nonspecific ST-T wave abnormalities; left ventricular hypertrophy. QRS complexes largest in midprecordial leads; Q waves in inferior (II, III, aVF) or precordial (V2 to V6) leads, or both.			

I	II	III	aVR	aVL	aVF

V1	V2	V3	V4	V5	V6

Disorder	ECG abnormality
Intracranial hemorrhage—May cause deep, wide T waves, bradycardia, prolonged QT interval, minor ST elevation (<3 mm), U waves	
Ischemia (including arteritis, Kawasaki aneurysm occlusion, or anomalous coronary artery)	With anomalous coronary arteries, resting ECG is often normal. Focal ST segment elevation or depression, Q waves, T wave inversion. Reciprocal changes.

Table 8-4 ECG Features of Disorders Associated with or Mistaken for Disease States[1] (*Continued*)

Disorder	ECG abnormality[1]
Kawasaki disease—Most with Kawasaki have ECG evidence of carditis.	The most common ECG findings are elevated ST-T segments, elevated Q/R ratio (55% each), followed by a prolonged QT interval (35%), elevated P waves, diminished R waves (V1), prolonged PR intervals and flat T waves. After coronary artery formation, classic myocardial ischemic findings can occur. • ECG findings are not part of current criteria in the diagnosis of Kawasaki disease • Echocardiogram is recommended when Kawasaki disease is considered Modified from: McCrindle BW, Rowley AH, Newburger JW, et al. Diagnosis, treatment, and long-term management of Kawasaki disease: a scientific statement for health professionals from the American Heart Association. *Circulation.* 2017;135(17):e927-e999.
Lyme Disease—Carditis occurs in 16%. Most are older than 10 years, have arthralgias or cardiopulmonary symptoms (pain, dyspnea, syncope)	The most common ECG findings in order of frequency are 1st degree AV block, then 2nd or 3rd degree AV block (usually transient), prolonged QT, and then ST-T wave changes. Modified from: Costello JM, Alexander ME, Greco KM, et al. Lyme carditis in children: presentation, predictive factors, and clinical course. *Pediatrics.* 2009;123(5):e835-e841.
Myocarditis—Patients may have ECG evidence of both myocarditis and pericarditis. In one study, 100% of patients with myocarditis had abnormal ECG, 73% had elevated CK, and 54% had elevated troponin. 90% had cardiomegaly, 15% pulmonary edema, and 5% an infiltrate. Shortness of breath occurred in 69%, vomiting in 48%, poor feeding in 40%, + URI 39%. *Source:* Durani Y, Egan M, Baffa J, et al. Pediatric myocarditis: presenting clinical characteristics. *Am J Emerg Med.* 2009;27(8):942-947.	Sinus tachycardia is most common, with frequent nonspecific ST-T wave changes, occasional ischemic changes, pathologic Q waves, and variable AV blocks. | *Most common ECG findings (in myocarditis)*	Frequency
Sinus tachycardia	46%
Ventricular hypertrophy	41%
ST wave abnormality	32%
T wave abnormality	31%
Bundle branch	10%
Arrhythmia	7%
AV block	5%
Prolonged QT interval	5%	

(*Continued*)

Table 8-4 ECG Features of Disorders Associated with or Mistaken for Disease States[1] (Continued)

Disorder	ECG abnormality[1]
Pericarditis—(1) Diffuse ST elevation. (2) ST depression in aVR ± II and V1. ST segment is typically concave upward or ≤ 5 mm height. Q waves are rare. PR segment depression is common inferior + lateral. (3) Sequence: (a) initial ST, (b) ST returns to baseline, (c) T waves flip ↓ and T wave amplitude is usually ≤ 5 mm, (d) T waves normalize. (4) Height of ST segment/T wave > 0.25 in V5, V6, or I	
Prolonged QT syndrome—QTc interval > 0.46–0.50 milliseconds, may need stress testing to uncover prolongation of QT. See www.qtdrugs.org for causes.	
Sudden unexpected death syndrome (SUDS) or Brugada syndrome—RBBB with ST segment elevation in V1 to V3 or incomplete RBBB with ST segment elevation in V1 and V2	
Wolff-Parkinson-White syndrome—Delta wave, wide QRS, short PR interval, wide complex AFib/SVT	

[1]The list is not all inclusive and only describes common ECG findings for diseases. [2]Epsilon wave = terminal notch in QRS complex.

ARRHYTHMIAS

Figure 8-1 Symptomatic Bradycardia[1]

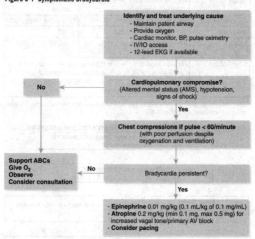

Identify and treat underlying cause
- Maintain patent airway
- Provide oxygen
- Cardiac monitor, BP, pulse oximetry
- IV/IO access
- 12-lead EKG if available

Cardiopulmonary compromise?
(Altered mental status (AMS), hypotension, signs of shock)

No

Yes

Chest compressions if pulse < 60/minute
(with poor perfusion despite oxygenation and ventilation)

Support ABCs
Give O₂
Observe
Consider consultation

No

Bradycardia persistent?

Yes

- **Epinephrine** 0.01 mg/kg (0.1 mL/kg of 0.1 mg/mL)
- **Atropine** 0.2 mg/kg (min 0.1 mg, max 0.5 mg) for increased vagal tone/primary AV block
- **Consider pacing**

[1]Shock—identify and treat possible causes: Hypovolemia, hypoxia, hydrogen ion (acidosis), hypo/hyperkalemia, hypoglycemia, hypothermia, toxins, tamponade (cardiac), tension pneumothorax, thrombosis (heart/lung), trauma (blood loss or increased intracranial pressure, or tamponade/pneumothorax).

Table 8-5 Differentiation of Sinus Tachycardia from Supraventricular Tachycardia

	Sinus tachycardia	Supraventricular tachycardia
History	Volume loss (dehydration, bleed), drugs, other stressor	Often vague and nondescript, if prolonged—CHF or shock
Heart rate < 1 year	< 220	≥ 220
Heart rate > 1 year	< 180–200	> 180–200
QRS width	Narrow for age	Narrow in 90%
P waves	Upright leads I, aVF	Rare, negative in II, III, aVF
HR and R-R variability	Beat-beat (R-R varies), responds to stimulation	No variability, no response to stimulation
HR changes	Slow increase or decrease	Abrupt onset and termination

Table 8-6 Wide Supraventricular Tachycardia (Aberrancy) vs. Ventricular Tachycardia[1]

	Supraventricular Tachycardia	Ventricular Tachycardia
History	Wolff Parkinson White (WPW) in up to 30% in infancy[2]	70% structural cardiac disease
Symptoms and BP	Not a useful differentiator	Not a useful differentiator
Heart rate	> 220 infant, > 180 child	> 120
P waves	Retrograde P waves possible	Dissociation of P and QRS
Other features	Features found useful in differentiating adult VT (*absence of RS in all precordial leads, QRS concordance in precordial leads, QRS ≥ 0.12–0.14 ms*) vs. SVT (*triphasic QRS with RBBB in V1 or V6*) have not been studied in children	

[1]During management, generally assume wide complex tachyarrhythmia is ventricular tachycardia. [2]Ebstein's anomaly esp. associated with WPW in 10–30%.

Table 8-7 Stable Tachycardia with a Pulse and Adequate Perfusion Management

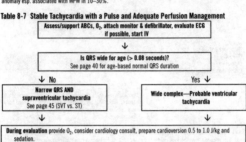

Assess/support ABCs, O₂, attach monitor & defibrillator, evaluate ECG if possible, start IV

↓

Is QRS wide for age (> 0.08 seconds)?
See page 40 for age-based normal QRS duration

↓ No   Yes ↓

Narrow QRS AND supraventricular tachycardia
See page 45 (SVT vs. ST)

Wide complex—Probable ventricular tachycardia

↓

During evaluation provide O₂, consider cardiology consult, prepare cardioversion 0.5 to 1.0 J/kg and sedation.
Identify/treat possible causes: ↓ O₂, ↓ volume, ↑ temperature, ↓ or ↑ K⁺, metabolic disorders, tamponade, tension pneumothorax, toxins/drugs, pain, & thromboebolism

↓

Consider vagal maneuvers

↓

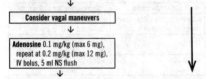

Adenosine 0.1 mg/kg (max 6 mg), repeat at 0.2 mg/kg (max 12 mg), IV bolus, 5 ml NS flush

↓

Consult pediatric cardiologist
Attempt cardioversion at 0.5 to 1 J/kg, with ↑ to 2 J/kg
Sedate if time permits

Consider medications[1]
Amiodarone 5 mg/kg IV over 20 to 60 minutes OR Procainamide 15 mg/kg IV over 30 to 60 minutes

[1]Consider MgSO₄ 25 mg/kg IV over 15 minutes if torsades. *Source: Circulation.* 2005;112:I-167.

Figure 8-2 Unstable Tachycardia Management[1, 2]

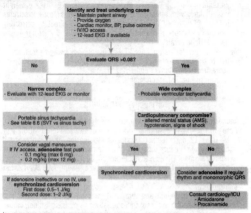

[1]See figure 2-11 for pulseless VF/VT, PEA management. *Source. PALS Card 2015.*
[2]Shock—identify and treat possible causes: Hypovolemia, hypoxia, hydrogen ion (acidosis), hypo/hyperkalemia, hypoglycemia, hypothermia, toxins, tamponade (cardiac), tension pneumothorax, thrombosis (heart/lung), trauma (blood loss or increased intracranial pressure, or tamponade/pneumothorax).
Modified from 2005 American Heart Association Guidelines for Cardiopulmonary Resuscitation and Emergency Cardiovascular Care, Circulation 2005; 112: I-167.

OTHER RHYTHM/ECG DISTURBANCES

Atrial flutter: Atrial rate of 250–350 beats/minute with variable but regular ventricular rate depending on degree of AV block (sawtooth pattern). Nearly always seen in children with congenital heart disease, especially after cardiac surgery. Can develop in newborns with normal cardiac anatomy. Treat if unstable with synchronized cardioversion—initially use 0.5 J/kg doubling to 1 J/kg, then 2 J/kg if needed. Digoxin, procainamide, and amiodarone are used in hemodynamically stable patients.

Atrial fibrillation: Atrial rate of > 300–600 with irregularly irregular ventricular rates often > 100–150 beats/minute. As with a flutter, most infants have structural heart disease. Management of unstable patients requires synchronized cardioversion. If stable, anticoagulation is usually required before converting rhythm.

Prolonged QT interval: (1) Inherited form may be associated with deafness, or (2) acquired due to class I antiarrhythmics (e.g., quinidine, procainamide), amiodarone, phenothiazines, lithium, cyclic antide-pressants, ↓ K+, ↓ Ca^{2+}, ↓ Mg^{2+}, myocarditis, liver disease, weight loss. Children with prolonged QTc may present with syncope or seizures [QTc = QT interval/(square root of RR interval)]. Treat by correcting underlying disorder or discontinuing drug. See Table 8-2 for age-based normal QTc intervals.

Torsades de pointes: Polymorphic VT with morphology swinging from nega-tive to positive direction in 1 lead. Etiology: see ↑ QT mentioned previ-ously. Treatment: Correct underlying disease, MgSO$_4$ 25–50 mg/kg slow IV, overdrive pacing, isoproterenol, lidocaine, phenytoin.

ANTIARRHYTHMIC AGENTS

Adenosine—Endogenous purine nucleoside used to treat SVT.

Dose—0.1 mg/kg IV push (max 6 mg), may double and repeat at 0.2 mg/kg (max 12 mg). If unsuccessful or hypotension, then synchronized cardioversion. Reduce dose 75% if carbamazepine/dipyridamole use or heart transplant (Thajudeen A, Stecker EC, Shehata M. Arrhythmias after heart transplantation: mechanisms and management. *J Am Heart Assoc.* 2012;1(2):e001461).

Contraindications—Sick sinus syndrome, second- or third-degree AV block, current use of digoxin and verapamil (may precipitate VFib), asthma (may precipitate bronchospasm especially if using theophylline), carba-mazepine/*Tegretol* use (may increase degree of heart block), denervated heart (post-transplant)

Select Side Effects—Flushing, palpitations, chest pain, bradycardia, heart block, headache, dyspnea, bronchoconstriction in asthmatics

Amiodarone—Class III antiarrhythmic with adrenergic inhibition, ↑ action potential/refractory period, ↓ AV conduction/sinus node function used for ventricular fibrillation, ventricular tachycardia, SVT, atrial fib/flutter.

Dose—(pulseless VF/VT) 5 mg/kg rapid IV/IO bolus (max 300 mg). (VT/SVT with pulse) 5 mg/kg IV/IO over 20–60 minutes (max 300 mg). May repeat up to maximum dose of 15 mg/kg/day. IV maintenance dose 5 mcg/kg/minute (max 15 mcg/kg/minute)

Contraindications—Sinus node disease, bradycardia, second- or third-degree AV block, age ≤ 30 days causes gasping syndrome: respiratory distress, acidosis, cardiac arrest

Select Side Effects—↓ HR resistant to atropine (may need isoproter-enol or pacer), ↓ BP, cardiac arrest, Torsades de pointes (↑ QT), ARDS/pneumonitis, hepatitis

Digoxin—Cardiac glycoside with inotropic and AV blocking effects. Obtain cardiology consult before administering this agent.

Total digitalizing dose (TDD) is given over 16–24 hours: 1/2 of dose initially IV, followed by 1/4 dose at both 8 and 16 hours. Oral doses are 20% greater, with maintenance dose 12.5% of TDD every 12 hours starting 12 hours after TDD complete.

Table 8-8 Unstable Tachycardia Management

Age	Total digitalizing dose IV	Maintenance (IV) daily dose
Premature neonate	15–25 mcg/kg	Maintenance dose is 20–30% of loading dose for premature neonate, and 25–35% of loading dose for others (divide above dose every 12 hours)
Term neonate	20–30 mcg/kg	
1–24 months	30–50 mcg/kg	
2–5 years	25–35 mcg/kg	
5–10 years	15–30 mcg/kg (max 1.5 mg)	

Contraindications—Ventricular dysrhythmias (esp. VF). In patients receiving digoxin, cardioversion or calcium infusion might precipitate ventricular fibrillation.

Select Side Effects—Atrial and supraventricular arrhythmias with or without block, bradycardia, vomiting, diarrhea, headache, confusion, and visual changes.

Esmolol—β1 selective blocker with short half-life (2 minutes). Used in SVT, hypertensive emergency/urgency. Consider cardiology or ICU consultation prior to use.

Dose—100–500 mcg/kg IV over 5 minutes with initial maintenance infusion of 50 mcg/kg/minutes. May increase infusion 50 mcg/kg/minutes every 5 minutes to maximum of 200 mcg/kg/minute (0.2 mg/kg/minute).

Contraindications—Sinus bradycardia, or heart block, CHF, cardiogenic shock

Select Side Effects—Low blood pressure, bradycardia, confusion, vomiting, bronchoconstriction

Lidocaine—Class IB antiarrhythmic. Used in shock-resistant VF, pulseless VT

Dose—1 mg/kg IV/IO or 2–3 mg/kg ET. Second bolus of 0.5–1.0 mg/kg IV/IO (2–10 × higher for ET) if needed. Infusion: 20–50 mcg/kg/minute

Contraindications—Amide anesthetic allergy, AV, SA, intraventricular heart block

Select Side Effects—↓ BP/HR, altered LOC, seizure, vomit, respiratory depression

Procainamide—Class IA antiarrhythmic with anticholinergic/anesthetic effects

Dose—15 mg/kg IV over ≥ 30 minutes. Infusion: 20–80 mcg/kg/minute (daily max 2,000 mg/24 hours)

Contraindications—Second- or third-degree heart block, Torsades de pointes, QT prolongation, myasthenia gravis, lupus, hypersensitivity to procaine

Select Side Effects—↓ BP, ↑ or ↓ HR, QT/QRS widening, confusion, vomiting, neutropenia, thrombocytopenia, anemia, ↑ LFTs, lupus-like syndrome

Verapamil—Calcium channel blocker with negative inotropic and chronotropic effect

Dose—0.1 mg/kg IV (max 5 mg). Repeat 0.2 mg/kg (max 10 mg) in 30 minutes if no effect. When used, needs expert consultation, continuous ECG, and IV calcium available.

Contraindications—Avoid in infancy as associated with hypotension and cardiac arrest. Other contraindications include sinus bradycardia, heart block, shock, ventricular tachycardia, wide complex SVT/AFib/Aflutter due to bypass tract.

Select Side Effects—↓ BP/HR, heart block, CHF, seizures, respiratory insufficiency in muscular dystrophy, ↑ LFTs, GI upset, constipation

CHEST PAIN

Table 8-9 Select Serious Causes of Chest Pain in Children

Ischemia from arteritis (Kawasaki's), coronary artery anomalies, HTN, ↓ O_2	*Arrhythmias* (↓ or ↑ HR)
	↓ BP with ↓ coronary perfusion
Structural anomalies (e.g., aortic stenosis), pulmonic stenosis, cardiomyopathy (HCM, dilated)	*Infectious* (pericarditis, myocarditis, endocarditis)
	Aortic dissection
	Sickle cell (chest syndrome)
Pulmonary (emboli, pneumothorax)	* Life-threatening conditions in only 1–6% of pediatric chest pain

Chest pain etiologies at a pediatric ED	Musculoskeletal	25–64%	Psychogenic	9–13%
	Respiratory	13–21%	Trauma	5%
	Idiopathic	2–21%	GI or cardiac	3–5% each

Modified from Steven M. Selbst et. Al., Pediatric Chest Pain: A Prospective Study, Pediatrics. 1988;82:319. Cerebral Blood Flow Abnormalities in Children With Sydenham's Chorea: A SPECT Study, Clin Pediatr. 2004;43:241.

CONGENITAL HEART DISEASE

Table 8-10 Most Common Congenital Defects Diagnosed at Different Ages[1]

0–6 Days		7–13 Days		14–28 Days	
D-Transposition of great arteries	19%	Coarctation—aorta	16%	VSD	16%
Hypoplastic LH	14%	VSD	14%	Coarctation—aorta	12%
Tetralogy of Fallot	8%	Hypoplastic LH	8%	Tetralogy of Fallot	7%
Coarctation—aorta	7%	D-Transposition of great arteries	7%	D-Transposition of great arteries	7%
VSD	3%	Tetralogy of Fallot	7%	Patent ductus	5%
Other defects	49%	Other defects	48%	Other defects	53%

[1]LH—left heart; VSD—ventricular septal defect.
Data from Marino BS, Bird GL, Wernovsky G. Diagnosis and management of the newborn with suspected congenital heart disease. *Clin Perinatol.* 2001;28(1):91-136.
Data from Flanagan MF, Fyler DC. Cardiac disease. In Avery GB, Fletcher MA, MacDonald M, eds. *Neonatology: Pathophysiology and Management of the Newborn.* Philadelphia, PA: J.B. Lippincott; 1994:524; with permission.

Table 8-11 Pulse Oximetry in Congenital Heart Disease (CHD)

Beyond first 24 hours of life, pulse oximetry can be used to screen for CHD
• < 90% SpO_2 in right hand or foot = positive screen (ECHO)
• 90–94% SpO_2 in right hand or foot OR > 3% difference → repeat screen in 1 hour (max 3 times)
• ≥ 95% in right hand or foot AND ≤ 3% difference → negative screen

Adapted from Kemper AR, Mahle WT, Martin GR, et al. Strategies for implementing screening for critical congenital heart disease. *Pediatrics.* 2011;128:e1259.

Table 8-12 Hyperoxia Test in Cyanotic CHD*

(1) Obtain arterial blood gas (ABG) on room air.

(2) Place patient on 100% oxygen for 10 minutes.

(3) Repeat ABG:
   - Cyanotic heart disease usually $PaO_2 < 50$ mm Hg following 10 minutes of 100% O_2 (see disorders and hyperoxia test results, which follows).
   - Those with lung disease usually can raise their $PaO_2 > 100$ mm Hg.

*Useful if echocardiography unavailable.

Table 8-13 Lesions with Ductal Dependent Systemic (S) or Pulmonary (P) Flow[1]

Tetralogy of fallot (P), Ebstein's anomaly (P), critical PS (P), tricuspid atresia (P), pulmonic valve atresia (P)	Hypoplastic left heart (S), interrupted aortic arch (S), critical coarctation of aorta (S), critical AS (S), d-TGA (P)

[1]Mostly disorders with failed hyperoxia test or shock in first 3 weeks of life are often responsive to prostaglandin E1 (see dose Table A-2).

Table 8-14 Specific Cardiac/Noncardiac Disorders and Hyperoxia Test Results[1,2]

Disorders	PaO₂ (%sat) FiO₂ 21%	PaO₂ (%sat) FiO₂ 100%	PaCO₂
No disease	> 70 (> 95%)	> 300 (100%)	35
Lung or neurologic disease	50 (85%)	> 150 (100%)	50
d-TGA ± VSD, tricuspid atresia + PS or atresia, critical PS, tetralogy of fallot	< 40 (< 75%)	< 50 (< 85%)	35
Truncus arteriosus, TAPVR, hypoplastic left heart, single ventricle	40–60 (75–93%)	< 150 (< 100%)	35
Persistent pulmonary HTN of newborn, LV outflow tract obstruct (AA hypoplasia, interrupted AA, critical coarctation, AS)	Pre 70 (95%)[3] Post < 40 (< 75%)	Variable	35–50
d-TGA + (coarctation of aorta or interrupted aortic arch) or + pulmonary HTN	Pre < 40 (< 75%) Post > 50 (< 90%)	Variable	35–50

[1]A failed hyperoxia test indicates ductal dependent systemic or pulmonary blood flow. [2]TGA—transposition of great arteries; PS—pulmonary stenosis; TAPVR—total anomalous pulmonary venous return; HTN—hypertension; AA—aortic arch; AS—aortic stenosis. [3]Defect is (pre) pre-ductal or (post) post-ductal.

Modified from Alex R. Kemper, William T. Mahle, Gerard R. Martin, W. Carl Cooley, Praveen Kumar, W. Robert Morrow, Kellie Kelm, Gail D. Pearson, Jill Glidewell, Scott D. Grosse and R. Rodney Howell. Strategies for Implementing Screening for Critical Congenital Heart Disease. *Pediatrics* November 2011; 128 (5): e1259-e1267. DOI: https://doi.org/10.1542/peds.2011-1317

Table 8-15 Chest Radiography in Acyanotic CHD

Normal pulmonary flow	PS, MS or MR, AS, coarctation of the aorta
↑ Pulmonary flow	ASD, VSD, PDA, left to right shunts with pulmonary HTN, AV canal

Table 8-16 Chest Radiography in Cyanotic CHD

↓ Pulmonary flow	Severe PS, pulmonary atresia, tetralogy of fallot (normal/boot-shaped heart), TGA with PS, tricuspid atresia, Ebstein's anomaly (massive heart), Eisenmenger's complex
↑ Pulmonary flow	TAPVR (Snowman sign—late finding, supracardiac venous return via dilated right and left superior vena cava), hypoplastic LH, TGA (egg-shaped heart tilted on its side with a narrow mediastinum "egg on a string") ± VSD, truncus arteriosus

ACYANOTIC HEART DISEASE

Cardiac lesions with flow of blood from high pressure left to right side of the heart.

Examples—(1) *Atrial septal defect* often asymptomatic until adulthood and can cause right atrial enlargement (RAE) and SVTs. (2) *Ventricular septal defects* (VSD) if small may cause loud holosystolic murmur at left sternal border. If moderate, CHF may develop after first few weeks as normal newborn pulmonary resistance drops, decreasing RV pressure, and increasing the left to right shunt. RVH > LVH ± left atrial enlargement (LAE) may be evident on ECG. (3) *Patent ductus arteriosus*—Early systolic/diastolic murmur at second, third left intercostal (IC) space, later becomes machinery type and radiates to the back. Progressive CHF may develop while ECG may show LVH if PDA is large.

Management of CHF—Elevate head of bed, O₂, furosemide (*Lasix*) 1 mg/kg IV, morphine 0.05 mg/kg IV, dopamine/dobutamine if shock, vasodilator if ↑ BP or vasoconstriction (e.g., nitroprusside), treat cause (e.g., prostaglandin E1 [PGE1; dose on Table A-2] if ductal dependent lesion—hypoplastic left heart, coarctation, interrupted aortic arch, TGA).

CYANOTIC HEART DISEASE WITH DECREASED PULMONARY FLOW

Obstruction of flow at the right side of the heart so there is less flow to the lungs

Example—Tetralogy of Fallot: VSD, RV outflow obstruction, RVH, overriding aorta—Acute shunting leads to ↑ RR, ↑ cyanosis, ↓ murmur, stroke, or death. Precipitants: crying, defecating, exercise, ↓ systemic vascular resistance (SVR), ↓ LV pressure, and RV outflow spasm.

Acute management of hypercyanotic "Tet spell"—O₂, knee-chest position (↓ venous return), morphine 0.1 mg/kg IV (↓ outflow spasm), NS 10–20 ml/kg

IV (SVR), phenylephrine (see dose on Table A-2, goal = ↑ SVR 20%), prostaglandin E1 (see dose on Table A-2) ± propranolol or esmolol (consult cardiology for these drugs). Use caution as they lead to ↓ BP/HR especially in neonates.

CYANOTIC HEART DISEASE WITH INCREASED PULMONARY FLOW

Example— (1) *d-Transposition of great arteries*: Aorta arises from RV and pulmonary artery from LV. Mixing of blood is via foramen ovale, patent ductus arteriosus ± VSD. Patients have cyanosis/CHF. CXR-cardiomegaly (egg on a string appearance). (2) *Total anomalous pulmonary venous return (TAPVR)*: All blood (systemic and pulmonary) returns to right atrium. ASD or patent foramen ovale must be present. CXR shows cardiomegaly and increased pulmonary vascular flow (Snowman sign).

Acute management—Treat as CHF, prostaglandin E1 for TGA and TAPVR patients with *infra*diaphragmatic venous return connection abnormalities (may worsen in patients with TAPVR) and abnormal *supra*diaphragmatic connections (see dose on Table A-2).

LEFT VENTRICULAR OUTFLOW OBSTRUCTION

Most common disorders presenting at ≤ 28 days old are hypoplastic left heart (HPLV) (51%), coarctation (CoA) (34%), and interrupted aortic arch (IAA) (13%).

Modified from: Rosenberg NM, Walker AR, Bechtel K, et al. Conscious sedation in the pediatric emergency department. *Pediatr Emerg Care*. 1998;14(6):436-439.

Table 8-17 Physiologic Murmurs

Murmur	Age	Location	Timing	Cause
Still's	3–6 years	Apex	Systole	Turbulent LV outflow
Pulmonary ejection	8–14 years	2nd left intercostal space (ICS)	Systole	RV outflow tract turbulence
Supraclavicular	4–14 years	Above clavicle	Systole	Brachiocephalic branching
Venous hum[1]	3–6 years	Base of neck	Entire	Venous return
Straight back pectus	All	Apex	Systole	RV filling with inspiration
Hemic exertion	All	Apex, left ICS	Systole	Rapid LV ejection
Neonatal pulmonary ejection	< 6 months	Right second ICS	Systole	Underdeveloped pulmonary arteries

[1]Venous hums decrease with supine position, turning head, and expiration.

PHYSIOLOGIC MURMURS

Murmur evaluation: Murmurs should be of concern if CHD, failure to thrive, frequent infections, asthma, chest pain, or syncope. Heart disease also is suggested if: (1) murmur is grade ≥ 3, holosystolic, diastolic, harsh/blowing, increased in upright position; (2) cyanosis or CHF; or (3) abnormal ECG, CXR, or blood pressure.

SYNCOPE

Table 8-18 Evaluation and Etiology of Pediatric Syncope

Evaluation (primarily based on clinical presentation)	ECG, pregnancy test females > 11–12; Hb, glucose, electrolytes, Holter if arrhythmia, CT head (abnormal neuro exam), CT chest (dissection, PE), ECHO (valvular heart disease)				
Etiology of syncope in infants and children presenting to a pediatric ED	Vasovagal	50%	Head trauma	5%
	Orthostasis	20%	Migraine	5%
	Atypical seizure	7%	Miscellaneous	13%

Modified from Pratt JL, Fleisher GR. Syncope in children and adolescents. *Pediatr Emerg Care.* 1989;5:80-82.

Table 8-19 Features Associated with Life-Threatening Cause of Syncope*

• Family history of cardiomyopathy or sudden death (HCM, prolonged QT)	• Abnormal ECG, examples Table 8-4
• Syncope during exercise or while supine (HCM, aortic + pulmonic stenosis, pulmonary hypertension)	• Abnormal cardiac examination
	• Recurrent syncope
	• Fall directly onto face (rapid onset)
• Syncope + chest pain or palpitations (HCM, ischemia, aortic stenosis)	• CHD
	• Drugs with cardiac effects
• Congenital deafness (long QT)	• Marfanoid appearance or collagen vascular disease in family

*The largest ED study to date of pediatric syncope found two or more of the following historical features to have 100% sensitivity for cardiac disease: (1) syncope with exercise, (2) chest pain preceding syncope during exercise, (3) no prodrome, and (4) palpitations preceding syncope.
Modified from Hurst D, Hirsh DA, Oster ME, et al. Syncope in the Pediatric Emergency Department—can we predict cardiac disease based on history alone?. *J Emerg Med.* 2015;49(1):1-7.

Table 8-20 Causes of Sudden Death in Young Athletes[1-3]

Cause	% of Total
Hypertrophic cardiomyopathy (HCM)	26%
Commotio cordis	20%
Coronary artery anomaly	14%
Left ventricular hypertrophy, not diagnostic of HCM	8%
Myocarditis	5%
Asthma, ruptured aortic aneurysm, arrhythmogenic right ventricular cardiomyopathy, tunneled (bridged) coronary artery, atherosclerotic coronary artery disease, dilated cardiomyopathy, myxomatous mitral valve, heat stroke, drug abuse, long Q-T, cardiac sarcoid, ruptured cerebral artery, trauma involving structural cardiac injury	≤ 1–3% each

[1]A history (especially family), exam, and ECG detects many disorders causing sudden death. A resting (± exercise) ECG in young adults and adolescents is standard in Europe while the American Heart Association does not endorse routine ECGs. An available automated external defibrillator at training/sport sites may save lives. [2]See ECG examples, Table 8-4.[3] The NCAA recommends screening all athletes for the sickle-cell trait due to death from exertional rhabdomyolysis (death within hours, days); for all strenuous exertion, ensure adequate rest, hydration, and recovery periods, and stop the workout if muscle cramping, swelling, weakness, inability to catch breath, or excess fatigue occurs.

Overall high school athlete risk is 1:50,000–80,000, with higher risk in males, African Americans, basketball athletes.

Adapted from Harmon KG, Drezner JA, Wilson MG, et al. Incidence of sudden cardiac death in athletes: a state-of-the-art review. *Heart.* 2014;100(16):1227-1234.

Data from Maron BJ. Sudden death in young athletes. *N Engl J Med.* 2003;349(11):1064-1075. doi:10.1056/nejmra022783

9 ■ DERMATOLOGY

Table 9-1 Rash Patterns and Etiology[1]

Acneiform	Acne vulgaris, drugs (steroid, Li, INH), Cushing's, chloracne
Acrodermatitis (extremity)	Papular acrodermatitis, smallpox, atopic dermatitis (infantile), tinea pedis, dyshidrotic eczema, poststreptococcal desquamation, Rocky Mountain Spotted Fever, drug rash
Clothing covered	Contact dermatitis, miliaria, psoriasis (summer), folliculitis
Flexural creases	Atopic dermatitis (childhood), infantile seborrheic dermatitis, intertrigo, candidiasis, tinea cruris, ichthyosis, inverse psoriasis
Linear Christmas tree distribution	Pityriasis rosea, secondary syphilis, drug reaction, guttate psoriasis, atopic dermatitis
Sun exposed	Phototoxic drug rash, photocontact dermatitis, lupus, viral exanthem, porphyria, xeroderma pigmentosum

[1]Vesiculobullous, petechial/purpuric, eczematous, papulosquamous rashes, see pages 60–65. Evaluation of patients with a petechial rash, see Table 18-7.

NEWBORN RASHES

Rash	Characteristics	Distribution	Course/Treatment
Erythema toxicum	Erythematous papules and sterile pustules surrounded by erythematous halo	Over entire body surface area, palms and soles spared, occurs in first few days of life	Self-limited
Transient neonatal pustular melanosis	Flaccid and superficial pustules, which disrupt easily, on a nonerythematous base, progress to hyperpigmented macules	Lesions may be present at birth, involves all areas including palms, soles, and genitalia	No treatment needed
Infantile acropustulosis	Intensely pruritic, discrete erythematous papules that become vesiculopustular within 24 hours and subsequently crust	Dense lesions over palms and soles and sides of feet, waxes (7–14 days) and wanes (2–4 months), may continue up to 2 years	Topical steroids and oral antihistamines

Rash	Characteristics	Distribution	Course/Treatment
Eosinophilic pustular folliculitis	Polymorphous eruption with pruritic vesiculopustules, coalesce to form exudative and crusted plaques	Mainly on scalp and face, but also on trunk and extremity Intermittent	High potency steroid cream
Miliaria	Tiny fragile, clear (crystallina) vesicles over healthy skin to pruritic erythematous papules (rubra)	In intertriginous areas, face, scalp, and trunk	Benign
Milia	1–2 mm white cysts	Forehead, cheeks, nose and upper lip, starting by days 4–5, resolves by 2 months	Self-limited
Transient benign vascular phenomena	Acrocyanosis	Blue, purple discoloration due to cold	Benign
	Cutis marmorata	Reticulated cyanosis/marbling of skin, symmetrically involving the trunk and extremity	
	Harlequin color change	Dependent part becomes bright red in contrast to pale upper half	

SCALING DERMATITIDES

	Characteristics	Distribution	Treatment
Irritant contact dermatitis	Lesions have erythema, oozing, weeping, and formation of microvesicles within epidermis	Over convex surfaces of perineum, lower abdomen, buttocks, and thighs sparing intertriginous areas	Removal of stimulus and temporary treatment with topical steroids and barrier pastes
Seborrheic dermatitis	Salmon-colored patches with greasy yellow scales	In intertriginous areas, diaper area, axilla, and scalp	Mild keratolytics, emollients, low potency steroids, antifungal shampoo

CUTANEOUS FUNGAL INFECTIONS

Rash		Characteristics	Treatment
Tinea versicolor (*Malassezia globosa*)		Reddish brown to hypopigmented macules covered with fine scales, enlarge to coalesce to form confluent patches No pruritus, area does not tan with exposure to sun	Antifungal shampoo, topical antifungal agents, oral antifungal if diffuse
Dermatophytoses (*Trichophyton, Microsporum, Epidermophyton*)	Tinea capitis	"Black dot ringworm", circular patches of alopecia with hair broken close to follicle or diffuse scaling with minimal hair loss	Oral griseofulvin, terbinafine, itraconazole with antifungal shampoo
	Kerion	Severe inflammatory response producing a boggy granulomatous mass often studded with small pustules	As above
	Tinea corporis	Elevated scaly plaque that spread centrifugally and clears centrally to form annular lesions	Topical antifungals
	Tinea unguium	Numerous white patches on the surface of the nail or thick, brittle, yellow nail that may separate from nail bed	Oral antifungals
Candida	Bright red with sharp borders, satellite red papules and pustules	In skin creases and areas of skin that are constantly moist or occluded	Topical antifungals

Select serious diseases causing rashes in the newborn period include:

Disease	Characteristics	Treatment
Congenital syphilis	Erythematous maculopapular or vesiculobullous lesions followed by desquamation involving hands and feet with mucous patches, persistent rhinitis, and condylomatous lesions also present. Systemic disease will manifest as lymphadenopathy, pneumonitis, nephritis, enteritis, pancreatitis, meningitis, or osteochondritis	Penicillin
Acrodermatitis enteropathica	Erythematous dry, scaly patches, and plaques may evolve into crusted, vesiculobullous, erosive lesions involving perioral, acral, and intertriginous areas, associated with diarrhea and hair loss	PO or IV Zinc
Herpes simplex	Presents at 5–11 days of life with small clustered pustules and vesicles that get denuded. May occur at site of trauma	Acyclovir

CHILDHOOD EXANTHEMS

Exanthems are eruptions of the skin associated with systemic illness.

Disease	Measles 1st disease	Scarlet fever 2nd disease	Rubella 3rd disease	Erythema infectiosum 5th disease	Roseola infantum 6th disease
Etiology	Paramyxovirus	Streptococcus pyogenes	Rubivirus	Parvovirus	Human herpes virus 6 and 7
Infectivity	Several days before to 4 days after rash	Until fever present, up to 24 hours of antibiotics	7 days before to 7 days after	Start at exposure to 4–14 days after	For 1–2 days after fever subsides
Morphology	Erythematous confluent maculopapular rash	Generalized erythematous, sandpaper, lasts 5–6 days	Rose-pink maculopapular	Slapped cheek, lacy reticular, worsens with sunlight	Rose-pink maculopapular, rash appears after fever falls
Distribution	Begins at hairline, spreads inferiorly	Begins on face and upper trunk, spreads inferiorly	Spreads inferiorly	Erythematous cheek Reticular extremities	Neck and trunk
Incubation period	8–12 days	2–5 days	14–21 days	4–21 days	10–15 days
Associated symptoms	Koplik spots, cough, coryza, conjunctivitis, Forchheimer spots	Pastia's lines, strawberry tongue, exudative pharyngitis, abdominal pain, rheumatic fever, circumoral pallor, Forchheimer spots	Tender occipital and posterior auricular lymph Nodes (LN), arthralgia, Forchheimer spots	Lymphadenopathy absent, rash waxes and wanes over weeks, arthritis, aplastic crisis	LN-cathy, febrile seizure may occur, Nagayama spots

Koplik spot: Clustered, white lesions on the buccal mucosa opposite the lower first and second molars.

Forchheimer spots: Fleeting small, red spots (petechiae) on the soft palate.

Pastia lines: Pink or red lines formed of confluent petechiae in skin creases.

Nagayama spots: Erythematous papules on the soft palate and uvula.

Enteroviruses: More than 30 exanthems are associated with coxsackievirus/ echoviruses. Rash = maculopapular, scarlatiniform, vesicular, or urticarial (e.g., hand-foot-mouth—fever, malaise, then vesicles in mouth, on palms, feet, lasts 3 to 6 days, reoccurs).

PAPULOSQUAMOUS AND ECZEMATOUS RASHES

ATOPIC DERMATITIS (AD)

Incessant pruritus is the only symptom of AD, characterized by intermittent flares and remission.

Essential features are pruritus, eczema (acute, subacute, chronic) with distribution on face, neck, and extensor involvement in infants and children and flexural involvement in any age, with sparing of groin and axilla, chronic relapsing history.

Diagnosis is supported by early age of onset, strong family and/or personal history of atopy or immunoglobulin E (IgE) reactivity, and xerosis.

Associated with:

1. Atypical vascular response (e.g., facial pallor)
2. Keratosis pilaris/pityriasis alba/hyper-linear palms/ichthyosis
3. Ocular and periorbital changes
4. Other findings (e.g., perioral changes or periauricular lesions, perifollicular accentuation/lichenification/prurigo)

No reliable biomarker exists for diagnosis, but IgE level can be helpful.

■ Treatment

Nonpharmacological Management

1. Petrolatum, Aquaphor, or newer agents such as Atopiclair, and Mimyx can reduce the severity of the disease, and are best when applied soon after bathing. There is strong evidence that application of moisturizers/emollients lubricate and soften the skin, occlusive agents retard evaporation, and humectants attract and hold water.
2. Hypoallergenic, neutral to low pH, fragrance-free soaps are recommended. Limit use of soaps.
3. Use of wet wraps with or without topical steroids is recommended in moderate to severe AD, especially during flares.

Pharmacological Treatment

1. **Topical corticosteroids (TCS):** Mid- to high-potency TCS appropriate for acute flare-ups; however, least potent TCS may be used for long-term management to reduce adverse effects. Use with caution on thin skin like the face, neck, and skin folds. Once daily application may be as effective as twice daily application.
2. **Immunomodulators:** Topical calcineurin inhibitors (TCI). Used if there is recalcitrance to steroids, long-term use of or atrophy of skin from steroids, or if required for sensitive skin, like the face, anogenital area, and skin folds. For children younger than 2 years, off-label use of tacrolimus

0.03% or 1% pimecrolimus can be recommended. Proactive use as maintenance therapy 2 to 3 times a week is recommended to reduce the need for a topical corticosteroid.

3. **Topical antibiotics and antiseptic:** In moderate to severe AD with signs of secondary infection, bleach baths and intranasal mupirocin may be recommended.

4. **Targeted biologic treatments:** Dupilumab (anti IL-4Rα monoclonal antibody).

5. **Topical phosphodiesterase inhibitor:** Crisaborole 2% for mild to moderate AD in adults and children older than 2 years of age.

6. **Other:** Probiotics, UV-A and UV-B can be tried. Oral antibiotics if secondary infection.

7. **Hydroxyzine/Benadryl:** For itching. Use humidifier to prevent excessive drying.

CONTACT DERMATITIS CAUSED BY IRRITANTS OR ALLERGENS

Diaper dermatitis (irritant): Patchy or confluent erythema in areas of occlusion and friction (convex surfaces). Spares inguinal folds. Blistering and erosion may occur. Consider Candida if red, pustular or papular lesions involving convex and concave surface.

Management: (a) Keep area dry. (b) Desitin or Bepanthen applied topically. (c) Occlusive barrier [e.g., zinc oxide ointment or Orlando butt balm (mix zinc oxide 30 g, Aquaphor 20 g, Burow's solution 10 ml)] after diaper change. (d) Topical antifungal if secondary fungal infection. (e) Low potency steroids can be used in recalcitrant cases. (f) Oral Mycostatin. (g) If breastfeeding treat mom's Candida.

Allergic dermatitis: Exhibits initial eczematous reaction with red papules or vesicles overlying area of edema (e.g., linear streaks for poison ivy, oak, sumac).

Management: Remove offending agent, Burow's solution, cool compresses, topical or brief systemic steroids.

Table 9-2 Other Papulosquamous and Eczematous Rashes

Disorder	Skin lesions	Treatment
Dyshidrotic eczema	Scaling vesicles, blisters, fissures Feet > hands, lateral digits, hyperhidrosis ± localized atopic dermatitis	High-dose topical steroids ± oral steroids first, cold compress. Calcineurin inhibitors, psoralen, PUVA, stress-reduction therapy have also been tried
Eczema herpeticum	Herpes clusters at site of atopic dermatitis	If young patient or moderate involvement, IV acyclovir. If well appearing and older, PO acyclovir

Table 9-2 Other Papulosquamous and Eczematous Rashes (*Continued*)

Disorder	Skin lesions	Treatment
Exfoliative dermatitis	General erythema and scaling with exfoliation head to toe, fluid loss, bullae, and sepsis, plus Nikolsky's sign	Mainstay of treatment aimed at maintaining skin hydration, avoid scratching, applying topical steroids, avoiding precipitating factors and treating underlying cause; compresses with Burow's solution or potassium permanganate also effective
Pityriasis rosea	Papules, scales Starts with a herald patch, erupts over 2–21 days over lines of cleavage of skin, Christmas tree pattern on back *(if African American, may spare trunk)*	Self-limiting, with a duration of 6–8 weeks Supportive care for pruritus
Psoriasis	Round or oval red plaques with silvery scales Scalp, trunk, extensor extremities, or areas of trauma; nail pitting, dystrophy, and fissuring of palms and soles may be present	Topical and systemic medication (MTX/cyclosporine), biologic agent, phototherapy, UV therapy, Psoralen, stress reduction, moisturizers, salicylic acid, urea, and climatotherapy
Seborrheic dermatitis	Mild patchy scaling to thick adherent scaling, intermittent active phases with burning, itching and scaling in winter and early spring with remission in summer, over oil-bearing areas of head and neck	Antifungal gels, calcineurin inhibitors, sulfur or sulfonamide combinations, or propylene glycol, low-potency shampoos containing salicylic acid, tar, selenium, sulfur, or zinc can be used. Selenium sulfide (2.5%), ketoconazole, and ciclopirox shampoos may help by reducing *Malassezia* yeast scalp reservoirs
Syphilis (secondary)	Diffuse/localized, maculopapular, nonpruritic, bilaterally symmetrical, with nontender LN-pathy, associated with constitutional symptoms and pain in bone and fatigue	Penicillin is drug of choice. Doxycycline is the next best alternative.
Tinea	Begins as erythematous scaly plaque, with central resolution giving it an annular appearance	Topical antifungals (azoles and allylamines) Systemic antifungals if severe

(*Continued*)

Table 9-3 Vesiculopustular Rashes[1]

Rash	Skin lesions/distribution	Management
Impetigo	Nonbullous: Honey-colored crust with moist erythematous base Bullous: Fragile, thin-roofed, flaccid, and transparent bullae with clear, yellow fluid that turns cloudy and dark yellow, on rupture there is no crusting, with a collarette of scales around the periphery over face, extremity, elbow, and trunk	Topical and systemic steroids
Staphylococcal scalded skin syndrome (SSSS)	Macular erythema with dermal exfoliation, generalized sunburn, circumoral erythema, periorifice crusting, Nikolsky's sign, sterile bullae affecting total body with sparing of mucosa	Fluid hydration, topical wound care, and antibiotics to treat infection
Herpes simplex	Vesicular lesions on the oral mucosa and tongue, which later rupture and coalesce and leave ulcerated plaques, with tender lymphadenopathy	Acyclovir
Herpes zoster	Self-limited grouped vesicular lesions covering one or two adjacent dermatomes	Wet dressing, Burow's solution, calamine lotion, pain medications, antiviral treatment. Tricyclic antidepressants (TCA), gabapentin, pregabalin, narcotic or non-narcotic pain meds can be used for post-herpetic neuralgia
Erythema multiforme	Papules, wheals, target lesions involving entire surface of the body. No mucosal involvement in minor. > 2 mucosal involvement in Stevens-Johnson syndrome	Oral antihistamines, analgesics, local skin care, and soothing mouthwashes, topical steroids, meticulous wound care and use of Burow's or Domeboro solution dressings, remove offending drug, treat infection
Toxic epidermal necrolysis	Widespread erythema, necrosis, and bullous detachment of the epidermis and mucous membranes, resulting in exfoliation and possible sepsis and/or death	Withdrawal of offending agent, isolation, fluid and electrolyte balance, nutritional support, protective dressing, pain management

[1]Other conditions that may mimic or have vesicular lesions—scabies (more often papular, excoriated, or scaling). Threadlike burrows are seen in the classic form, dyshidrosis, ID reaction, insect bites, molluscum contagiosum (simulates vesicles), coxsackievirus (hand, foot, mouth).

Table 9-4 Petechial and Purpuric Rashes[1-3]

Rash	Skin lesions	Treatment
Idiopathic thrombo-cytopenic purpura (and thrombotic thrombocytopenic purpura [TTP])	Petechiae, ecchymosis, hema-tomas on exposed sites, bony prominences, and mucosa	Mild: no treatment Moderate to severe: +/- intra-venous IG (IVIG), +/- steroids
Henoch-Schönlein purpura	Petechiae, purpura typically symmetrical in dependent body areas +/- joint pain, abdominal pain, +/- renal involvement	Adequate hydration, treat pain, steroids/immunosuppressive drugs if complications
Acute leukemia	Petechiae, purpura, (general-ized or localized), adenopathy, hepatosplenomegaly, sternal tenderness	Treat as per protocol
Aplastic anemia	Petechiae, purpura, ecchymosis, generalized or at sites of injury	Supportive care, immunosuppressive therapy, or HCT
DIC	Generalized petechiae (tend to be palpable with *meningo-coccemia*), purpura, areas of skin necrosis	Replacement of platelets, cryoprecipitates, and/or fresh frozen plasma
Factor deficiency (e.g., hemophilia)	Easy bruising, abnormal bleeding under the skin and mucous membrane +/- involvement of muscle and joints	Replacement of factor

[1]See "Bleeding Disorders," pages 120-123, and "Evaluation of Patients with Petechiae," Table 18-7.
[2] Other purpuric rashes: vasculitis, *Rickettsia* (RMSF), histiocytosis X, scurvy, trauma, medicines (steroids, thiazides), dysproteinemias, Kaposi's sarcoma, pyogenic granuloma.
[3]See etiology and differential for fever and petechiae, Table 18-8.
Eichenfield LF, Tom WL, Chamlin SL, et al. Guidelines of care for the management of atopic dermatitis: section 1. Diagnosis and assessment of atopic dermatitis. *J Am Acad Dermatol.* 2014;70(2):338-351.

Table 10-1 Developmental Milestones

Age	Milestones			
	Social	Language	Fine motor	Gross motor
2 months	Social smile	Coos, gurgling sounds	Follows object 180 degrees	Holds head up
4 months	Spontaneous smile	Turns to voice, laughs	Brings objects to midline	Rolls front to back
6 months	Knows familiar faces	Babbles	Passes object from one hand to the other	Sits independently
9 months	Stranger anxiety	Says "mama/dada" nonspecifically	Uses immature pincer	Crawls, pulls to stand
12 months	Separation anxiety	Follows one-step command with gesture, 3 words	Uses mature pincer	Walks
18 months	Independence	Says 10–25 words	Builds four-cube tower	Runs stiffly, walks up stairs with assistance
2 years	Parallel play	Says 2–3-word sentences	Displays handedness	Runs
3 years	Cooperative play	States first name, follows command with 2–3 steps	Builds eight-cube tower, undresses	Rides tricycle
4 years	Cooperative play	Tells stories	Uses scissors	Hops and stands on one foot up to 2 seconds
5 years	Wants to please and be like friends	Speaks clearly	Can print some letters and numbers	Stands on one foot more than 10 seconds

Table 10-2 Weight, Height, Head Circumference—5th, 50th, and 95th Percentiles

Age	Males			Females		
	Height (cm)	Weight (kg)	Head circum. (cm)	Height (cm)	Weight (kg)	Head circum. (cm)
1 month	51.4-55.9-59.7	—	—	50.8-54.3-58.4	—	—
3 months	58.3-61.9-66.6	5.35-6.95-8.45	39.7-41.7-43.1	56.7-61.0-64.8	5.40-6.30-7.75	39.0-40.3-42.6
6 months	64.8-68.2-71.9	7.00-8.39-10.70	42.4-44.0-46.8	63.3-66.7-70.9	6.58-7.55-8.96	40.8-42.6-45.0
9 months	67.9-72.6-76.6	8.05-9.30-10.89	43.6-45.4-47.4	66.8-71.0-75.5	7.40-8.73-10.45	42.6-44.3-46.2
12 months	72.9-77.3-82.9	8.90-10.55-12.35	44.7-47.0-49.4	70.0-76.2-80.5	8.28-9.80-11.57	43.5-45.6-48.0
18 months	77.8-83.7-90.2	9.98-11.91-15.45	45.5-48.0-50.1	76.1-81.6-87.5	9.15-10.95-13.50	44.0-46.5-49.2
2 years	83.0-89.1-95.5	10.95-12.93-15.77	46.4-49.0-51.2	82.4-88.0-94.4	10.25-12.36-15.08	45.0-47.8-49.9
3 years	90.5-96.7-103.3	12.47-14.95-18.00	—	89.1-95.7-102.9	11.75-14.40-18.03	—
4 years	96.9-104.2-111.8	13.75-17.01-21.00	—	95.7-103.2-110.2	13.72-16.44-20.87	—
5 years	103.1-111.1-118.8	15.76-19.16-24.10	—	101.9-109.9-117.2	14.60-18.48-25.65	—

Modified from Kuczmarski, R. J., 2000 CDC Growth Charts for the United States: Methods and Development. *Vital and Health Statistics.* May 2002;11(246).

OTHER GROWTH MILESTONES

- *Dentition*—1st teeth to erupt: Lower central incisors (6–10 months), upper central incisors (8–12 months), lateral incisors (9–16 months), first molars (13–19 months), cuspids (16–23 months), 2nd molars (23–33 months). Most children have a full set of primary teeth by 3 years. Permanent teeth begin to erupt at 6 years, continues until 12 years.
- *Fontanelle*—Posterior fontanelle closes by 1–2 months. Anterior fontanelle, closes at 9–18 months.
- *Sinuses*—The ethmoid and maxillary sinuses are aerated at birth, while the sphenoid sinus becomes aerated by 5 years. Frontal sinus appears at 7–8 years with complete development in adolescence.
- *Menarche*—Median age at menarche for US girls is 12.43 years. Primary amenorrhea: No menarche and has no secondary sex characteristics at 14 years OR no menarche but has secondary sex characteristics at 16 years.

11 ■ ENDOCRINOLOGY

ADRENAL CRISIS (INSUFFICIENCY)

Presentation: Fever, vomiting, altered mental status, $\downarrow$ BP, shock, $\downarrow$ Na+, $\uparrow$ K+, $\downarrow$ glucose, $\uparrow$ eosinophils.

Associated with chronic steroid use or unidentified adrenal disease [e.g., Addison's, congenital enzyme defects (e.g., congenital adrenal hyperplasia with ambiguous genitalia)].

Laboratory assessment may reveal hyponatremia with or without hyperkalemia, metabolic acidosis, and hypoglycemia.

The table that follows lists the common steroid preparations and their potency relative to hydrocortisone. Hydrocortisone is the least potent preparation commonly prescribed. A hydrocortisone dose of 20 mg is roughly equivalent in potency to a prednisone dose of 5 mg. Note that cortisol and hydrocortisone should be considered to have equivalent potencies.

Glucocorticoid	Approximate equivalent dose (mg)	Physiologic dose $(mg/m^2/day)$
Hydrocortisone	20	6–12
Prednisone/Prednisolone	5	1.5–3
Methylprednisolone	4	1.2–2.4
Dexamethasone	0.75	0.2–0.4

ADRENAL CRISIS THERAPY

- Assess hydration, BP, and blood glucose. If possible, draw and store blood sample [glucose, electrolytes, creatinine, ACTH, cortisol, aldosterone, and plasma renin activity (low aldosterone and high plasma renin seen in primary adrenal insufficiency)] for later steroid-level analyses.
- 20 ml/kg normal saline bolus IV to correct shock (may repeat as needed).[1]
- Dextrose 2 ml/kg of 25% dextrose in water ($D_{25}W$) or 4 ml/kg 10% dextrose in water ($D_{10}W$) IV should correct hypoglycemia.[2]
- Patients with suspected adrenal crisis should undergo immediate treatment with a parenteral injection of 100 mg (older than 2 years of age), or 50 mg (younger than 2 years of age) hydrocortisone, after which, appropriate fluid resuscitation should be administered, as well as 200 mg ($50–100$ mg/m^2 for children) of hydrocortisone/24 hours (by way of continuous IV therapy or 6-hourly injection). If hydrocortisone is unavailable, prednisolone may be used. Dexamethasone is least-preferred, as its onset of action is slow.

- Antibiotics if suspicion of sepsis (e.g., ceftriaxone 50 mg/kg).
- Exert caution if associated hypothyroidism is treated, as thyroxine increases cortisol clearance.

DIABETES MELLITUS

INSULIN GUIDELINES

- All dosing should be coordinated with the patient's endocrinologist if available.
- Basal/maintenance insulin (typical total daily requirements):
  a. Prepubertal: 0.7 units/kg/day
  b. Midpubertal: 1 unit/kg/day
  c. Late pubertal: > 1–2 units/kg/day
     **If *newly* diagnosed, initial dosing is usually 60–70% of these values

Insulin regimens:

- **Basal-bolus concept:** (i.e., a pump or intermediate-acting/long-acting insulin/basal analog once or twice daily and rapid-acting or regular boluses with meals and snacks) has the best ability of mimicking physiologic insulin profile.
- **Different therapeutic strategies:**
  a. **Glucose and meal-adjusted regime:** 30–45% of total daily insulin given as basal insulin, the rest given preprandial with rapid-acting/regular insulin adjusted for meal, glycemia, and activity.
  b. **Less intensive regime:**
     - Three times daily: Mix of short/rapid + intermediate before breakfast, rapid/regular before afternoon snack or dinner, intermediate-acting before bed
     - Two times daily: Mix of short/rapid/intermediate before breakfast and the main evening meal
     - Prandial insulin: adjusted by glucose and carbohydrate content, extra injections when needed
  c. **Fixed insulin dose regime:** limited flexibility, more challenging.
  d. **Insulin pump regimes** are gaining popularity with a fixed or variable basal rate and adjusted bolus doses with meals.
  e. **Sensor augmented therapies:** Continuous glucose monitoring (CGM) used with pump therapy or MDI (pen/syringe), well tolerated in children, but use decreased with time in different studies. Intermittently viewed CGM (iCGM) is being increasingly used in children older than 4 years in countries where it is available.

Table 11-1 Insulin Preparations

Insulin[1]	Preparation	Onset (hours)	Peak (hours)	Duration (hours)	
Ultra-rapid acting analog	Faster aspart	0.1–0.2	1–3	3–5	Better intended to match the time-action profile of prandial insulin. Useful for pumps and closed-loop approaches.
Rapid-acting analog (quicker effect than regular insulin to treat hyperglycemia)	Aspart, glulisine, lispro	0.15–0.35	1–3	3–5	Give immediately before meals (in exception of cases such as infants and toddlers who are reluctant to eat, give after food). Most often used as prandial or snack boluses in combination with longer-acting insulins (see basal-bolus regimens). Most used in insulin pumps.
Regular/Soluble (short acting) (identical to human insulin)	Short acting	0.5–1	2–4	5–8	Used either with intermediate-acting insulin in a twice daily regimen or as a premeal bolus injection in basal-bolus regimen (given 20–30 minutes before meals) together with intermediate-acting insulin 2 to 3 (or even 4) times daily or a basal analog given once or twice daily.
Intermediate	Isophane NPH	2–4	4–12	12–24	Suitable for twice daily regimens, tailored basal substitution and for pre-bed dosage in basal-bolus regimens.
Long	Detemir[2] 100 units/ml (Levemir)	1–2	6–12	20–24	Basal analogs have a more predictable insulin effect and less of a peak than NPH and allow basal dosing independent of meal time, once or twice a day. 30–45% of total daily dose.
	Glargine[2] (Lantus)	2–4	Prolonged	24	
	Glargine 300 units/ml[3]	2–6	Minimal peak	30–36	
	Degludec[4]	0.5–1.5	Minimal peak	> 42	

[1]Previous numbers and timing based on *International Society for Pediatric and Adolescent Diabetes* data and may not reflect true pediatric values. [2]Detemir and Glargine are not approved for use in children younger than 2 years old. [3]Approved for use in children less than the 1-year-old to 5 years. [4]Approved for use in children as young as 1 year of age. Data from Bangstad, H. J., Danne, T., Deeb, L., Jarosz-Chobot, P., Urakami, T., & Hanas, R. (2009). Insulin treatment in children and adolescents with diabetes. Pediatric diabetes, 10, 82-99.

Premixed insulins (fixed ratio mixtures of pre meal and basal insulins) are used in some countries particularly for prepubertal children on twice daily regimens.

Recently, premixed insulins have also become available with rapid-acting analogs. Biphasic insulin aspart 30 (30% aspart and 70% aspart bound to NPH) given for three main meals combined with NPH at bedtime was equally efficient as premixed human insulin (70% NPH) given for morning and bedtime with regular insulin for lunch and dinner in adolescents.

Premixed insulins with regular (or rapid acting): NPH in different ratios, for example, 10:90, 15:85, 20:80, 25:75, 30:70, 40:60, and 50:50 are available in various countries from different manufacturers. Premixed insulins are suitable for use in a pen injector device.

Biosimilar: Glargine insulin LY2963016, a first biosimilar insulin, has been approved in several countries also for pediatric use. A biosimilar insulin lispro is under production.

DIABETIC KETOACIDOSIS (DKA), INTERNATIONAL SOCIETY FOR PEDIATRIC AND ADOLESCENT DIABETES GUIDELINES

Diagnosis requires all three criteria: glucose > 200, pH < 7.3, or bicarb < 15, ketosis (blood or urine).

Evaluate according to PALS guideline (including mental status, cardiorespiratory status, history of polyuria, polydipsia, weight loss, polyphagia, vomiting).

Check blood glucose and urine acetone (>3 mmol confirms ketoacidosis).

Use current weight for all calculations.

Assess for dehydration: Prolonged cap refill (>2 seconds) and abnormal skin turgor are considered most useful signs for predicting 5% dehydration. Weak pulses, hypotension, oliguria suggest >10% dehydration.

Evaluate mentation: If obtunded, secure airway (avoid intubation as far as possible); empty stomach if required.

■ Management
- Place oxygen if in shock
- CR monitor
- 2 IV lines (fluids + draw blood)
- Draw blood: POC glucose, blood glucose, blood gas, BMP, Ca, Mg, phosphorus, +/− CBC, urine hCG, HbA1c
- Fluids:
  - First hour: fluid resuscitation 10–20 ml/kg of 0.9 NS or RL over 1 to 2 hours (can repeat up to three times until circulation restored).
  - If intravenous/osseous access is not available, rehydrate with nasogastric tube, give same volume of fluid with normal saline (0.9%), half-strength Darrow's solution or oral rehydration solution (ORS) until perfusion improves. This can be done at a constant rate over 48 hours. If a nasogastric tube is not available, give ORS by oral sips at a rate of 5 ml/kg per hour.

- Important: Shock must be adequately treated before proceeding. There should be good peripheral perfusion and adequate blood pressure.
- At start of second hour: Rehydrate 0.9 NS+20 mEq/l K Phos + 20 mEq/l KCl or K acetate (if K < 5 mEq/l).
- Hydrate with maintenance + replacement of deficit over 24 to 48 hours (approximately 1.5 to 2 times daily requirement).
- When BG = 250–300 mg/dl (13.9–16.7 mmol/l): Change fluids to D5 0.45 NS + 20 K Phos + KCl (increases chloride load and metabolic acidosis) or K-Acetate (preferred) at same rate above.
- If glucose 100, change dextrose to 10 or 12.5%.

When using two-bag method: Bag 1 has no glucose and bag 2 has 10% glucose.[3]

At BG > 350, 100% of the fluid should be fluid with no dextrose.
At 300 to 349, bag 2 will provide 25% of the fluid to achieve 2.5% solution.
At levels 250 to 299, bag 2 will provide 50% of the fluid to achieve 5% solution.
At levels 200 to 249, bag 2 will provide 75% of the fluid to achieve 7.5% solution.
At levels < 200, bag 2 will provide 100% of fluid to achieve 10% dextrose solution.

Insulin: Start insulin 0.05 to 0.1 units/kg/hour at least 1 hour after starting fluid replacement (initial volume expansion) until resolution of DKA (pH) > 7.30, serum bicarbonate > 15 mmol/l, beta-hydroxybutyrate (BOHB) < 1 mmol/l, closure of anion gap. Aim to decrease glucose at 100 ml/dl/hour or 5.6 mmol/l/hour and rise in pH at 0.03 units/hour.
When DKA resolves: Start oral fluids. Administer SC insulin 15 minutes before discontinuing IV insulin, check BG every hour until BG stable on SC insulin.
https://cdn.ymaws.com/www.ispad.org/resource/resmgr/Docs/ispad-lfac-pocketbook-final.pdf
If insulin cannot be given intravenously by a side drip or infusion pump, use deep subcutaneous or intramuscular insulin: Give 0.1 unit/kg of short-acting (regular, soluble) or rapid-acting insulin SC or IM into the upper arm, and repeat this dose every 1 to 2 hours.
Potassium: For a child being rehydrated with ORS, no added potassium is needed as ORS contains potassium. Serum potassium should be monitored every 6 hours or more frequently if indicated. If intravenous potassium is not available, potassium could be replaced by giving fruit juice, bananas, or coconut water orally.
Bicarbonate: Only administer if hyperkalemia or epinephrine-resistant shock or with cardiac dysfunction with a pH < 6.9 or severe hyperkalemia.
Monitoring: BG every 1 hour, electrolytes and BOHB every other hour. Ca, Mg, and phosphorous every 4 hours.
Discharge: When able to tolerate per os (P.O.), no vomiting, bicarbonate ≥ 17, normal electrolytes and appropriate follow-up scheduled.

COMPLICATIONS OF DIABETES AND THERAPY

Cerebral edema: Occurs 4 to 12 hours after the start of therapy; is the leading cause of death and morbidity in diabetic ketoacidosis (DKA) (https://www.chop .edu/clinical-pathway/diabetes-type1-with-dka-clinical-pathway).

■ Diagnosing Clinically Significant Cerebral Edema[4]
Presence of either of the following has a sensitivity of 92% for detecting cerebral edema in the setting of DKA:
  1 Diagnostic criteria plus 2 major criteria *or*
  1 Major criteria and 2 minor criteria

Diagnostic criteria	• Abnormal motor or verbal response to pain • Decorticate or decerebrate posture • Cranial nerve palsy (especially III, IV, and VI) • Abnormal neurogenic respiratory pattern (e.g., grunting, tachypnea, Cheyne-Stokes respiration, apneusis)
Major criteria	• Altered mentation/fluctuating level of consciousness (GCS ≤ 13) • Sustained heart rate deceleration (decline > 20 bpm) not attributable to improved intravascular volume or sleep state • Age-inappropriate incontinence
Minor criteria	• Vomiting • Headache • Lethargy or not easily arousable from sleep • Diastolic blood pressure > 90 mm Hg • Age younger than 5 years

- Treat with mannitol, reduce fluids to $1\times$ maintenance fluid, intubation. Target PCO_2 should approximate patient's baseline PCO_2 preintubation if patient was able to maintain normal ventilator response to acidosis (unless herniating).
  Hypertonic saline (3%) 5 ml/kg over 30 minutes may be an alternative to mannitol, especially if there is no initial response to mannitol.
- **Consider ICU**: Age younger than 2 years, pH < 7, shock, altered mental status, glucose > 1,000, Na > 160.

High risk of complications: In children younger than 3 years, very severe acidosis, pH < 7, low $PaCO_2$, elevated BUN, bicarbonate therapy, administration of insulin in the first hour, initial glucose > 1,000 mg/dl, Na > 160 (https:// www.chop.edu/clinical-pathway/diabetes-type1-with-dka-clinical-pathway).

Hyperosmolar coma is rare in children and is associated with preexisting neurologic disorders. Blood glucose is typically > 600 mg/dl, serum osmolality is > 330, and ketosis is minimal or absent. The corrected sodium is usually high. Aggressive fluids management and management of underlying cause and treatment of complications (e.g., rhabdomyolysis, renal failure, electrolyte abnormalities, infections) are primary treatment modalities. Insulin boluses are not recommended. Use only when serum glucose concentration is no longer declining at the rate of < 3 mmol/l (approximately 50 mg/dl) per hour with fluid administration alone.

Sources: Carchman et al.[5] and Glaser.[6]

HYPOGLYCEMIA

Hypoglycemia is defined as a blood glucose <40–55 mg/dl (<30–45 mg/dl in neonate). Values of 55–70 mg/dl may indicate mild hypoglycemia (especially in diabetics). It is most commonly due to poor nutrition or overmedication with insulin, toxins (see Table 31-3), or hypoglycemic agents.

Table 11-2 Etiology of Hypoglycemia

Neonatal	Prematurity, SGA, infant of diabetic mother, birth asphyxia	
Decreased intake	Vomiting, malnutrition	
Decreased absorption	Diarrhea, malabsorption	
Glucose underproduction	Prematurity, SGA, malnutrition	
	Ketotic hypoglycemia	Ketonemia and ketonuria, high BOHB and normal plasma lactate
Inborn errors of metabolism	Glycogen storage disease	High plasma lactate and high BOHB
	Fatty acid oxidation defect	Low BOHB but elevated FFA
Hyperinsulinemia	Endogenous (high C-peptide level)/exogenous (low C-peptide level)	Low BOHB and FFA IGFBP-1 level decrease or remain stable with increased insulin
Endocrine disorder	Panhypopituitarism, GH deficiency, cortisol deficiency	Evaluate levels of specific hormones
Drug: ingestion/ toxins/alcohol	Ethanol, salicylates, propranolol	Elevated level of medication present

FFA—free fatty acid; BOHB—beta-hydroxybutyrate; GH—growth hormone; IGFBP—insulin-like growth factor-binding protein; SGA—small for gestational age.
Modified from Gandhi, Kajal. "Approach to hypoglycemia in infants and children." Translational pediatrics 2017;6(4):408.

Symptoms: Sweating, dry mouth, nausea, trembling, flushing, hunger, anxiety, decreased concentration, fatigue, confusion, drowsiness, weakness, and lack of coordination.

Labs: Glucose, insulin and C-peptide, lactate, beta-hydroxybutyrate, FFA, IGFBP, GH, and cortisol level. Urine organic acids. May require PET scan with dihydroxyphenylalanine (DOPA) for evaluation of focal versus diffuse tumors or MRI for pituitary or hypothalamic abnormality.

Treatment: Treat if symptomatic or <45 in asymptomatic patients.

Table 11-3 Management of Hypoglycemia

Age	Dose and concentration	Other treatment[1]
0–30 days	5–10 ml/kg of $D_{10}W$ IV	Glucagon 0.02–0.03 mg/kg if < 20 kg, 1 mg if > 20 kg, administer IM, SC, or IV; Diazoxide IV if severe
1–24 months	2–4 ml/kg of $D_{25}W$ IV	
> 2 years	1–2 ml/kg of $D_{50}W$ IV	

[1]Octreotide may be used IV if hyperinsulinemia or sulfonylurea overdose (Table 31-44).

In patients with DM
  If normal mentation: treat with oral glucose.
  If altered mentation and at home: SC glucagon can be used.
  If in hospital: IV dextrose 25–50% can be used.
  If hyperinsulinism: treat with frequent feeding, followed by diazoxide. Octreotide is the second line of medical therapy. Glucagon infusion at rates of 0.005–0.02 mg/kg/hour should be used as a temporary treatment in children with hyperinsulinism in whom adequate amounts of dextrose cannot be given.

Growth hormone and cortisol replacement are specific treatments for children with hypoglycemia and hypopituitarism or adrenal insufficiency.

REFERENCES

1. Tafuri K. Pediatric adrenal insufficiency (Addison disease). Medscape. https://emedicine.medscape.com/article/919077-overview. Updated December 7, 2018.
2. Kirkland L. Adrenal crisis. Medscape. https://emedicine.medscape.com/article/116716-overview. Updated February 14, 2018.
3. Velasco JP, Fogel J, Levine RL, Ciminera P, Fagan D, Bargman R. Potential clinical benefits of a two-bag system for fluid management in pediatric intensive care unit patients with diabetic ketoacidosis. Pediatr Endocrinol Diabetes Metab. 2017;23(1):6-13. doi:10.18544/PEDM-23.01.0068.
4. Muir AB, Quisling RG, Yang MC, Rosenbloom AL. Cerebral edema in childhood diabetic ketoacidosis: natural history, radiographic findings, and early identification. Diabetes Care. 2004;27(7):1541-1546.
5. Carchman RM, Dechert-Zeger M, Calikoglu AS, Harris BD. A new challenge in pediatric obesity: pediatric hyperglycemic hyperosmolar syndrome. Pediatr Crit Care Med. 2005;6(1):20-24.
6. Glaser N. Pediatric diabetic ketoacidosis and hyperglycemic hyperosmolar state. Pediatr Clin North Am. 2005;52:1611-1635.

12 ■ ENVIRONMENTAL DISORDERS

HYPERTHERMIA

Table 12-1 Minor Heat Illness

- *Heat syncope*: Postural hypotension from vasodilation, volume depletion, and ↓ vascular tone.
  - Management: Rehydrate with salt containing fluids, remove from heat and evaluate for serious disease.
- *Heat cramps*: Painful, contractions of large muscle groups of the legs, abdomen, or arms in those who are sweating liberally and drinking hypotonic solutions (e.g., water).
  - Management: Replace fluids—Oral or IV rehydration. Do not use salt tablets.
- *Heat tetany*: Hyperventilation that may result in respiratory alkalosis, positive Chvostek sign, laryngospasm, or carpopedal spasm.
  - Management: Move to cooler environment. Persistent hyperventilation may require partial rebreather oxygen mask set below 5 l/minute.
- *Heat exhaustion*: Salt and water depletion causing orthostasis, and hyperthermia [usually < 104°F (40°C)]. *Mental status and neurologic exam are normal.* Lab: high hematocrit, electrolytes normal, sodium may be decreased in some.
  - Management: Initiate treatment with NS 10–20 ml/kg IV and continue to hydrate as needed.

Table 12-2 Heatstroke

Clinical features	Risk factors
• Hyperpyrexia (temp. > 104–105.8°F) • Central nervous system dysfunction (seizures, altered mentation, decreased plantar responses, hemiplegia, ataxia) • Loss of sweating (variably present)	• Very young or old age • Drugs that limit sweating (anticholinergics, amphetamines, cocaine, antihypertensive agents)

Complications of heatstroke: Rhabdomyolysis, hypoglycemia, renal or liver failure, ↓ or ↑ Na, ↓ Ca, ↓ phosphate, ↓ or ↑ K, and disseminated intravascular coagulation.

Table 12-3 Heatstroke Management

- Administer oxygen and protect airway if comatose or seizing. Check blood glucose, and treat hypoglycemia. Measure temperature with continuous rectal probe or Foley catheter temperature sensor that is accurate at high temperatures.
- Begin IV NS cautiously as pulmonary edema is common and the mean fluid requirement in heat stroke is > 20 ml/kg in the first 4 hours. Consider central venous pressure monitoring to guide fluid resuscitation.

(Continued)

Table 12-3 Heatstroke Management (Continued)

- Begin immediate cooling by: (1) *Evaporation*: spray with tepid water and direct fan at patient (leads to 0.1–0.3°C/minute temp. drop). For shivering, IV lorazepam 0.05–0.1 mg/kg IV. (2) *Ice water (or 60°F) tub immersion*: may complicate resuscitation and monitoring (leads to temperature drop ~ 0.16°C/minute). (3) *Ice packs (to neck, axilla, groin), cooling blankets, peritoneal dialysis, and gastric lavage* with cold water are slow or unproven. (4) Avoid aspirin (contributes to hyperpyrexia). Avoid repeat acetaminophen doses (possible liver damage and ineffective in heatstroke).
  Stop the previous measures at temperatures of 100.4 to 101.3°F to avoid overcorrection.
- Most effective but invasive method is internal cooling. Cardiopulmonary bypass requires specialized institutions; gastric, rectal, and/or bladder lavage have not been shown to be more effective than evaporative cooling alone.
- Place a temperature-sensing Foley catheter to monitor urine output and temperature (see rhabdomyolysis, which follows).
- Obtain CBC, electrolytes, renal function, glucose, liver enzymes, LDH/CPK, PT, and PTT, arterial blood gas, and fibrin degradation products; ECG and CXR.
- Exclude other causes of fever: infection, malignant hyperthermia, hyperthyroidism, drugs, etc.

Table 12-4 Other Heat-Related Disorders

- **Malignant hyperthermia (MH):** Autosomal dominant. Fever (late sign), hypercarbia, + muscle rigidity after anesthetics or succinylcholine. *Treatment*: Stop agent, correct hypercarbia, give loading bolus of dantrolene 2.5 mg/kg IV (max 10 mg/kg).
- **Neuroleptic malignant syndrome:** Similar to MH (with *F*ever, *E*ncephalopathy, *V*itals unstable, *E*levated enzymes, *R*igid muscle) but due to antipsychotics (e.g., haloperidol, phenothiazines). *Treatment:* stop agent, cool patient—see heatstroke (see page 77) and administer bromocriptine 2.5–10 mg PO or NG three times per day. Benzodiazepines may be useful for agitation. Some experts recommend dantrolene 2.5 mg/kg IV (max 10 mg/kg) although this is more effective in malignant hyperthermia. Avoid phenothiazines.
- **Rhabdomyolysis:** Syndrome with release of contents into circulation due to tissue hypoxia, direct injury, exercise, enzyme defects, metabolic disease (DKA, ↓ K, ↓ Na, or ↓ phosphate, thyroid), toxins, infections, heatstroke. *Complications*: renal failure, ↓ K, ↑ or ↓ Ca, ↑ or ↓ phosphate, ↑ uric acid, compartment syndrome, DIC. *Treatment*: (1) IV NS to keep urine output > 2–3 ml/kg/hour, (2) alkalinize urine, (3) ± mannitol if poor urine output: 0.25–0.5 g/kg IV, + add 12.5 g to each L NS, (4) dialyze ↑ K, or uremia.

HYPOTHERMIA

Table 12-5 Hypothermia

Severity	Temp. °F (°C)	Features
Mild	90–95 (32–35)	Shivering, vasoconstriction, + slurred speech at < 95°F
Moderate	82–90 (28–32)	At < 89°F altered mental status, mydriasis, shivering ceases, muscles are rigid, incoordination, bradypnea
Severe	≤82 (≤28)	Bradycardia in 50%, Osborne waves on ECG, voluntary motion stops, pupils are fixed and dilated
	79 (26)	Loss of consciousness, areflexia, no pain response
	77 (25)	No respirations, appear dead, pulmonary edema
	68 (20)	Asystole

Table 12-6 Management of Hypothermia

- Evaluate for cause (e.g., sepsis, hypoglycemia, CNS disease, adrenal crisis).
- **Mild hypothermia** (<32°C): Administer humidified warmed O_2. Passive external rewarming (warm blankets, hot packs) and treatment of underlying disease is often the only treatment needed.
- **Moderate hypothermia** (29–32°C): Passive rewarming + active internal rewarming. Drugs and cardioversion for cardiac arrest may be ineffective. Warm humidified O_2 and warm IV fluids with gastric or peritoneal lavage if poor response to warm fluids/O_2 (<1°C/hour temperature rise). Perform CPR and ALS (e.g., defibrillation) as needed with meds at longer intervals.
- **Severe hypothermia** (≤29°C): (1) Warm humidified O_2, and warm IV fluids. (2) If no cardiac arrest, warmed peritoneal dialysis (41°C dialysate), or (3) pleural irrigation (41°C). (4) If core temp. <25°C consider venous–venous bypass or extracorporeal membrane oxygenation. (5) Consider open pleural lavage for direct cardiac rewarming if core temp <28°C after 1 hour bypass in an arrest rhythm. If signs of life, and no cardiac arrest, avoid CPR and ALS. If cardiac arrest, CPR and ALS are OK (only defibrillate once, consider withholding medications until temperature >29–30°C). (6) Do not treat atrial arrhythmias. (7) Use NS to treat ↓ BP. Use vasopressors cautiously as needed. (8) Consider D_{10}/D_{25}, naloxone, hydrocortisone 1 mg/kg IV, antibiotics as needed.

ENVENOMATIONS

PIT VIPER (CROTALIDAE) BITE

- **Emergency Treatment for Crotalid Envenomation**
  - Decrease movement, remove jewelry or clothing, and immobilize extremity at or below the level of the heart.
  - Avoid incision and drainage and tourniquets. Avoid early fasciotomy, and instead administer antivenin with close observation of response.
  - If snake is brought to the ED, treat with respect, decapitated snakes can bite reflexively for up to an hour.
  - Perform exam, measure envenomation site, and administer fluids, pressors prn.
  - If no signs of envenomation, clean wound, administer tetanus, and observe for a minimum of 6 hours. Consider antibiotics (e.g., Augmentin × 5 days).
  - If significant envenomation, obtain CBC, electrolytes, renal and liver function tests, PT, PTT, fibrinogen, urinalysis, ECG, and type and cross.

- **Ovine–Crotalidae Polyvalent Immune Fab Antivenin (FabAV; CroFab)**
  Sheep derived and more potent than equine antivenin (AVCP), which is no longer available, + less allergy (17% acute, 12% delayed). Allergy to FabAV, papaya, or papain is a relative contraindication.

  - Administer first dose of 4 to 6 vials (some double-dose if low BP, airway compromise).
  - Repeat 2 to 6 vials every hour until no progression.
  - Administer an additional 2 vials at 6, 12, and 18 hours if no progression.
  - Dilute FabAV to a total of 250 ml in NS (less if < 10 kg). Infuse IV over 1 hour.
  - The manufacturer, BTG International Inc., states, "Pediatric CroFab dose = adult dose" (https://www.crofab.com/Treatment-With-CroFab /Dosing-and-administration).
  - Polyvalent equine F(ab')2 antivenin (ANAVIP) is approved by the FDA for adults and children.

Sources: National Highway Traffic Safety Administration. Crash Injury Research and Engineering Network (CIREN): an update. *Ann Emerg Med.* 2001;38:181-182; Goto CS, Feng SY. Crotalidae polyvalent immune Fab for the treatment of pediatric crotaline envenomation. *Pediatr Emerg Care.* 2009;25(4):273-279; quiz 280-282.

Table 12-7 Evaluation and Management of Crotalidae Envenomation

Grade	Features of *Crotalidae* Envenomation	Laboratory
None	± Fang marks, no pain, erythema or systemic symptoms.	None
Mild	Fang marks, mild pain/edema, ±vesicles, all within 10–15 cm of bite. No systemic symptoms.	No abnormalities
Moderate	Fang marks, all local signs extend beyond wound site. + systemic symptoms (vomiting, paresthesias), mild coagulopathy (without bleeding).	Hemoconcentration, thrombocytopenia, hypofibrinogenemia
Severe	Fang marks, severe pain/edema, severe symptoms (↓ BP, respiratory distress), coagulopathy with bleeding.	Significant anemia, prolonged clotting time, metabolic acidosis

CORAL SNAKE (ELAPIDAE) BITE

Southeast United States and Arizona. These snakes must bite and chew. Local effects + bite marks may be minimal. *Symptoms are systemic:* altered level of consciousness (LOC), descending flaccid paralysis, cranial nerve deficits, weakness/respiratory failure, and may be delayed 24 hours. Admit for respiratory or neurologic deterioration. All symptomatic patients require coral snake antivenin. *Dosing*: potentially associated with severe allergic reactions and should only be administered in a continuously monitored setting. Sonoran (Arizona) coral snake venom is less toxic, no deaths have been reported, and coral snake antivenin is ineffective.

SPECIAL SITUATIONS

Mojave rattlesnake: May cause muscle weakness, paralysis, or respiratory failure with few local symptoms. FabAV is effective.
Exotic snakes: Call 800-222-1222 for information regarding available antivenin.
Serum sickness will develop in many receiving >5 vials of antivenin within 5–20 days causing joint pain, myalgias, and possibly rash. Warn patient and treat with diphenhydramine (Benadryl) 1 mg/kg orally every 4–6 hours and prednisone 1–2 mg/kg orally daily.

SPIDER BITES

Table 12-8 Salient Characteristics of Black Widow Spider Bites

Black widow spiders	Features of black widow bites
• Found in all of the United States, mostly South • Females ~ 5 cm with legs and 1.5 cm without legs • Only females are toxic • 1/5 have red hourglass on abdomen	• Mild to moderately painful bite. • In 1 hour, redness, swelling, and cramping at bite, which later spreads. • Often no local symptoms are appreciated. Pain is felt in the abdomen, flank, thighs, and chest and is described as cramping. • ↓ BP, shock, coma, respiratory failure.

Table 12-9 Management of Black Widow Spider Bites

Management of black widow spider bites	
• Lorazepam (Ativan) 0.05–0.1 mg/kg IV • Consider *Latrodectus* antivenin. Dose: 1–2 vials IV in 50–100 ml NS Skin test prior to using • Allergy and serum sickness can occur • Calcium is ineffective	Indications[1] for admission/antivenin • Respiratory or cardiac symptoms • Severe cramping or pain despite lorazepam use • History of ↑ BP or cardiac disease

[1] Controversial as no deaths have occurred in 30 years. Allen C. Arachnid envenomations. *Emerg Med Clin North Am.* 1992;10(2):269-298.

Table 12-10 Brown Recluse Spiders

Brown recluse spiders	Management
• Live mostly in the southern and midwestern United States. Bites are mild or painless. • Characterized by a brown violin-shaped mark on the cephalothorax. • Bites are often innocuous resulting in a delay in seeking care. • At first, lesions are red with central blister/pustule. • Later discoloration appears and pustule drains creating an ulcer. • Fever, chills, arthralgias, GI upset, DIC, or shock. • Hemoglobinuria (renal failure).	• Wound care, tetanus • Refer to surgeon for possible excision if > 2 cm and well-circumscribed border. • ± Hyperbaric oxygen (controversial). • Dapsone limited to adults with proven brown recluse bites. Dapsone not recommended in children due to risk of methemoglobinemia. • Antivenom not commercially available.

MARINE ENVENOMATION

Table 12-11 Marine Puncture Wounds

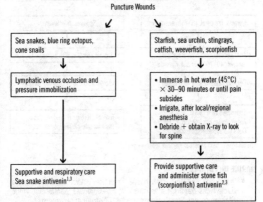

Puncture Wounds

Sea snakes, blue ring octopus, cone snails	Starfish, sea urchin, stingrays, catfish, weeverfish, scorpionfish
↓	↓
Lymphatic venous occlusion and pressure immobilization	• Immerse in hot water (45°C) × 30–90 minutes or until pain subsides • Irrigate, after local/regional anesthesia • Debride + obtain X-ray to look for spine
↓	↓
Supportive and respiratory care Sea snake antivenin[1,3]	Provide supportive care and administer stone fish (scorpionfish) antivenin[2,3]

[1] *Sea snakes.* Bites are painless, causing paralysis + muscle necrosis. Administer polyvalent sea snake antivenin (Commonwealth Serum Laboratories, Australia) within 36 hours. If unavailable, tiger snake and polyvalent Elapidae antivenin are effective. [2] *Stone fish (a type of scorpionfish).* Venom causes muscle toxicity, with paralysis of cardiac, skeletal, and involuntary muscles. Pain is immediate and intense. The wound is ischemic, cyanotic, and may lose tissue. Heat (45°C) partially inactivates venom. Follow package insert for antivenin (Commonwealth Serum Laboratories, Australia). [3] In the United States, call (619) 222-6363 or (415) 770-7171 for antivenin.

Table 12-12 Marine Exposures Causing Urticaria or Vesicles

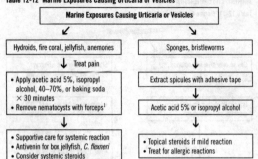

Marine Exposures Causing Urticaria or Vesicles

Hydroids, fire coral, jellyfish, anemones

↓ Treat pain

- Apply acetic acid 5%, isopropyl alcohol, 40–70%, or baking soda × 30 minutes
- Remove nematocysts with forceps[1]

↓

- Supportive care for systemic reaction
- Antivenin for box jellyfish, *C. flexneri*
- Consider systemic steroids

Sponges, bristleworms

↓

Extract spicules with adhesive tape

↓

Acetic acid 5% or isopropyl alcohol

↓

- Topical steroids if mild reaction
- Treat for allergic reactions

[1] Do not rinse in fresh water but may rinse in ocean water.

MARINE INFECTIONS

- Organisms causing soft-tissue infection: *Aeromonas hydrophila*, *Bacteroides fragilis*, *Escherichia coli*, *Pseudomonas*, *Salmonella*, *Vibrio*, *Staphylococcus/Streptococcus* species, *Clostridium perfringens*.
- Irrigate, debride, explore, and obtain X-rays to exclude foreign bodies.
- Antibiotic agents for treating soft-tissue infection or prophylaxis:
  - *Parenteral agents*: Third-generation cephalosporin and/or an aminoglycoside.
  - *Oral agents*: Septra, cefuroxime, tetracycline if older than 8 to 12 years.

13 ■ FLUID AND ELECTROLYTES

ELECTROLYTE DISORDERS

Table 13-1 Formulas

Anion gap	• $Na^+ - (Cl^- + HCO_3^-)$ *Normal* = 8–16 mEq/l
Osmolal gap	• Measured − calculated osmolality *Normal* = 0–10 mOsm/L
Calculated osmolality (285–295 mOsm/kg)	• $(Na \times 2) + (Glucose/18) + (BUN/2.8)$

BUN—blood urea nitrogen.

See pages 197-198 for an evaluation of organic acidurias and other metabolic disorders.

Table 13-2 Causes for the Increase in the Anion Gap, Normal Anion Gap, and Osmolal Gap

Causes of ↑ anion gap	Causes of normal anion gap (hyperchloremic acidosis)
Methanol, metformin	**F**istula (biliary/pancreatic)
Uremia	**U**retrogastric conduit
Diabetes	**S**aline administration
Paraldehyde	**E**ndocrine: Addison's, hyper-parathyroidism
Iron, INH	**D**iarrhea
Lactate	**C**arbonic anhydrase inhibitor
Ethanol, ethylene glycol	**A**mmonium chloride
Salicylates, starvation, seizure	**R**enal tubular acidosis
Toluene, cyanide, carbon monoxide, colchicine	**S**pironolactone

Causes of ↑ osmolal gap
Alcohols (methanol, ethylene glycol, isopropanol)
Sugars (glycerol, mannitol)
Ketones (acetone, diabetic ketoacidosis)

Reproduced from Kliegman, R. M., Behrman, R. E., Jenson, H. B., & Stanton, B. M. (2015). Nelson textbook of pediatrics e-book. Elsevier Health Sciences.

Appropriate compensation during simple acid base disorder

Metabolic acidosis	$PCO_2 = 1.5 \times (HCO_3^-) + (8 \pm 2)$
Metabolic alkalosis	PCO_2 increases by 7 mm Hg for each 10 mEq/l increase in serum HCO_3^-
Respiratory acidosis	
Acute	(HCO_3^-) increases by 1 for each 10 mm Hg increase in PCO_2
Chronic	(HCO_3^-) increases by 3.5 for each 10 mm Hg increase in PCO_2
Respiratory alkalosis	
Acute	(HCO_3^-) falls by 2 for each 10 mm Hg decrease in PCO_2
Chronic	(HCO_3^-) falls by 4 for each 10 mm Hg decrease in PCO_2

Normal pH   7.35–7.45
       HCO_3 20–28 mEq/l
       PCO_2 35–45 mm Hg

Interpreting acid base disturbance:
1. pH: <7.35 = acidosis, >7.45 = alkalosis
2. PCO_2: If pH and PCO_2 in opposite directions = respiratory disorder
        If pH and PCO_2 in same direction = metabolic disorder
3. HCO_3: High in metabolic alkalosis or compensated respiratory acidosis
        Low in metabolic acidosis or compensated respiratory alkalosis
4. Suspect mixed acid base disorder if:
   a. Normal pH with abnormal PCO_2 or HCO_3
   b. Inappropriate compensatory response (greater or lesser)
   c. Shift of both pH and HCO_3 toward acidosis or alkalosis

CALCIUM

Hypocalcemia: Total calcium < 8.5 mg/dl or ionized Ca^{+2} < 2.0 mEq/l (1.0 mmol/l)
Hypercalcemia: Total calcium > 10.5 mg/dl or ionized Ca^{+2} > 2.7 mEq/l (1.3 mmol/l)

Table 13-3 Hypoalbuminemia Correction

Hypoalbuminemia correction	• For each change in serum albumin of 1 g/dl ↑ or ↓, serum calcium changes 0.8 mg/dl in same direction.

Table 13-4 Hypocalcemia—Clinical Features

Symptoms	Physical findings	Electrocardiogram
Paresthesia, fatigue, seizures, tetany, vomiting, weakness, laryngospasm	• Hyperactive reflexes • Chvostek-Trousseau (C-T) signs[1] • Low blood pressure • Congestive heart failure	• Prolonged QT, > 450 msec (especially Ca^{+2} < 6 mg/dl) • Bradycardia • Arrhythmias

[1]C = muscle twitch with tap facial nerve. T = carpal spasm after forearm BP cuff up for 3 minutes.

Table 13-5 Hypocalcemia Etiology[1,2]

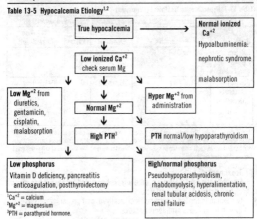

[1]Ca^{+2} = calcium
[2]Mg^{+2} = magnesium
[3]PTH = parathyroid hormone.

Table 13-6 Drugs That Cause Hypocalcemia

• Cimetidine	• Glucagon	• Phosphates
• Cisplatin	• Glucocorticoids	• Protamine
• Citrate (transfusion)	• Heparin	• Norepinephrine
• Dilantin, phenobarbital	• Loop diuretics (Lasix)	• Na^+ nitroprusside
• Gentamicin, tobramycin	• Magnesium sulfate	• Theophylline

Table 13-7 Hypocalcemia Treatment

Check serum electrolytes, BUN, creatinine, albumin, magnesium, arterial pH				
Drug	Preparation	Elemental	Route	Drug dose (max. dose)[3]
Ca gluconate	10% solution—100 mg/ml	9.8 mg/ml	IM, IV[1,2]	0.5–1 mg/kg (5–10 ml)
Ca chloride	10% solution—100 mg/ml	27 mg/ml	IV[1,2]	0.2–0.3 ml/kg (5–10 ml)
Ca gluconate	500, 650, 975, 1,000 mg		PO	100 mg/kg four times per day (500 mg/kg)

(Continued)

Table 13-7 Hypocalcemia Treatment (*Continued*)

Check serum electrolytes, BUN, creatinine, albumin, magnesium, arterial pH				
Drug	Preparation	Elemental	Route	Drug dose (max. dose)[3]
Calcium glubionate (calcionate)	1,800 mg/5 ml	115 mg/5 ml	PO	
Calcium carbonate (Oyster Cal, Caltrate, Tums)	400–1,177 mg	400 mg/1 g	PO	200–1,300 mg/day

[1]Administer IV calcium (Ca) slowly (over ≥ 5–10 minutes) while patient on cardiac monitor. IV calcium may cause hypotension, tissue necrosis, bradycardia, or digoxin toxicity. [2]Consider central administration to prevent tissue damage. Local infiltration of hyaluronidase reverses necrosis. [3]All are doses of salt (listed drug) and not of elemental calcium.

■ Treatment

Symptomatic hypocalcemia should always be treated because it has serious neuronal and cardiac effects.

IV calcium indicated if seizures, if critically ill, or if preparing for surgery.

Switch to oral once symptoms improve.

Treat with magnesium if hypomagnesemia present.

Treat with phosphate-lowering drug if associated with hyperphosphatemia.

Do not completely treat if associated with rhabdomyolysis and pancreatitis.

Treat acidosis first before treating the hypocalcemia.

Diet should be high in calcium and low in phosphate (4:1). Patients with renal failure should be given a low-solute, low-phosphate formula (e.g., Similac 60/40)

Table 13-8 Hypercalcemia—Clinical Features

Clinical Features	
General	• Weakness, polydipsia, dehydration
Neurologic	• Confusion, irritability, hyporeflexia, headache
Skeletal	• Bone pain, fractures
Cardiac	• Hypertension, QT shortening, wide T wave, arrhythmia
GI	• Anorexia, weight loss, constipation, ulcer, pancreatitis
Urologic	• Polyuria, renal insufficiency, nephrolithiasis

Table 13-9 Hypercalcemia[1]

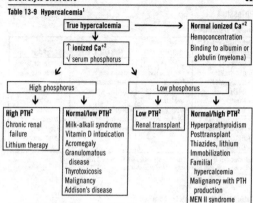

[1]Ca^{+2} = calcium. [2]PTH = parathyroid hormone.

Table 13-10 Hypercalcemia Management

- Especially important for $Ca^{+2} > 12$ mg/dl, hypotension, or cardiac arrhythmias.
- IV NS 20 ml/kg with 30 mEq/l of potassium chloride with repeat boluses to keep urine output $> 2–3$ ml/kg/hour and increase calcium excretion.
- Furosemide 1–2 mg/kg can be used to promote urinary calcium excretion (after adequate hydration) but rarely necessary.
- Calcitonin SC (2–4 units/kg every 24 hours) or IV along with bisphosphonate acids like etidronate, ibandronate, risedronate, clodronate, alendronate, pamidronate, and zoledronic act by inhibiting bone resorption.
- Consider glucocorticoid steroid if sarcoid, vitamin A or D toxicity, or leukemia, mithramycin, metastatic bone disease. Dialysis may also be useful.

POTASSIUM

Etiology of Hypokalemia

Total body deficit (chronic)	Total body deficit (acute)	Shift ECF to ICF	Other
• Prolonged diuretic use • Inadequate K intake • Laxative use • Diuretics • Hyperhidrosis • Hypomagnesemia • RTA • Dengue	• DKA • Severe GI loss • Dialysis and diuretic treatment • Alcohol intoxication and overdose	• Alkalosis • Insulin use • Catecholamine use • Sympathomimetic use • Diuretic therapy • Alkalinization • Hyperthermia	• Mineralocorticoid excess • Renal disease, RTA, periodic hypokalemic paralysis • Increased aldosterone • Celiac disease

Acute decrease in pH will increase K⁺ (a ↓ pH of 0.1 will ↑ K⁺ 0.3–1.3 mEq/l).
Acute metabolic acid–base disorders cause most changes.

Table 13-11 Hypokalemia (< 3.5 mEq/l)

• **Labs:** Electrolytes, blood gas, drug screen. ACTH, cortisol, renin, aldosterone, insulin, and C-peptide based on clinical suspicion of diagnosis.

Clinical features of hypokalemia	Treatment of hypokalemia
• Lethargy, confusion, weakness • Areflexia, difficult respirations • Autonomic instability, low BP	• Ensure good urine output first • If mild, replace orally only • Parenteral K⁺ if severe hypokalemia (e.g., cardiac or neuromuscular symptoms or DKA) • Administer K⁺ no faster than 0.5–1 mEq/kg/hour using ≤40 mEq/l (cautiously while continuously on cardiac monitor) unless life-threatening hypokalemia, give no more than 20 mEq/dose.
ECG findings in hypokalemia	
• Examples Table 8-4, page 42 • K⁺ ≤ 3 mEq/l: low-voltage QRS, flat T waves, ↓ ST segment, prominent P and U waves. • K⁺ ≤ 2.5 mEq/l: prominent U waves • K⁺ ≤ 2 mEq/l: widened QRS	

Table 13-12 Hyperkalemia

Hyperkalemia: K > 5.5 in child and > 6 in newborn in nonhemolyzed sample.	
Etiology 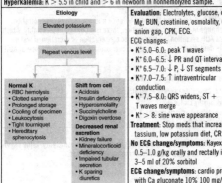	**Evaluation:** Electrolytes, glucose, calcium, Mg, BUN, creatinine, osmolality, CBG, anion gap, CPK, ECG. ECG changes: • K^+ 5.0–6.0: peak T waves • K^+ 6.0–6.5: ↓ PR and QT intervals • K^+ 6.5–7.0: ↓ P, ↓ ST segments • K^+ 7.0–7.5: ↑ intraventricular conduction • K^+ 7.5–8.0: QRS widens, ST + T waves merge • K^+ > 8: sine wave appearance **Treatment:** Stop meds that increase potassium, low potassium diet, CR monitor **No ECG change/symptoms:** Kayexalate 0.5–1.0 g/kg orally and rectally in 3–5 ml of 20% sorbitol **ECG change/symptoms:** cardio protect with Ca gluconate 10% 100 mg/kg IV max of 2 g, slowly (lowers K 1.2 mEq/l in 4–6 hours) Move K from ECF to ICF: Insulin + glucose (0.5–1.0 g/kg IV) + insulin (1 unit/3 g glucose IV) Nebulized albuterol (2.5 mg in children < 25 kg, 5 mg in children > 25 kg) Sodium bicarbonate: 1–2 mEq/kg IV, may repeat **Lower total body potassium** Diuretics: Furosemide 1 mg/kg IV Kayexalate 1 g/kg orally/rectally (lowers K 1.2 mEq/l in 4–6 hours) Hemodialysis

Clinical features
- Paresthesia, weakness
- Ascending paralysis sparing head, trunk, and respiration
- Life-threatening arrhythmias

Modified from Van Mieghem, C., Sabbe, M., & Knockaert, D. (2004). The clinical value of the ECG in noncardiac conditions. Chest, 125(4), 1561–1576.

SODIUM

Daily Na^+ requirements: In newborn, 1–2 mEq/kg/day, and in premature, 3–4 mEq/kg/day.

Serum Na is determined by water balance and not sodium concentration.

With change in sodium concentration, there is a change in osmolality, which influences ADH secretion, which leads to conservation or excretion of water.

Volume depletion takes precedence over osmolality in the influence of ADH, even if there is hyponatremia.

■ Hyponatremia (Serum Na < 135)

Table 13-13 Clinical Features of Hyponatremia

• Lethargy, apathy, confusion	• Cerebral edema
• Depressed reflexes, muscle cramps	• Seizures
• Pseudobulbar palsies	• Hypothermia

Labs: Serum Na, electrolytes, blood sugar, BUN, serum osmolality, urine osmolality and specific gravity, urine Na, creatinine, blood gas.

Table 13-14 Algorithm for Evaluation of Hyponatremia

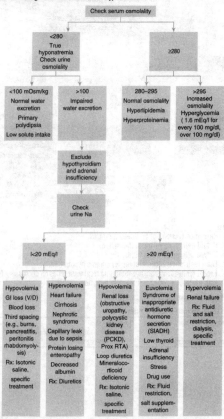

Management of hyponatremia

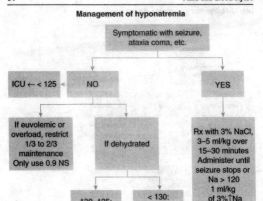

Rules:
1. Rate of correction not to exceed 8 mmol/l.
2. If fluid deficit, Rx with isotonic saline.
3. If hypervolemic, restrict fluids.
4. Fluid restriction is cornerstone for chronic hyponatremia.
5. Except for hypovolemic, hyponatremia treatment relies on decreasing free water intake +/− renal free water excretion.

■ **Hypernatremia (Serum Na > 145)**

Table 13-15 Clinical Features of Hypernatremia

• Lethargy, irritability, coma	• Doughy skin
• Seizures	• Late preservation of intravascular volume
• Spasticity, hyperreflexia	(and vital signs)

Table 13-16 Hypernatremia Etiology, Diagnosis, Management[1]

Na$^+$ + H$_2$O loss with low total body Na$^+$		H$_2$O loss with normal total body Na$^+$		Excess Na$^+$ with increased total body Na$^+$
↓	↓	↓	↓	↓
Renal losses osmotic diuresis (mannitol, glucose, urea)	*Extrarenal loss* excess sweat, diarrhea	*Renal loss* diabetes insipidus (nephrogenic, central) Serum osm > 295 mOsm/l Serum Na$^+$ > 145 mEq/l U$_{osm}$ < 150 mOsm/l	*Extrarenal loss* Respiratory and skin loss	Primary hyperaldosteronism, Cushing's syndrome, hypertonic dialysis, hypertonic Na$^+$ bicarbonate, NaCl tablets, improperly mixed formulas
↓	↓	↓	↓	↓
Diagnostic Tests				
U Na$^+$ > 20 mEq/l, U$_{osm}$ hypotonic	U Na$^+$ < 10 mEq/l, U$_{osm}$ > 600–800 mOsm/l	U Na$^+$ varies U$_{osm}$ often < 100–150 mOsm/l	U Na$^+$ varies U$_{osm}$ > 600–800 mOsm/l	U Na$^+$ > 20 mEq/l U$_{osm}$ isotonic or hypertonic
↓	↓	↓	↓	↓
Management				
Hypotonic saline	Hypotonic saline	Water replacement D$_5$W	Water replacement D$_5$W	Diuretic+H$_2$O replacement D$_5$W

[1]U—urine, U$_{osm}$—urine osmolality.

Management of Hypernatremia

Correct hypernatremia slowly over approximately 48 hours. Over-vigorous rehydration causes cerebral edema, seizures, coma, or death. Lower Na$^+$ no faster than 1–2 mEq/l/hour.

In hypernatremia with dehydration, first restore intravascular volume with isotonic fluid, normal saline preferred. Most patients do well with 3–4 ml/kg of water for each 1 mEq/l that the sodium level exceeds 145 mEq, with Na concentration of half normal saline at a rate of 20–30% greater than maintenance fluid. Patients with pure water loss may require a more hypotonic (0.2 NS) fluid.

With endogenous Na$^+$ overload, treatment consists of salt restriction and correction of the primary underlying disorder. If there is excess exogenous mineralocorticoid, restrict salt and modify replacement therapy.

Desmopressin (DDAVP) is indicated in children with diabetes insipidus. Intranasal DDAVP dose is 0.05–0.3 ml daily, bid.

DEHYDRATION

Dehydration is total water depletion with respect to sodium, and volume depletion is the decrease in the circulation volume. It is usually associated with
metabolic acidosis (excess HCO_3 loss in stool with diarrhea, or urine with RTA,
or glycogen depletion causing ketosis, or poor tissue perfusion causing lactic
acidosis, or H^+ ion retention from poor tissue perfusion). Sometimes there may
be alkalosis from vomiting with loss of gastric contents containing chloride, sodium, and potassium causing hypochloremic, hypokalemic metabolic alkalosis.
Dehydration:

Mild (3–5%): Normal HR, pulse, capillary refill, BP, and respiration.

Moderate (6–10%): Listless, irritable, prolonged capillary refill, ↑ HR and
RR, ↓ UO.

Severe (> 10%): Lethargy, altered mental status, ↑ HR and RR, sunken
eyes, no tears, oliguria or anuria.

Table 13-17 Dehydration—Classification and Management

Classification	Isotonic	Hypotonic	Hypertonic[1]
Na⁺ (mEq/l)	130–150	<130	>150
Cause	Usually GI[2] and ECF[3] fluid loss	Dilute fluid (water) replacement	Too dilute formula, ↑ Na⁺ intake, ICF[3] > ECF[3] loss
Deficit	Na⁺ = water loss	Na⁺ > water loss	Water > Na⁺ loss
BP	Depressed	Very depressed	May be preserved
RR	Increased	Increased	Minimal increase
Skin/Turgor	Dry/Poor	Clammy/Very poor	Doughy/Fair
Mentation	Lethargy	Coma or seizure	Irritable or seizure
Rehydrate[4]	Normal saline	Normal saline	D₅ 1/2 NS with K⁺
Unique feature (*exclude hypoglycemia in all patients*)	Most common. Oral rehydration is appropriate for children if <5–10% dehydration if able to take liquids PO.	Consider 3% NS if seizures, life-threatening symptoms (see page 94 for indication/dosing).	NS can paradoxically ↑ Na⁺. Lower Na⁺ < 2 mEq/l/hour or < 10 mEq/l/day. Too rapid Rx = congestive heart failure, CNS edema, renal damage. ± ↓ Ca⁺²

[1]4 ml/kg free water deficit for each 1 mEq/l Na > 145. [2]GI—gastrointestinal. [3]ICF—intracellular fluid; ECF—extracellular fluid. [4]Use NS to reverse shock in all cases.

■ **Dehydration—Further Management**

Severe dehydration: Rapid correction with normal saline or Ringer's lactate 20 ml/kg over 20 minutes can repeat as needed (monitoring for improved HR, BP, urine output, perfusion, and mentation). Slow rate in patients with cardiac insufficiency, congestive heart failure, pulmonary edema, and diabetic ketoacidosis.

With isonatremic or hyponatremic dehydration, correct entire deficit over 24 hours.

Deficit is determined by degree of dehydration.

For second phase, the child requires 1/2 of remaining deficit and 1/3 of maintenance fluid over 8 hours.

Third phase consists of 1/2 of the deficit and 2/3 of maintenance fluid over 16 hours.

With hypernatremic dehydration, correct slowly over 48 hours; may need to correct over 72 to 84 hours if very severe hypernatremia.

Add potassium after the patient voids and normal renal function is documented.

Replacement (usually over 8 hours) is maintenance plus deficit volume plus ongoing losses, usually 1.25 to 1.5 times maintenance.

Do IV hydration if ill, patient needs to stay NPO, severe dehydration (> 10%), cannot take oral fluids, or serious lab abnormality.

Other treatment options:

(1) Intraosseous (if severely ill, see page 11); (2) Subcutaneous—recombinant human hyaluronidase (rHuPH$_2$0; Hylenex, Baxter International) increases subcutaneous fluid absorption 1.6- to 3.3-fold. Apply LMX or FMLA to skin; in 30 minutes insert 24–25 gauge angiocatheter or needle into mid-anterior thigh or interscapular; 1 ml (150 units) is injected SC through needle followed by continuous pump facilitated SC infusion of 20 ml/kg NS over 1 hour, may repeat (50% swell locally); OR (3) NG/feeding tube: 50 ml/kg Pedialyte over 3 hours.

Table 13-18 IV Maintenance Fluid Calculation

By Body Weight	4 ml/kg/hour (100 ml/kg/day) for 1st 10 kg, + 2 ml/kg/hour (50 ml/kg/day) for 2nd 10 kg, + 1 ml/kg/hour (25 ml/kg/day) for each kg above 20 kg
Maintenance Na^+ requirements = 2–3 mEq/100 ml maintenance fluid administered	
Maintenance K^+ requirements = 2 mEq/100 ml maintenance fluid administered	

Some experts (not all) recommend isotonic saline (normal saline/NS) over hypotonic saline (e.g., 1/2 NS) with appropriate potassium, etc., for maintenance fluids to decrease iatrogenic hyponatremia.

Modified from Montanana, P. A., i Alapont, V. M., Ocon, A. P., Lopez, P. O., Prats, J. L. L., & Parreño, J. D. T. (2008). The use of isotonic fluid as maintenance therapy prevents iatrogenic hyponatremia in pediatrics: a randomized, controlled open study. Pediatric Critical Care Medicine, 9(6), 589-597. Beck CE. Hypotonic versus isotonic maintenance intravenous fluid therapy in hospitalized children: a systematic review. Clin Pediatr (Phila). 2007;46(9):764-770.

Table 13-19 Composition of Oral and Intravenous Solutions

Solution	Sodium (mEq/l)	Potassium (mEq/l)	Chloride (mEq/l)	Bicarbonate (mEq/l)[1]	Glucose (g/dl)
Extracellular fluid	142	4	103	27	~0.1
0.9 NS	154	0	154	0	0
D5NS	154	0	154	0	5
5% albumin	130–160	0	130–160	0	0
Hypertonic 3% NS	513	0	513	0	0
0.45 NS	77	0	77	0	0
0.3 NS	51	0	51	0	0
0.2 NS	34	0	34	0	0
LR	130	4	109	28	0
Infant Carvajal's[2]	81	0	61	20	4.65
Child Carvajal's[2]	132	3.8	109	27	4.8
WHO solution[3]	90	20	80	—	2.0
Pedialyte	45	20	35	30	2.5
Rehydralyte	75	20	65	30	2.5
Resol	50	20	50	34	2.0
Ricelyte	50	25	45	10	3.0
Infalyte	50	20	40	—	2.0
Gatorade	28	2	—	—	2.1
Ginger ale	4	0.2	—	—	9.0
Coke/Pepsi	3/2	0.1/0.9	13.4/7.3	10.0/10.0	10.5/10.5
Apple/Grape juice	1–4	15–30	—	—	12.0/15.0
Jell-O	24	1.5	—	—	15.8

[1]Or citrate or lactate. [2]Used for burns and contains 12.5 g/l albumin. [3]Excess World Health Organization (WHO) formula causes ↑ Na, give with free water.

Table 13-20 Treatment of Dehydration by Oral Rehydration

Oral rehydration	WHO recommendations
Wheat- and rice-based oral electrolyte solutions are superior to glucose solutions for rehydration, ↓ stool frequency volume.	• First, hydrate with 100 ml/kg WHO formula over 4 hours. • Then, 50 ml/kg of water or breastmilk over next 2 hours. • If still dehydrated, 50 ml/kg WHO formula next 6 hours. • Then, 100 ml/kg of WHO formula over next 24 hours, then 150 ml/kg/day of WHO formula. Give additional free H_2O with WHO formula or hypernatremia may occur.

The latest improved ORS formula contains less glucose and sodium (245 mOsm/l compared with the previous 311 mOsm/l). The lower concentration of the new formula allows for a quicker absorption of fluids, reducing the need for intravenous fluids and making it easier to treat children with acute noncholera diarrhea without hospitalization.

According to UNICEF and WHO, oral rehydration therapy should be combined with guidance on appropriate feeding practices. Provision of zinc supplements (20 mg of zinc per day for 10–14 days) and continued breastfeeding during acute episodes of diarrhea protect against dehydration and reduces protein and calorie consumption that have the greatest impact on reducing diarrhea and malnutrition.

MEDICINES

Table 14-1 Common GI Therapeutic Agents

Drug	Available forms	Dosing
Bisacodyl (Dulcolax)	Suppository: 10 mg Tab: 5 mg	Oral (≥3–10 years): 5 mg/day Oral (>10 years): 5–15 mg/day Rectal (2–10 years): 5 mg every day Rectal (>10 years): 5–10 mg every day
Cimetidine	Solution: 300 mg/5 ml Tab: 200, 300, 400, 800 mg	Infant: 5–10 mg/kg/day div every 6 hours to every 12 hours Child: 20–40 mg/kg/day div every 6 hours to every 8 hours, max 400 mg/dose Adolescents (≥16 years): 400 mg 4×/day or 800 mg bid
Docusate sodium (Colace)	Syrup: 60 mg/15 ml Solution: 12.5 mg/5 ml, 50 mg/5 ml, 50 mg/15 ml Cap/Tab: 50, 100, 250 mg Cap as calcium: 240 mg Suppository: 100 mg/5 ml; 283 mg/5 ml	Oral (6 months–2 years): 12.5 mg three times per day Oral (≥2–12 years): 50–150 mg/kg/day div every day or four times per day Oral (≥12 years): 500 mg/day div bid or three times per day Rectal (2–12 years): 100 mg/day Rectal (≥12 years): 283 mg every day
Famotidine (*Pepcid*)	Suspension: 40 mg/5 ml Cap/Tab: 10, 20, 40 mg Chewable tab: 10, 20 mg Injectable: 20 mg/2 ml	**Peptic ulcer:** 1–16 years: 0.25 mg/kg IV bid OR 0.5 mg/kg PO QHS (maximum of 40 mg/day) **GERD:** < 3 months: 0.5 mg/kg PO daily × 8 weeks ≥ 3–12 months: 0.5 mg/kg PO every 12 hours × 8 weeks 1–16 years: 1 mg/kg div bid (maximum of 40 mg/dose)
Glycerin	Infant suppository	Insert + retain > 15 minutes (bid or daily prn)
Lactulose	Solution: 10 g/15 ml	1–2 g/kg/day (1.5–3.0 ml/kg/day)
Lansoprazole (Prevacid)	Cap/Dissolving tab: 15, 30 mg	**GERD:** ≥ 3 months: 7.5 mg bid or 15 mg daily 1–11 years: If ≤ 30 kg, 15 mg once daily. If > 30 kg, 30 mg once daily ≥ 12 years: 15 mg once daily

Table 14-1 Common GI Therapeutic Agents (*Continued*)

Drug	Available forms	Dosing
Metoclopramide (Reglan)	Injectable: 5 mg/1 ml Syrup: 5 mg/5 ml Tab: 5, 10 mg	<6 years: 0.1 mg/kg 6–14 years: 2.5–5 mg once >14 years: 10 mg once Max dose: 10 mg
Omeprazole (Prilosec)	Cap: 10, 20, 40 mg	5–10 kg: 5 mg daily 10 kg to < 20 kg: 10 mg daily ≥ 20 kg: 20 mg daily
Ondansetron (Zofran)	Injectable: 2 mg/ml Oral solution: 4 mg/5 ml Tab/ODT tab: 4, 8 mg	*Intravenous:* < 6 months: safety not known ≥ 6 months: 0.10–0.15 mg/kg IV (max 4 mg) *Oral:* 8–15 kg: 2 mg PO 15–30 kg: 4 mg PO > 30 kg: 8 mg PO
Polyethylene glycol (PEG) 3350 (Miralax)	PEG 14 oz or 26 oz (1 cap = 17 g)	*Fecal impaction:* 1.0–1.5 g/kg/day for 3–6 days, max 100 g/day. Follow with maintenance dose 0.4 g/kg daily for 2 months *Constipation:* 0.2–0.8 g/kg/day (divided bid), max 17 g/day (mix with 4–8 oz fluid)
Ranitidine (Zantac)	Syrup: 15 mg/1 ml Tab: 75, 150, 300 mg Cap: 150, 300 mg Injectable: 25 mg/ml or 150 mg/6 ml	*IV prophylaxis for GI bleed* Infants: 2–4 mg/kg/day every 8 hours Children/adolescents: 3–6 mg/kg/day div every 6 hours, max 300 mg/day *GERD:* Oral ≤ 16 years: 5–10 mg/kg/day div twice a day, max 300 mg/day > 16 years: 150 mg twice a day
Simethicone (Mylicon, GasX)	Drops: 40 mg/0.6 ml Tab: 80, 125, 180 mg	< 2 years: 20 mg 4×/day (max 240 mg/day) 2–12 years: 40 mg 4×/day (max 480 mg/day) > 12 years: 40–160 mg 4×/day (max 480 mg/day)
Sodium phosphate (Fleet Enema)	Solution: 66 mL, 133 ml	*Constipation, rectal:* 1–18 years: 2.5 ml/kg, max 133 ml/dose
Sucralfate (Carafate)	Suspension: 1 g/10 ml Tab: 1 g	*Peptic ulcer disease:* 40–80 mg/kg/day div every 6 hours, max 1 g/dose *Esophagitis:* < 6 years: 500 mg/dose 4×/day ≥ 6 years: 1 g 4×/day

COLIC AND CRYING

Table 14-2 Etiologies for Crying in Infants*

Diagnosis	Frequency (percentage) Total n = 237
Crying with no other diagnosis	65 (27)
Viral illness	49 (21)
Gastroesophageal reflux	30 (13)
Colic	14 (6)
Other[1]	14 (6)
Gastroenteritis	12 (5)
Atypical colic (not meeting formal definition below)	11 (5)
Constipation	11 (5)
Bronchiolitis	8 (3)
Feeding disorder/difficulty	7 (3)
Otitis media	7 (3)
Vaccine adverse event	3 (1)
Reducible inguinal hernia	3 (1)
Clavicle fracture	2 (< 1)
Urinary infection (UTI)	2 (< 1)

[1]One each of acute lymphoblastic leukemia, bacteremia + UTI, cellulitis, cholecystitis, dermatitis, epidural hematoma, gas, infantile spasms, intussusception, nephrolithiasis, nursemaid's elbow, toe trauma, thrush, spinal muscular atrophy.
Modified from Freedman SB, Al-Harthy N, Thull-Freedman J. The crying infant: diagnostic testing and frequency of serious underlying disease. *Pediatrics.* 2009;123(3):841-848.

Colic: Defined as paroxysms of crying that last >3 hours and occur >3 days/week for at least 3 weeks. Colic is a behavioral syndrome usually occurring in otherwise healthy infants aged 2 weeks to 4 months. Crying is more common in the evenings, and in bottle-fed infants. Variable associations with excess feeding (>125 kcal/kg/day), food allergy, reflux, incomplete burping after feeds, maternal smoking, abnormal intestinal microflora, and low birth weight have been found.

Evaluation—Serious diseases are uncommon (5.1% according to the study mentioned previously), with UTI being the most common serious diagnosis). Approximately 99% of all diagnoses made based on history and physical examination. Evaluation is directed at excluding serious disorders (congenital heart anomalies including anomalous left coronary artery from the pulmonary artery); infection; occult trauma of the head, torso, or extremity; corneal abrasion; surgical disorders (intussusception, hernia, volvulus, Hirschsprung's disease, testicular torsion); hair tourniquet; ingrown eyelash; child abuse; etc. After serious disease excluded, ensure that proper feeding techniques are used [e.g., volume of feeding (~115–125 kcal/kg/day), burping, upright status continued after feedings, appropriate formula, see page 209]. In breastfed infants, maternal diets that avoid dairy, soy, eggs, peanuts, wheat, and shellfish may improve symptoms. In formula-fed babies, changing to a hydrolyzed formula may improve symptoms.

Management—For those without serious disorders and a final diagnosis of colic, reassure parents that colic is self-limited. Do not use dicyclomine as this can cause apnea, seizures, and syncope. *Lactobacillus reuteri*, strain DSM17398, 5 drops daily, may decrease symptoms in breastfed infants.* Oral hypertonic glucose was found in one study to be an effective remedy; however, more randomized studies are required to recommend this therapy. Studies on herbal treatment, physical therapy, acupuncture, and massage do not show sufficient evidence and have conflicting results.**

Sources:

*Sung V, D'Amico F, Cabana MD, et al. *Lactobacillus reuteri* to treat infant colic: a meta-analysis. *Pediatrics.* 2018;141(1). pii: e20171811.

**Biagioli E, Tarasco V, Lingua C, Moja L, Savino F. Pain-relieving agents for infantile colic. *Cochrane Database Syst Rev.* 2016;9:CD009999.

CONSTIPATION

Table 14-3 Organic Causes of Constipation in Children

Anatomic malformation	Imperforate anus, anal/colonic stenosis, anteriorly displaced anus, spinal cord dysplasia
Drugs/Environmental exposures	Opiates, anticholinergics, antidepressants, antacids, laxative abuse, chemotherapy, lead poisoning, botulism
Metabolic/Endocrine	Diabetes, hypercalcemia, hypokalemia, hypothyroidism, porphyria, multiple endocrine neoplasia type 2B
Neurogenic	Hirschsprung's disease, anal sphincter achalasia, pseudo-obstruction (e.g., visceral myopathy, visceral neuropathy)
Spinal cord abnormalities	Myelomeningocele, spinal cord tumor, trauma, tethered cord
Systemic disease/other	Celiac disease, cystic fibrosis, milk protein intolerance, connective tissue disorders [e.g., scleroderma, systemic lupus erythematosus (SLE), Ehlers-Danlos], psychiatric disorder (e.g., anorexia nervosa), pelvic mass

Consider the items in the table if there is failure to thrive, pilonidal dimples/hair tuft, sacral agenesis, flat buttocks, anteriorly displaced anus, tight empty rectum with palpable abdominal fecal mass, gush of liquid stool and air from rectum after digital exam, occult blood, absent anal wink, absent cremasteric reflex, or decreased low extremity tone/strength/relaxation phase of DTRs.

Table 14-4A Diagnosis/Management of Functional Constipation in Children <6 Months

Alarming signs and symptoms: onset of symptoms <1 month, delayed passage of meconium by 48 hours of life, failure to thrive, abdominal distension, bloody stool (gross or occult), empty rectum, explosive stool evacuation after digital rectal exam, tuft of hair or dimple at lumbosacral region. Refer to pediatric GI specialist if there are alarming signs.

Constipation diagnosed per Rome III/Rome IV criteria,[1] symptom duration > 1month, absence of organic pathology, no alarming signs

↓

Exclusively breastfed >2 weeks old?

↓

If yes, likely to be normal. Reevaluate after 2–4 weeks.
If not exclusively breastfed, verify proper formula preparation, keep a diary, education regarding stool patterns in infants.

↓

If patient continues to be symptomatic, and there is *no fecal impaction*, consider *maintenance therapy* (see the following).

If patient continues to be symptomatic, and/or there is *fecal impaction*, start medications.
First line:
• Oral PEG with or without electrolytes: 1–1.5 g/kg/day, max 100 g/day, × 3–6 days
Alternative:
• If PEG is not available, 1 enema/day (bisacodyl or sodium docusate) × 3–6 days.

Then start *maintenance therapy* for at least 2 months until symptom-free for 1 month.
First line:
• Oral PEG 0.4 g/kg/day, max 17 g/day. Mix with 4–8 oz fluid.
Alternative:
• If PEG is not available, oral lactulose 1–2 g/kg/day.

↓

If medications are not effective, refer to GI specialist.
If symptoms return after a symptom-free period, may restart medications. Refer to GI specialist after two relapses.

---

[1]Russo M, Strisciuglio C, Scarpato E, Bruzzese D, Casertano M, Staiano A. Functional chronic constipation: Rome III criteria versus Rome IV criteria. *J Neurogastroenterol Motil.* 2019;25(1):123–128.
Modified from Russo, M., Strisciuglio, C., Scarpato, E., Bruzzese, D., Casertano, M., & Staiano, A. (2019). Functional chronic constipation: Rome III criteria versus Rome IV criteria. Journal of neurogastroenterology and motility, 25(1), 123. Tabbers MM, DiLorenzo C, Berger MY, et al. Evaluation and treatment of functional constipation in infants and children: evidence-based recommendations from ESPGHAN and NASPGHAN. JPGN. 2014;58: 258–274.

Table 14-4B Diagnosis/Management of Functional Constipation in Children ≥ 6 Months

Constipation diagnosed per Rome III criteria, symptom duration >2 months if age ≥4 years, absence of organic pathology, no alarming signs.

If there is no fecal impaction, start with maintenance therapy (see the following), education, diary, and toilet training. Reevaluate after 2 weeks.

If there is *fecal impaction*, start medications.

First line:
• Oral PEG with or without electrolytes: 1–1.5 g/kg/day, max 100 g/day, ×3–6 days.

Alternative:
• If PEG is not available, 1 enema/day (bisacodyl or sodium docusate) ×3–6 days.

If treatment for fecal impaction is not effective, refer to a pediatric gastroenterologist.

If treatment is effective for fecal impaction, continue with maintenance therapy, education, diary, and toilet training. Reevaluate after 2 weeks.

Maintenance therapy:
First line:
• PEG 0.4 g/kg/day mixed with 4–8 oz fluid.

Alternative:
• If PEG is not available, lactulose 1–2 g/kg/day.

If maintenance therapy is effective, continue for 2 months until symptom free for 1 month. If symptoms return, refer to pediatric GI specialist.

If maintenance therapy is not effective, titrate medication dosages, reeducate and reassess. If symptoms persist, refer to GI specialist. If symptoms resolve after medication adjustment, continue maintenance therapy until symptom free for 1 month. If symptoms return, refer to pediatric GI specialist.

Modified from Tabbers MM, DiLorenzo C, Berger MY, et al. Evaluation and treatment of functional constipation in infants and children: evidence-based recommendations from ESPGHAN and NASPGHAN. *JPGN.* 2014;58: 258-274.

DIARRHEA

Acute gastroenteritis (AGE) is defined as frequent loose or watery stools (three or more within 24 hours) that may occur with or without vomiting, nausea, or fever. Symptoms usually resolve in less than 7 days but can last up to 14 days. Excess fluid losses can lead to dehydration in children.

Viruses are the most common cause of AGE in resource-rich countries. Rotavirus was once the leading cause of persistent or severe diarrhea in children. With the introduction of rotavirus vaccines, norovirus is now the leading cause of AGE. Other viruses that cause AGE include sapovirus, astrovirus, and enteric adenovirus. Clinical features of viral AGE may include nonbloody stools, vomiting, and respiratory symptoms.

Common bacterial causes of AGE include *Salmonella enterica* subspecies, *Campylobacter, Shigella, Yersinia,* and *Escherichia coli* O157:H7. Clinical features often include high fever (>40°C), blood or mucus in stool, and abdominal pain.

Source: Shane AL, Mody RK, Crump JA, et al. 2017 infectious diseases Society of America Clinical Practice guidelines for the diagnosis and management of infectious diarrhea. *Clin Infect Dis.* 2017;65(12):e45-e80.

Secretory diarrhea is enterotoxin induced (e.g., *Escherichia coli,* Vibrio, clostridia, some staphylococcal species, *Shigella,* Salmonella). Enterotoxins cause fluid and electrolyte secretion from crypt cells and block absorption of Na^+ and Cl^- by the carrier mechanism. Glucose coupled Na^+ absorption is not blocked. Fecal Na^+ is >60 mOsm/l, and stool osmotic gap $(290 - 2 + [stool\ Na^+ + stool\ K^+]) < 100$ mOsm/l.

Cytotoxic diarrhea is usually due to viral agents (e.g., rotavirus) and is characterized by the destruction of villous mucosa. Shortened villi decrease the intestinal surface area available for fluid absorption.

Osmotic diarrhea is usually due to malabsorption (e.g., lactose intolerance). Osmotically active agents retain fluid in the bowel. Osmotic diarrhea exacerbates cytotoxic and secretory diarrhea via impaired absorption of nutrients and electrolytes. Oral Mg and sorbitol cause osmotic diarrhea. Fecal Na^+ is < 70 mOsm/l, and stool osmotic gap $(290 - 2 \times [stool\ Na^+ + stool\ K^+]) > 100$ mOsm/l. Fecal pH < 5.5 or reducing substances > 0.25–0.5% Σ carbohydrate malabsorption.

Dysenteric diarrhea is due to invasion of mucosa and submucosa of the colon and terminal ileum by infectious agents (e.g., Salmonella, *Shigella, Yersinia, Campylobacter,* enteroviruses). Edema, bleeding, and leukocyte infiltration typically occur.

CLINICAL EVALUATION OF THE CHILD WITH DIARRHEA

Clinical history should include the patient's age, onset, frequency, and duration of diarrhea, characteristics of emesis and diarrhea (bilious, bloody, presence of mucous), weight prior to illness, recent oral intake, changes in urine output, and systemic signs such as fever and mental status.

Physical examination should assess for the degree of dehydration quickly and accurately. Acute weight loss is the gold standard of determining dehydration status, although the original weight prior to illness is often unavailable. Important components are general appearance (active, listless, less responsive), capillary refill time (≤2 seconds is normal), abnormal skin turgor, and abnormal respiration patterns (may indicate underlying metabolic acidosis). Other features to consider include the presence of tears, sunken eyes, mucous membranes, radial pulse, and tachycardia.

Laboratory testing is not necessary for children presenting with AGE. However, in the presence of bloody or mucoid stools, fever, severe abdominal pain, or signs of sepsis, stool cultures should be sent to evaluate for Salmonella, Shigella, Campylobacter, Yersinia, Shiga-toxin E. coli and Clostridium difficile (if age is greater than 2 years with history of antibiotic use). If there is a history of voluminous rice water stools, eating undercooked shellfish, exposure to salty waters, stool culture should also evaluate for Vibrio. If patients are younger than 3 months old, blood cultures should be obtained. In patients with bloody diarrhea and fever, it is also important to obtain complete blood count and serum electrolytes to monitor for possible signs of hemolytic uremic syndrome related to E. coli O157 infections.

Sources: Colletti JE, Brown KM, Sharieff GQ, Barata IA, Ishimine P; ACEP Pediatric Emergency Medicine Committee. The management of children with gastroenteritis and dehydration in the emergency department. *J Emerg Med.* 2010;38(5):686-698; Guarino A, Ashkenazi S, Gendrel D, Lo Vecchio A, Shamir R, Szajewska H. European Society for Pediatric Gastroenterology, Hepatology, and Nutrition/European Society for pediatric infectious diseases evidence-based guidelines for the management of acute gastroenteritis in children in Europe. *JPGN.* 2014;59:132-152; Shane AL, Mody RK, Crump JA, et al. 2017 infectious diseases Society of America Clinical Practice guidelines for the diagnosis and management of infectious diarrhea. *Clin Infect Dis.* 2017;65(12):e45-e80.

DIARRHEA THERAPY

First-line therapy for mild to moderate dehydration due to AGE is with a reduced osmolarity oral rehydration solution. Oral rehydration therapy (ORT) is often effective in AGE, as cotransport of sodium with glucose remains intact. WHO solution can be used in all ages and in those with hypotonic, isotonic, or hypertonic dehydration. For patients with severe dehydration who have signs of sepsis, shock, or altered mental status, first-line therapy is resuscitation with IV isotonic fluids. Once the patient is rehydrated, maintenance fluids should be started to replace ongoing losses. See Table 14.5 for the American Academy of Pediatrics' guidelines for managing acute gastroenteritis.

Drug therapy: Kaolin-pectin (Kaopectate) is an adsorbent. Bismuth subsalicylate (Pepto-Bismol) inhibits intestinal secretions and is useful in traveler's diarrhea.

Antibiotics are indicated for Shigella and Vibrio cholerae. Azithromycin, ciprofloxacin, or ceftriaxone may be used to treat Shigella. Vibrio cholerae is treated with doxycycline (first line) or with ciprofloxacin, azithromycin, or ceftriaxone. Yersinia enterocolitica is treated with trimethoprim-sulfamethoxazole. Azithromycin is effective for Campylobacter. Antibiotics for Salmonella are not indicated unless the patient is younger than 3 months old, toxic appearing, or immunocompromised.

See pages 143-169 for antibiotic recommendations and dosing for specific organisms and exposures.

Recent studies have shown that the use of probiotics, specifically *Lactobacillus rhamnosus* GG, does not decrease the duration of diarrhea in acute gastroenteritis.

Chronic diarrhea: Culture the stool and test for lactose intolerance (reducing substances > 0.25–0.50% and pH < 5.5). If lactose intolerance suspected, discontinue dairy products for 2 weeks.

SPECIFIC AAP RECOMMENDATIONS

- Use oral rehydration therapy for mild to moderate dehydration. If oral rehydration fails, nasogastric hydration may be preferred to IV hydration. (See pages 97-99 for IV fluid recommendations, intraosseous, and NG options.)
- Children who require rehydration should continue to be fed age-appropriate diets after rehydration (early feeding will decrease the duration of diarrhea).
- As a general rule, pharmacologic agents should not be used for acute diarrhea (opiates/atropine are contraindicated; anticholinergic agents/ bismuth subsalicylate, adsorbents, lactobacillus compounds are not recommended).

Sources: Subcommittee on Acute Gastroenteritis, Provisional Committee on Quality Improvement. Practice parameter: the management of acute gastroenteritis in young children. *Pediatrics*. 1996;97(3):424-435; Guarino A, Ashkenazi S, Gendrel D, Lo Vecchio A, Shamir R, Szajewska H. European Society for Pediatric Gastroenterology, Hepatology, and Nutrition/European Society for pediatric infectious diseases evidence-based guidelines for the management of acute gastroenteritis in children in Europe. *JPGN*. 2014;59:132-152; Shane AL, Mody RK, Crump JA, et al. 2017 Infectious diseases Society of America Clinical Practice guidelines for the diagnosis and management of infectious diarrhea. *Clin Infect Dis*. 2017;65(12):e45-e80.

Table 14-5 American Academy of Pediatrics Practice Guideline for Managing Acute Gastroenteritis

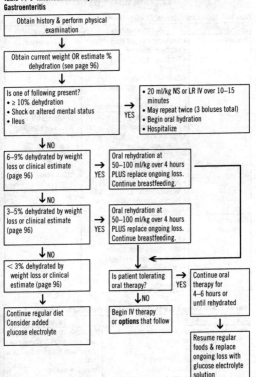

Ondansetron (Zofran) 1.6 mg (6–12 months), 3.2 mg (1–3 years), 4 mg (4–12 years) orally every 8 hours × 6 doses leads to ↓ vomiting/IV fluid use/admission rates.

GASTROINTESTINAL BLEEDS

Table 14-6 Upper Gastrointestinal Bleeding—Etiology

Age	Most frequent causes	Features
Newborn/Infants	• Swallowed maternal blood • Vitamin K deficiency • Stress ulcers (hospitalized infants) • Gastritis/Esophagitis • Intestinal duplications and vascular anomalies • Milk protein allergy (rarer cause)	See Apt-Downey test, which follows
Toddlers	• Mallory-Weiss tears • Foreign body ingestion • Accidental ingestion of caustic chemicals • Gastritis • Frequent NSAID use • *Helicobacter pylori* infection • Henoch-Schönlein purpura • Hemolytic uremic syndrome (HUS) • Perianal streptococcal cellulitis • Varices	Mallory-Weiss tears: history of cough, retching, or vomiting Varices: look for liver cirrhosis, portal vein thrombosis, portal hypertension
Older children/adolescents	• Gastric ulcer, gastritis, esophagitis, varices • Pill esophagitis • Inflammatory bowel disease (Crohn's, ulcerative colitis) • Enteric infections • Anal fissures, hemorrhoids • Hemophilia	

Table 14-7 Most Common Causes of Lower GI Bleed Presenting to a Pediatric ED

Age	Most frequent causes	Features
Newborn/infant	• Cow's milk protein allergy • Anal fissures • Volvulus • Necrotizing enterocolitis • Hirschsprung's disease • Intussusception • Intestinal duplications, vascular lesions	Milk protein allergy: associated with proctocolitis, hematochezia, may also be allergic to soy protein Volvulus: bilious emesis, prematurity Intussusception: lethargy, currant jelly stools (late sign) Vascular lesion: Dieulafoy lesion, AVM, hemangioma

Table 14-7 Most Common Causes of Lower GI Bleed Presenting to a Pediatric ED (*Continued*)

Age	Most frequent causes	Features
Children	• Enteric infection • Meckel's diverticulum • Intussusception • Vasculitis (Henoch-Schönlein) • Hemolytic uremic syndrome • Lymphoid hyperplasia • Polyps • Rectal prolapse • Streptococcal perianal infection • Food coloring	HUS: after infection of *E. coli* O157:H7 Lymphoid hyperplasia: common in IgA-deficient patients or hypogammaglobulinemia Food coloring: fruit punch, beet, candies, licorice, blueberries spinach, iron
Adolescents	• Inflammatory bowel disease (Crohn's, ulcerative colitis) • Enteric colitis • Hemorrhoids • Anal fissure • Frequent NSAID use • Vascular malformations	

EVALUATION AND MANAGEMENT OF SIGNIFICANT GI BLEEDING

- Place cardiac monitor, administer O_2, and insert two large bore IVs.
- Draw CBC, comprehensive metabolic panel, coagulation studies, type and cross at least 15 ml/kg of packed RBCs.
- Administer 20 ml/kg NS bolus and repeat to correct hypotension or shock.
- Consider blood transfusion if there is no response to first two fluid boluses.
- Consider plain radiograph for suspicion of foreign body ingestion; abdominal ultrasound for suspicion of portal hypertension.
- **Pharmacotherapy:** For severe GI bleeding, start proton pump inhibitors. For children < 40 kg, pantoprazole IV 0.5–1.0 mg/kg/day may be used. For children ≥ 40 kg, pantoprazole 20–40 mg/day may be used. For variceal bleeding in addition to symptoms previously mentioned, consider vasopressin (0.002–0.005 units/kg/minute, titrate to maximum of 0.01 unit/kg/minute) or octreotide (1–2 mcg/kg IV bolus, followed by 1–2 mcg/kg/hour continuous infusion). Multiple serious side effects can occur with either medication; therefore, intensive monitoring is required if either is administered.
- **Endoscopy and specialty consult:** Considered first line in diagnostic and intervention management. Endoscopy identifies bleeding site in 75–90% of upper GI and 48–90% of lower GI bleeds. It also provides therapeutic management by coagulating or sclerosing the site of the bleeding.

- **Urgent surgery indications:** Unrelenting hemorrhage, >50–75 ml/kg blood transfused in 2 hours, perforation, vascular compromise, unable to identify GI bleeding site with endoscopy
- **Contrast studies** are not indicated acutely. Angiography can detect a bleeding site if the bleeding rate is >0.5–2.0 ml/minute. Embolization can ensue but carries major risks including femoral artery thrombosis and bowel ischemia.
- **Radionuclide scanning (Tc-99):** May detect low-grade GI bleeding from a Meckel's diverticulum. Tc-99 has an affinity for parietal cells present in gastric mucosa and in 90% of Meckel's diverticulum. It has a sensitivity of 85–97% and specificity of 95% in pediatric patients. A positive scan consists of a persistent focus of uptake in the right lower quadrant or lower abdomen. This test is indicated for any child younger than 3 years who presents with persistent painless lower GI bleeding.

Erroneous stool guaiac testing: Acidic pH lowers the sensitivity of guaiac, so use specific gastric test cards (e.g., Gastroccult) when evaluating blood from an upper gastrointestinal source.

- *False positive:* Iron, red fruits, meats, iodine, bromide, horseradish, turnips, tomatoes, fresh red cherries, or chlorophyll
- *False negative:* Dried stool specimens, outdated reagent or guaiac card, bile, vitamin C, or certain antacids

Apt-Downey Test for Fetal vs. Maternal Blood: Mix stool in a test tube with an equal quantity of tap water. Centrifuge or filter out solids. Add one part 1.0% NaOH to five parts of supernatant. Read in 2 minutes. Fetal Hb resists alkali denaturation. A persistent pink color indicates the presence of fetal Hb. If supernatant turns yellow, Hb is adult and thus maternal.

NEONATAL JAUNDICE

Over 80% of newborn infants will develop jaundice in the first few days of life. This is due to increased RBC breakdown and increased enterohepatic circulation of bilirubin. Jaundice can be visibly detected at 2.5–3.0 mg/dl. Physiologic jaundice can last up to 2 weeks of life.

Persistent severe unconjugated hyperbilirubinemia (≥25 mg/dl) can lead to acute and chronic bilirubin encephalopathy. Acute bilirubin encephalopathy causes lethargy, hypotonia, poor suck, irritability and can eventually lead to opisthotonus, arching of neck, apnea, seizure, and death. Chronic bilirubin encephalopathy (kernicterus) leads to cerebral palsy, auditory and visual dysfunction, and intellectual disability.

Conjugated (direct) hyperbilirubinemia is always abnormal [perinatal infections, biliary/liver disease, inborn metabolic errors (galactose, tyrosine, thyroid)], and requires further evaluation. Direct bilirubin should be ≤ 15% of the total bilirubin level.

Unconjugated (indirect) hyperbilirubinemia is abnormal and requires evaluation if risk factors (see Table 14-8), presenting features (see the above discussion of neonatal jaundice), or specific levels are present (Table 14-10).

Table 14-8 Risk Factors for Severe Hyperbilirubinemia[1]

• Predischarge total serum bilirubin or transcutaneous bilirubin in the high-risk or high-intermediate risk zone (see chart on page 114).
• Lower gestational age or jaundice in first 24 hours.
• Exclusive breastfeeding (especially if nursing poorly or excess weight loss [> 8–10%]).
• Isoimmune or other hemolytic disease (G6PD deficient, hereditary spherocytosis)
• Prior jaundiced sibling, cephalohematoma or excess bruising, or East Asian race.
• Maternal diabetes, oxytocin use, and male sex are minor risk factors.

[1]Neurotoxic risk: Isoimmune, G6PD deficient, asphyxia, sepsis, acidosis, albumin <3 mg/dl.

Table 14-9 Evaluation of Neonatal Jaundice >35-Week Gestation

Indication	Investigations
Jaundice ≤ 24 hours old	• Transcutaneous bilirubin (TcB) and/or total serum bilirubin (TSB)
Excessive jaundice for age	• TcB and/or TSB
Jaundice requiring phototherapy, or rapidly rising TSB not explained by history and physical examination	• Blood type, Coombs' test (if cord blood not tested) • CBC, peripheral smear • Direct or conjugated bilirubin • *Depending on age, TSB level:* Repeat TSB 4–24 hours • *Optional:* Reticulocyte count, G6PD, and end tidal carbon monoxide (ETCO)
TSB nearing exchange levels or no phototherapy response	• Reticulocyte count • G6PD • Albumin • ETCO *if available*
High direct/conjugated bilirubin (above lab normal cutoffs)	• Urinalysis and urine culture • Evaluate for sepsis, bowel or biliary disease if indicated by history and physical examination
Jaundice ≥ 3 weeks of age or sick infant	• Direct or conjugated bilirubin • *Direct bilirubin elevated* assess for cholestasis • Check thyroid, galactosemia screens, assess for hypothyroidism

Subcommittee on Hyperbilirubinemia. Management of hyperbilirubinemia in the newborn infant 35 or more weeks of gestation. *Pediatrics.* 2004;114(1):297-316; Varvarigou A, Fouzas S, Skylogianni E, Mantagou L, Bougioukou D, Mantagos S. Transcutaneous bilirubin nomogram for prediction of significant neonatal hyperbilirubinemia. *Pediatrics.* 2009;124(4):1052-1059.

Table 14-10 Transcutaneous Bilirubin (TcB) Cutoffs for High, Low, and Minimal Risk[1] for Significant Hyperbilirubin[2,3] Levels in Newborns Born at ≥35 Weeks

Hours since birth	High risk level (mg/dl)	Low risk level (mg/dl)	Minimal risk level (mg/dl)
12	6.5	4.5	4.2
18	7.7	5	4.8
24	8	5.8	5.3
36	9.3	8	7.8
48	11	9.5	8.8
60	12.5	11	10
72	13.5	13	12.5

[1]High-risk bilirubin level [likelihood ratio (LR) > 10 that serum bilirubin is high], low risk (LR < 0.1), minimal risk (LR = 0) . [2]Significant = any serum bilirubin that exceeds the threshold for phototherapy. [3]Most studies indicate that the TcB can underestimate the TSB (especially at high levels). Therefore, always measure the TSB if (1) TcB is at 70% of the level recommended for use of phototherapy, (2) therapeutic intervention is being considered, (3) TcB is above the 95th percentile on a TcB nomogram or 75th percentile on a TSB nomogram, or (4) upon follow-up after discharge in an infant where the TcB was > 13 mg/dl.
Modified from Varvarigou A, Fouzas S, Skylogianni E, Mantagou L, Bougioukou D, Mantagos S. Transcutaneous bilirubin nomogram for prediction of significant neonatal hyperbilirubinemia. *Pediatrics*. 2009;124(4):1052-1059.

Table 14-11 Bilirubin Cutoffs (mg/dl) for Initiating Therapy in Jaundiced Newborns Born at ≥35 Weeks

Age	24 hours	48 hours	72 hours	96 hours	5–7 days
Cutoff for starting phototherapy[1,2]	Total serum bilirubin in mg/dl				
Low risk (≥38 weeks and well)	12	15	17.5–18	20	21
Medium risk (≥38 weeks + risk, 35–37 6/7 weeks + well)	10	13	15.5	17	18
High risk (35–37 6/7 weeks + risk)	6.5–7	11	13.5	14.5	15
Cutoff for starting exchange transfuion[1,3]	Total serum bilirubin in mg/dl				
Low risk	19	22	24	25	25
Medium risk	16.5	19	21	22	22
High risk	15	17	18.5	19	19

[1]Risk factors include isoimmune hemolytic disease, G6PD deficiency, asphyxia, lethargy, temperature instability, sepsis, acidosis, and albumin <3 g/dl. [2]It is an option to provide home phototherapy for levels 2–3 mg/dl below cutoffs, but do not use home therapy for any newborn with risk factors. [3]Immediate consult for exchange transfusion is indicated for signs of encephalopathy, or TSB ≥ 5 mg/dl above cutoffs, or total bilirubin (μmol/l) to albumin (μmol/l) ratio level is ≥ 0.94 for low-risk, ≥ 0.84 for medium-risk, or ≥ 0.8 for high-risk newborn. Modified from Petrova A, Mehta R, Birchwood G, Ostfeld B, Hegyi T. Management of neonatal hyperbilirubinemia: pediatricians' practices and educational needs. *BMC Pediatr.* 2006;6:6; Varvarigou A, Fouzas S, Skylogianni E, Mantagou L, Bougioukou D, Mantagos S. Transcutaneous bilirubin nomogram for prediction of significant neonatal hyperbilirubinemia. *Pediatrics*. 2009;124(4):1052-1059.

ANEMIA

Table 15-1 Normal RBC Indices (Mean ± 2 Standard Deviations)

Age	Hb (g/dl)	Hct (%)	MCV (fl)	MCH (pg)	MCHC (g/dl)
Birth	16.5 ± 3.0	51 ± 9	108 ± 10	34 ± 3	33 ± 3
1–3 days	18.5 ± 4.0	56 ± 14	108 ± 13	34 ± 3	33 ± 4
1 week	17.5 ± 4.0	54 ± 12	107 ± 19	34 ± 6	33 ± 5
2 weeks	16.5 ± 4.0	51 ± 12	105 ± 19	34 ± 6	33 ± 5
1 month	14.0 ± 4.0	43 ± 12	104 ± 19	34 ± 6	33 ± 4
2 months	11.5 ± 2.5	35 ± 7	96 ± 19	30 ± 4	33 ± 4
3–6 months	11.5 ± 2.0	35 ± 6	91 ± 17	30 ± 5	33 ± 3
0.5–2 years	12.0 ± 1.5	36 ± 3	78 ± 8	27 ± 4	33 ± 3
2–6 years	12.5 ± 1.0	37 ± 3	81 ± 6	27 ± 3	34 ± 3
6–12 years	13.5 ± 2.0	40 ± 5	86 ± 9	29 ± 4	34 ± 3
12–18 years (female)	14.0 ± 2.0	41 ± 5	90 ± 12	30 ± 5	34 ± 3
12–18 years (male)	14.5 ± 1.5	43 ± 6	88 ± 10	30 ± 5	34 ± 3

CAUSES OF ANEMIA BY AGE

Neonate: Blood loss, isoimmunization, or congenital hemolytic anemia. *3 to 6 months:* Congenital disorder of hemoglobin (e.g., thalassemia), blood loss. *6 months to 2 years:* Iron deficiency is associated with early or excessive cow's milk.

Hereditary hemolytic anemia (spherocytosis, hemoglobinopathy, or red cell enzyme deficiency) suggested by a family history of anemia, jaundice, gallstones, or splenectomy. B_{12} deficiency suggested by tortuous retinal vessels (hemoglobinopathy), glossitis, and diminished vibratory/position sense. RBC distribution width (RDW) reflects cell heterogeneity. Variable RDW sizes are seen in hemolysis or reticulocytosis. Markedly high WBC counts, high glucose, sodium, and triglycerides falsely elevate RBC counts.

Table 15-2 Anemia Differential Diagnosis

Microcytic	Iron deficiency (RDW > 14%), thalassemia (RDW < 14%), chronic inflammation, sideroblastic anemia, lead poisoning, B_6 deficiency.
Macrocytic	Folic acid or B_{12} deficiency, Fanconi's syndrome, hepatic disease.

(Continued)

Table 15-2 Anemia Differential Diagnosis (Continued)

Normocytic (high reticulocyte count)	*Extrinsic disorders:* Antibody-mediated hemolysis, fragmentation hemolysis, DIC, hemolytic uremic syndrome, artificial heart valves, liver and renal disease. *Intrinsic disorders:* Membrane disorders (spherocytosis, elliptocytosis), enzyme deficiencies (glucose-6-phosphate dehydrogenase or pyruvate kinase deficiency), hemoglobin disorders (SS, SC, S-thalassemia).
Normocytic (low reticulocyte count)	Diamond-Blackfan, transient erythroblastopenia of childhood, aplastic crisis, bone marrow infiltrate (leukemia, metastatic disease), renal disease, infection, malnutrition.

SICKLE CELL ANEMIA

DIAGNOSIS AND EVALUATION OF PATIENTS WITH SICKLE CELL DISEASE

- Most children are diagnosed by newborn screening, which is available in every state.
- Sickle cell screen may be negative up to 4 to 6 months of age and in sickle trait.
- A routine Hb is recommended to assess severity or change of anemia.
- Consider a reticulocyte count to screen for aplastic crisis. Mean reticulocyte for sickle cell patient is 12%; in aplastic crises it may be <3%.
- Urine-specific gravity is not a useful test for dehydration, as it may be low from isosthenuria (inability to concentrate the urine).
- Profound and sudden decrease in Hb combined with increased reticulocyte count is suggestive of splenic sequestration or hemolytic crisis.

FEVER IN SICKLE CELL ANEMIA

Penicillin prophylaxis decreases the incidence of sepsis and death for sickle cell children aged 6 months to 5 years. However, as these children are susceptible to invasive infections, all children with SCD with fever >38.5°C should be rapidly triaged and examined. Urgent complete blood count, reticulocyte count, blood culture, urine culture, and possibly lumbar puncture (based on the clinical exam) must be performed. Children with respiratory symptoms and signs should be investigated with a chest radiograph to rule out pneumonia and chest syndrome. Broad-spectrum antibiotics such as ceftriaxone or cefotaxime should be initiated even before any laboratory results or chest X-ray results. For severe cases such as meningitis, vancomycin should be added. The presence of a focal infection does not obviate the need for urgent delivery of antibiotics. A subset of children who meet ALL the following low-risk criteria and do not appear toxic may be managed as outpatients after a dose of parenteral ceftriaxone (75 mg/kg) in the ED after consultation with a hematologist, and with close 24-hour follow-up and retreatment.

Table 15-3 Low-Risk Criteria for Outpatient Management of Fever in Sickle Cell Patients

>12 months	Chest X-ray without infiltrate
Well appearing	No ceftriaxone in past 8 weeks
Fever < 39.5°C	No history of bacteremia or sepsis
Normal vital signs	No splenic sequestration in past 4 weeks
Tolerating PO	No recurrent visits for febrile illness
No concern for sequestration, vaso-occlusive crisis or chest syndrome	No history of noncompliance in past
No hypoxia	Fully immunized
No central venous device in place	High likelihood of follow-up (has transportation and phone, not currently in shelter, no missed clinic appointments in past)
Baseline hemoglobin levels	No allergy to cephalosporin
Reticulocyte > 1%, platelets >100,00/µl	Remain clinically stable 3 hours after antibiotic is received
WBC 5,000–30,000, negative urinalysis	Endemic *Streptococcus pneumoniae* in the community is sensitive to antibiotics

Modified from Yawn BP, Buchanan GR, Afenyi-Annan AN, et al. Management of sickle cell disease: summary of the 2014 evidence-based report by expert panel members. JAMA. 2014;312(10):1033-1048; NIH/NHBLI Division of Blood Diseases and Resources. *The Management of Sickle Cell Disease.* 4th ed. Publication No. 02-2117; revised 2002.

MANAGEMENT OF SICKLE CELL DISEASE COMPLICATIONS

Acute chest syndrome (ACS) is a complex of pulmonary symptoms and a lung infiltrate. ACS is one of the most common serious complications of sickle cell anemia and the second most common cause of admission. Patients present with sudden cough, fever, and findings of lower respiratory tract infection such as rales and hypoxia. Chest X-ray reveals a pulmonary infiltrate. While there are no distinctive laboratory findings, the hemoglobin may drop below the baseline value during ACS. Treatment includes admission, oxygen, broad-spectrum antibiotics (cefotaxime or cefepime PLUS a macrolide), and fluids. Exchange blood transfusion is indicated for children with severe respiratory distress, multilobar infiltrates, inability to maintain oxygen saturation above 95% with supplemental oxygen, or the presence of pleural effusions.

Source: Howard J, Hart N, Roberts-Harewoood M, et al. Guideline on the management of acute chest syndrome in sickle cell disease. Br J Haematol. 2015;169(4):492-505.

Table 15-4 Causes of Acute Chest Syndrome

Cause	0–9 years	10–19 years
Infarction without known precipitant	15.9%	22.9%
Viral	10.9%	2.7%
Mycoplasma	8.8%	3.7%
Fat embolism +/− infection	7.3%	8.5%
Chlamydia	5.8%	8%
Mixed infections	4.9%	1.6%
Bacteria	4%	6.4%
Mycobacteria (TB and avium complex)	0.9%	0
Unknown	41.3%	42%

Modified from Vichinsky EP, Neumayr LD, Earles AN, et al. Causes and outcomes of the acute chest syndrome in sickle cell disease. National Acute Chest Syndrome Study Group. *N Engl J Med*. 2000;342(25):1855-1865.

Splenic sequestration (SS) crisis (1 to 6 years): Defined as a sudden enlargement of the spleen and a fall in hemoglobin by at least 2 g/dl below the baseline value. Second only to sepsis as a cause of death in children with sickle cell anemia. The reticulocyte count and circulating nucleated red blood cells are elevated. Platelet count is decreased due to trapping in the spleen. Sequestration may occur without any prior warning or a cause, and typically occurs between 1 and 4 years of age. However, cases have been reported in younger children. Less commonly seen in older children due to autosplenectomy. Abdominal pain, shock, left upper quadrant tenderness (or mass), and hypotension may occur. Infants may develop severe anemia and shock precipitously. Patients are usually younger than 6 years if SS disease, but older if SC or S-β-thalassemia variants. Obtain CBC, type and cross, and reticulocyte count. Admit and treat hypovolemia with intravenous fluids. If symptomatic or Hg < 5g/dl, perform PRBC transfusion with 5–10 cc/kg. Be aware that some blood will be mobilized from the spleen after the resolution of sequestration, which can result in hypercoagulability.

Aplastic crisis (6 months to young adulthood): Common especially in children with HbSS. Gradual fatigue, shortness of breath, fever, and syncope may occur. On examination, tachycardia or heart failure may occur. Hemoglobin is between 3 and 6 g/dl, and hallmark is a reduced reticulocyte count (<3%). Parvovirus B19 is the most common identified precipitant. Other causes include drug toxicity (phenylbutazone) and folate deficiency. Obtain complete blood count, reticulocyte count, and type and screen. Assess all children whose Hb is <6 or 2 g less than their baseline (if known) for aplastic crisis, SS, or ACS. Transfuse PRBCs to restore Hb to a safe level (but not necessarily to baseline levels).

Bone complications: Avascular necrosis of the femoral head occurs in 12% of patients. Osteomyelitis secondary to salmonella is more common in patients with HbSS. Sickle dactylitis can cause small lytic lesions in the digits and is more common in patients with HbSC disease.

Cardiac complications: Patients may develop congestive heart failure or compensatory cardiac dilation. There may be left ventricular hypertrophy on electrocardiography. Chest radiography may demonstrate a large cardiac silhouette.

Abdominal complications: Liver, splenic, and mesenteric infarctions may occur. Bilirubin gallstones are common, although <10% are symptomatic. Abdominal pain in children with sickle cell disease should be managed conservatively with fluids, pain control, and assessment for splenic and liver sequestration besides gallstones.

Source: Rhodes MM, Bates DG, Andrews T, Adkins L, Thornton J, Denham JM. Abdominal pain in children with sickle cell disease. *J Clin Gastroenterol.* 2014;48(2):99-105.

Genitourinary complications: Priapism is a sustained unwanted erection lasting more than 4 hours with pain and a soft glans. Stuttering priapism is multiple self-limited episodes that last <3 hours that can be a harbinger of more prolonged events. Priapism lasting >3 hours is unlikely to resolve spontaneously. Prompt medical treatment is essential to reduce complications. Early consultation of urology and hematology is imperative. Treatment of priapism consists of hydration, pain management, oxygen, and sedation (if required). If symptoms persist after the previous medical management, use of oral agents (e.g., pseudoephedrine, PDE5 inhibitors), penile aspiration and corporal irrigation using α adrenergic agents (epinephrine, pseudoephedrine) may be effective. Current guidelines recommend against the routine use of transfusions in priapism. These patients are less likely to require surgery to correct priapism than patients without sickle cell disease although surgical interventions such as shunting have been used with variable results when all other medical treatments have failed. Other genitourinary complications include painless hematuria and renal papillary necrosis and isosthenuria (difficulty concentrating urine).

Source: Yawn BP, Buchanan GR, Afenyi-Annan AN, et al. Management of sickle cell disease: summary of the 2014 evidence-based report by expert panel members. *JAMA.* 2014;312(10):1033-1048.

Hand-foot syndrome (dactylitis, 6 months to 6 years): Due to vaso-occlusion in hands and feet. This syndrome is the most common presentation of sickle cell anemia at 6 to 24 months, and often the first crisis experienced. Nonpitting edema from symmetric infarction of the metacarpals/metatarsals occurs. Treat as pain crisis.

Pain crisis (all ages): Most common sites of pain in order of decreasing frequency: lumbosacral spine, thigh and hip, knee, abdomen, shoulder, chest. Mild cases can be managed with acetaminophen or NSAIDs. Intravenous opioids is the treatment of choice in severe cases and should be titrated. Meperidine is not recommended (especially in high or repeated doses), as a metabolite (normeperidine) it can cause CNS excitation and seizures. Hydration (oral or IV) and oxygen are commonly accepted adjuncts. A PCA pump may be helpful for pain control.

Source: Puri L, Nottage KA, Hankins JS, Anghelescu DL. State of the art management of acute vaso-occlusive pain in sickle cell disease. *Paediatr Drugs.* 2018;20(1):29-42.

Sickle stroke (all ages): Occurs in 10 to 20% of children with sickle cell disease. Strokes are usually ischemic. Transcranial Doppler (TCD) screening decreases incidence by 1 to 2%. Patients should start TCD screening at 2 years of age up to 16 years of age. If screening is positive, treat with exchange transfusion to keep HbS < 20–30% of total and Hct < 35%. Mean age when strokes occur is 10 years although bleeds occur in older children. Presenting complaints may include headache, weakness, seizures, or coma. Any child with sickle cell anemia with symptoms of stroke should have an IV established and CBC, reticulocyte count, and type and screen ordered. An immediate exchange transfusion should be performed. A CT scan followed by an MRI/MRA will be required to confirm diagnosis. Consider admission to the intensive care unit to ensure close monitoring of vitals to prevent further neurological damage.

Source: Yawn BP, Buchanan GR, Afenyi-Annan AN, et al. Management of sickle cell disease: summary of the 2014 evidence-based report by expert panel members. *JAMA.* 2014;312(10):1033–1048.

BLEEDING

Table 15-5 Causes of Abnormal Bleeding Tests[1]

Lab value	Causes
Thrombocytopenia Low platelet count (<150,000/ml)	• Spurious clotted sample • Pseudothrombocytopenia secondary to response to EDTA occurs in 1:1,500 people. This will correct if repeated with heparin tube. • Decreased production of platelets (due to drugs, toxins, or infections), splenic sequestration or platelet pooling, platelet destruction (due to collagen vascular disease, drugs, post-transfusion, infection, ITP, DIC, TTP, HUS, or vasculitis)
Platelet dysfunction (with normal count)	• Adhesion defects (e.g., von Willebrand disease) or aggregation defects (e.g., thrombasthenia)
↑ BT (>9 minutes) Abnormal PFA-100 (platelet function test)	• All platelet disorders, DIC, ITP, uremia, liver failure, aspirin, abnormal PFA-100
↑ PTT (>35 seconds)	• Coagulation pathway defects (common factors II, V, X, intrinsic VIII, IX, XI, XII, von Willebrand), DIC, liver failure, heparin
↑ PT (> 12–13 seconds)	• Coagulation pathway defects (common factors II, V, X, extrinsic VII) DIC, liver failure, warfarin, circulating anticoagulants (i.e., lupus anticoagulant)

Bleeding

Table 15-5 Causes of Abnormal Bleeding Tests[1] *(Continued)*

Lab value	Causes
↑ TT (> 8–10 seconds)	• DIC, liver failure or uremia, heparin, hypofibrinogenemia
↓ Fibrinogen, ↑ Fibrin split products (FSP)	• DIC

[1]BT—bleeding time; TT—thrombin time; PTT—partial thromboplastin time; PT—prothrombin time; DIC—disseminated intravascular coagulopathy; ITP—idiopathic thrombocytopenic purpura; TTP—thrombotic thrombocytopenic purpura; HUS—hemolytic uremic syndrome.

Table 15-6 Replacement Factors

Medication	Dose (Consult hematology for dosing recommendations, see recommendations for factor 8, 9 deficiencies on page 123)
Amicar	Aminocaproic acid: 25–100 mg/kg PO/IV every 6–8 hours for up to 7 days.
Cryoprecipitate	Cryoprecipitate: 2–4 bags/10 kg, 1 bag = 50–100 units factor VIII activity.
DDAVP	*Desmopressin:* 0.3 mcg/kg in 50 ml NS IV over 30 minutes OR via nasal spray (1 puff if < 50 kg, 2 if > 50 kg); useful if baseline activity > 10%.
Activated factor VIIa	Recombinant activated human factor VII (recombinant FVIIa) 90–120 mcg/kg every 2–3 hours IV.
Factor VIII	Standard half-life products include: Advate, Hemofil-M, Koate, Kovaltry, Novoeight, Nuwiq, Recombinate, and Xyntha. There are now longer half-life products available that include: Adynovate, Afstyla, and Eloctate. Refer to prescribing information in the product insert for the use of factor replacement. Consult hematology. 1 unit/kg factor VIII ↑ activity level by 2% (factor VIII half-life = 12 hours)
Factor IX	Standard half-life products include: AlphaNine SD, BeneFIX, Ixinity, Mononine, and Rixubis. There are now longer half-life products available that include Alprolix and Idelvion—refer to the product information for the use of factor replacement.
Bispecific factor VIII	Emicizumab is a bispecific monoclonal antibody used to replace activated factor VIII in patients who have hemophilia A without factor VIII inhibitors. *Source:* Mahlangu J, Oldenburg J, Paz-Priel I, et al. Emicizumab prophylaxis in patients with hemophilia A without inhibitors. *N Engl J Med.* 2018;379(9):811-822. Emicizumab (ACE910) is an activated factor VIII used in patients with hemophilia A with factor VIII inhibitors. *Source:* Oldenburg J, Mahlangu JN, Kim B, et al. Emicizumab prophylaxis in hemophilia A with inhibitors. *N Engl J Med.* 2017;377(9):809-818.

(Continued)

Table 15-6 Replacement Factors (*Continued*)

Medication	Dose (Consult hematology for dosing recommendations, see recommendations for factor 8, 9 deficiencies on page 123)
von Willebrand factor (VWF)	Three plasma-derived VWF include: Humate-P, Alphanate, Wilfactin. Vonvendi is a recombinant human VWF. Recommendations for replacement doses of VWF are empirical, since no laboratory tests adequately predict the hemostatic effects. The dose given is also dependent on the site and the degree of bleeding.
Activated prothrombin complex	Used for treatment of acute breakthrough bleed in patients with inhibitors. Dose: 50–11 international units/kg every 6–12 hours IV.

Modified from Callaghan MU, Sidonio R, Pipe SW. Novel therapeutics for hemophilia and other bleeding disorders. *Blood*. 2018;132(1):23-30.

Table 15-7 Treatment of von Willebrand Disease (VWD)

Nose bleed	Nasal DDAVP on side not bleeding. If no response in 1 hour, IV DDAVP. If no response, pack, ENT consult, VWF
Major bleed	CNS or GI bleed, major trauma: VWF
Menorrhagia	DDAVP injection. Consider Amicar + DDAVP: 1 spray each nostril one time during acute episode
Oral bleed	Nasal DDAVP and aminocaproic acid
Surgery	*Minor*: DDAVP SC/IV + Amicar *Major*: VWF

Table 15-8 Factor VIII Deficiency Treatment

Bleed type	% activity desired	Dose[3] (units/kg)	Duration of therapy
Severe[1]			
CNS injury	80–100	40–50	14 days
GI bleed	80–100	40–50	3 days more than bleed
Major trauma	80–100	40–50	Depends on injuries
Retroperitoneal	80–100	40–50	6 days
Retropharyngeal	80–100	40–50	4 days
Pending surgery	80–100	40–50	Variable
Moderate[2]			
Mild head trauma	40–50	20–25	Variable
Deep muscle	40–50	20–25	Every day until resolution
Hip or groin injury	40–50	20–25	Repeat once in 1–2 days

Table 15-8 Factor VIII Deficiency Treatment (*Continued*)

Bleed type	% activity desired	Dose[3] (units/kg)	Duration of therapy
Mouth, lip, dental[3]	40–50	20–25	Variable
Hematuria	40–50	20–25	3–5 days
Mild[2]			
Laceration[4]	40–50	20–25	Until sutures out for 24 hours
Common joint	40–50	20–25	Recheck in 1–2 days
Soft tissue, small muscle[5]	40–50	20–25	Variable

[1]If baseline activity is 0%. Assume all severe bleeding cases have baseline of 0%. [2]Desmopressin (DDAVP) 0.3 mcg/kg IV or intranasal or subcutaneous has been used for mild and moderate bleeding states, especially useful if baseline factor is >10%. [3]To prepare for dental/oropharyngeal procedures, consider aminocaproic acid (Amicar) 100 mg/kg PO every 6 hours for 6 days or cyklokapron 25 mg/kg every 6 hours for 6 days. Also consider topical epinephrine, surgicel, or avitene. Cautery may worsen bleeding. [4]Epistaxis and minor lacerations may not need replacement. [5]Consider admission to observe for compartment syndrome.

OTHER TREATMENT OPTIONS IN HEMOPHILIA

Fresh frozen plasma (FFP) contains all coagulation factors and is used for un-known bleeding disorders. FFP or cryoprecipitate can be used to treat VWD. FFP 40 ml/kg raises activity of any factor to 100%. May cause fluid overload.

Cryoprecipitate: 5 to 10 units factor VII activity/ml (1 bag = 10 ml, 50–100 units factor VIII activity).

Desmopressin (DDAVP): 0.3 mcg/kg in NS IV over 30 minutes. Mild to moderate bleeding in VWF and hemophilia A. Causes seizures/↓ Na in those younger than 4 years.

Source: Ozgonenel B, Rajpurkar M, Lusher JM. How do you treat bleeding disorders with desmopressin? *Postgrad Med J.* 2007;83(977):159-163.

Prothrombin complex (factors II, VII, IX, X) can be used to treat hemophilia B but can precipitate thrombi and/or DIC.

HEMOLYTIC UREMIC SYNDROME (HUS)

HUS—A post-infectious disorder causing (1) nephropathy, (2) microangiopathic hemolytic anemia, and (3) thrombocytopenia. It commonly occurs in those younger than 5 years following a URI or gastroenteritis (esp. *E. coli* 0157:H7, *Shigella, Salmonella*). Organisms produce toxin that kills GI organ cells; 30% reoccur. *Treatment:* Admit and manage complications: (1) dialysis if congestive heart failure, BUN > 100, encephalopathy, anuria > 24 hours or hyperkalemia. (2) If hypertension, treat with antihypertensives. (3) Administer fluids and blood (especially if Hb < 8 g/dl) for hypotension. (4) If seizures, treat with appropriate medications and obtain CT or MRI. (5) Plasma exchange or plasmapheresis is indicated for CNS involvement or severe renal involvement.

(6) Platelet transfusion has the potential to worsen disease causing further organ damage.

Modified from Picard C, Burtey S, Bornet C, Curti C, Montana M, Vanelle P. Pathophysiology and treatment of typical and atypical hemolytic uremic syndrome. *Pathol Biol.* 2015;63(3):136-143.

Clinical features of HUS	
Prodrome	Upper-respiratory infection or gastroenteritis
Blood pressure	Hypertension in up to 50%
Gastrointestinal	75% have pain
Urinary	Decreased urination, gross hematuria is rare
Skin	Pallor, petechia, purpura
Central Nervous System	Seizures, coma, encephalopathy
Laboratory features of HUS	
Urine	Hematuria, proteinuria, casts
Hematology	
Low hemoglobin, low platelets, low WBC count, peripheral smear abnormalities (schistocytes, helmet cells)	
Chemistry	Hyponatremia, acidosis, hyperkalemia, elevated BUN/creatinine
PT/PTT	Are usually normal

HENOCH-SCHÖNLEIN PURPURA (HSP)

OVERVIEW

HSP is a systemic vasculitis with skin, joint, GI, or renal involvement. Scrotal, CNS, heart, and lung involvement are less common. HSP peaks at 4 to 5 years, can occur at any age. It is more common in winter and early spring. *Precipitants:* streptococci, mycoplasma, hepatitis B, salicylates, antibiotics, and food allergens. HSP is pathophysiologically a small vessel vasculitis, with WBCs infiltrating and necrosing the walls of capillaries, arterioles, and venules. *Evaluation:* CBC, creatinine/BUN/electrolytes. Rule out meningococcemia/sepsis/DIC. *Treatment:* Supportive care and steroids are used for abdominal pain and renal involvement, although their benefit has not been clearly established.

CLINICAL FEATURES

- *Skin*—Involved in most. Petechiae, coalesce to large ecchymoses. Purpura are gravity dependent occurring on the buttock and legs.
- *Painless edema*—25 to 35% (usually at dorsum of hands and feet), with painful edema of face, scalp.

- *GI tract*—50 to 90% with vomiting, or bleeding. Intussusception (3 to 6%), pancreatitis, or bowel infarcts occur.
- *Joint*—Involvement in 50 to 75%, usually knees/ankles, transitory periarticular swelling, nonmigratory. This is first site in 25% and resolves with rest.
- *Renal*—50% and may be the only site that is permanent. Episodic gross hematuria occurs in 30 to 40%.

Modified from Hetland LE, Susrud KS, Lindahl KH, Bygum A. Henoch-Schönlein purpura: a literature review. *Acta Derm Venereol.* 2017;97(10):1160–1166.

IDIOPATHIC THROMBOCYTOPENIC PURPURA (ITP)

OVERVIEW

ITP is an autoimmune disorder with antibodies vs. platelets. ITP is the most common platelet disorder in children, often between ages of 1 year and 4 years; 70% have prior viral infection (e.g., rubella, rubeola). Bone marrow has normal WBCs and RBCs. Eosinophilia and megakaryocytes (immature/basophilic stippling) may be present.

Treatment may be indicated if bleeding or platelets < 10,000–20,000/mm^3. Debate exists as to treatment indications.

CLINICAL FEATURES

- *Skin*—Bruising and petechiae are most common.
- *Mucous membranes*—Epistaxis, gum and GYN bleeding, and hematuria are less common than skin manifestations.
- *Hematologic*—Platelets usually < 20,000/mm^3, ± anemia.
- *GI*—Liver, spleen, and lymph nodes are not enlarged.
- *CNS*—Most common threat to life.
- *Systemic*—±HIV, lupus, lymphoma.

ITP Treatment: (1) *Steroids*—(1a) If active bleed and platelets <20,000, methylprednisolone 30 mg/kg (max dose, 1 g) IV over 30 minutes every 24 hours × 2–3 doses, OR 6 mg/kg IV over 30 minutes every 8 hours × 2–4 days; (1b) Prednisone 2 mg/kg/day × 2 weeks then tapered over third week. (2) *IV immune globulin*—1 g/kg/day over 4 hours × 1–2 days. (3) *IV anti-D immune globulin*—50 to 75 mcg/kg (Ig vs. D antigen of RBCs) over 5 minutes × 1 dose—leads to Hb drop of 0.5–2 g/dl. Only effective if Rh positive. (4) *Plasmapheresis*. (5) *Platelet transfusion*—10 to 30 ml/kg and platelet count should be assessed 10–20 minutes following infusion. Patients with ITP require larger-than-normal doses of platelets in transfusion due to rapid destruction. (6) *Splenectomy, rituximab, thrombopoietin receptor agonists* (TPO-RAs), or immunosuppressive therapy is appropriate for patients who continue to have clinically significant bleeding, patients with platelet counts <10,000 to 20,000/microL after first-line therapy has failed.

Modified from George JN, Woolf SH, Raskob GE, et al. Idiopathic thrombocytopenic purpura: a practice guideline developed by explicit methods for the American Society of Hematology. *Blood.* 1996;88(1):3-40.

THROMBOEMBOLISM

Underlying disorders leading to thromboemboli include protein S, protein C, antithrombin, antiphospholipid antibodies (e.g., lupus anticoagulant, anticardiolipin, anti-β2-glycoprotein), factor V Leiden (especially if on estrogens), prothrombin G20210A, elevated factor VIII, hyperhomocysteinemia, high lipoprotein(a), dysfibrinogenemia, and hypo/dysplasminogenemia. There is ↑ risk of clotting if genetic thrombophilia is four times higher than general population. Healthy children with thrombophilias rarely develop thrombi unless additional genetic disorders or exogenous risk factors are present (see the table that follows). *Presenting clinical features* are not defined, and adult scoring systems have not been reproduced in children. Deep venous thrombi may not cause symptoms. In admitted children who die from pulmonary embolism (PE), up to 50% have no symptoms attributable to the PE, and the diagnosis is only suspected in 15%.

Table 15-9 Risk Factors for Pulmonary Emboli and Deep Venous Thrombi in Children

Central venous catheter	33%	Birth control pill, abortion/miscarriage	5%
Cancer	23%	Obesity	3%
Congenital heart disease	15%	Lupus	2%
Trauma	15%	Sickle cell anemia	2%
TPN administration	8%	Liver failure	2%
Infection	7%	Other	4%
Nephrotic syndrome	6%	No risk factor identified	4%
Recent surgery	6%		

Modified from Monagle P, Chan AKC, Goldenberg NA, et al. Antithrombotic therapy in neonates and children: Antithrombotic Therapy and Prevention of Thrombosis, 9th ed: American College of Chest Physicians Evidence-Based Clinical Practice Guidelines. *Chest.* 2012;141(2 Suppl):e737S–e801S.

ONCOLOGIC EMERGENCIES

FEVER AND NEUTROPENIA (INFECTIOUS DISEASE SOCIETY GUIDELINES)

Fever—Single oral temp ≥ 38.3°C (101°F) or ≥ 38°C (100.4°F) over at least 1 hour.

Neutropenia—Neutrophils < 500/mm^3 or < 1,000/mm^3 with predicted ≤ 500/mm^3.

Evaluation—Blood culture (peripheral and catheter), culture lesions, urine and stool, CXR, CBC with differential, liver function tests, electrolytes.

Table 15-10 Antimicrobials for Neutropenia

Alternate dosing may be needed if < 3–6 months old.
(1) Cefepime 50 mg/kg (max 6 g/day) IV every 8 hours, OR (2) ceftazidime 150 mg/kg/day (max 6 g/day) IV divided every 8 hours, OR (3) imipenem 60–100 mg/kg/day divided every 6 hours (max 4 g/day), OR (4) aminoglycoside PLUS antipseudomonal β-lactam ADD vancomycin 10 mg/kg (max 500 mg) IV every 6 hours if any of the following: low BP, central catheter, chemotherapy + any mucosal damage (e.g., oral ulcerations), prophylaxis with quinolones before fever, known colonization with penicillin-resistant pneumococci, known gram-positive blood culture before susceptibility testing.

Modified from Lehrnbecher T, Robinson P, Fisher B, et al. Guideline for the management of fever and neutropenia in children with cancer and hematopoietic stem-cell transplantation recipients: 2017 update. *J Clin Oncol.* 2017;35(18):2082-2094.

Table 15-11 Hyperviscosity (Hyperleukocytosis) Syndrome

Etiology	Diagnosis
• ↑ Serum proteins with sludging and ↓ circulation. Common causes: leukemia (especially ALL).	• WBC (esp. blasts) > 100,000 cells/mm³ • ↑ Serum viscosity—Ostwald viscometer • Serum protein electrophoresis
Clinical features	**Management**
• Fatigue, headache, somnolence • Dyspnea, interstitial infiltrates, hypoxia, RV failure, renal failure • ↓ Vision, seizure, deafness, myocardial infarction • Retinal bleed and exudates	• IV Normal Saline (NS), plasmapheresis • Platelets if count < 20,000/mm³ • Phlebotomy with NS, and exchange transfusion (keep Hb ≤ 10 g/dl) • Antileukemic therapy

Table 15-12 Passive Hepatomegaly

Clinical features	Management
• Associated with tumor infiltrate (esp. neuroblastoma and <4 weeks old) • May cause mechanical compromise of lungs, heart, GI/renal systems, or disseminated intravascular coagulation	• Treat persistent emesis, hypoxia, leg edema, renal insufficiency, or DIC • Chemotherapy • Low-dose radiation 150 cGy/day × 3 • Surgical enlargement of abdominal wall

Table 15-13 Spinal Cord Compression[1]

Back pain	80%	*Diagnosis*—Stat MRI is diagnostic study of choice. Plain films are abnormal in only 35%, bone scan in 54%. Use CT and MRI instead.
Weakness	67%	
Local back tenderness	67%	
Paraplegia	57%	*Management*—(1) Dexamethasone 1 mg/kg IV, then 0.25 to 0.5 mg/kg PO every 6 hours, (2) surgical decompression (esp. previously unknown tumor type), (3) radiation or chemotherapy depending on cancer sensitivity.
Loss of bowel or bladder control	57%	
Sensory abnormality	14%	

[1] ≥ 90% due to sarcomas (rhabdomyosarcoma, Ewing's, osteogenic), neuroblastoma, and lymphoma. Modified from Klein SL, Sanford RA, Muhlbauer MS. Pediatric spinal epidural metastases. *J Neurosurg.* 1991;74(1):70-75; Lewis DW, Packer RJ, Raney B, Rak IW, Belasco J, Lange B. Incidence, presentation, and outcome of spinal cord disease in children with systemic cancer. *Pediatrics.* 1986;78(3):438-443; Kelly KM, Lange B. Oncologic emergencies. *Pediatr Clin North Am.* 1997;44:809.

Table 15-14 Superior Vena Cava Syndrome[1]

Clinical features	Management
Headache, swollen face, altered mental status, syncope, dyspnea, plethora, and venous distention of the face, neck, and arms with trachea compression	• Radiation (can ↑ swelling, cause resp. deterioration, distort histology). • Diuretics/steroids are unproven but are often used. • Cyclophosphamide ± vincristine and anthracycline if non-Hodgkin's or Hodgkin's lymphoma suspected. • Consult for stent of SVC.
Diagnosis	
CXR first, then CT or MRI. Obtain an ECG and echo if possible cardiac involvement and pulmonary function testing if lung involvement.	

[1] Anterior > middle mediastinal mass (most common lymphoma, Hodgkin's, ALL) or clot (e.g., central venous catheter) obstructing superior vena cava.

TUMOR LYSIS SYNDROME/TLS GUIDELINES

Cairo-Bishop definition (≥ 2 of following within 3 days prior or 7 days after cytotoxic chemotherapy, esp. leukemia/lymphoma): Uric acid ≥ 8 mg/dl, K+ ≥ 6 mEq/l, P ≥ 2 mmol/l, Ca ≤ 1.75 mmol/l (or ↑ 25% of any of these from baseline). Clinical TLS is present if arrhythmia, seizures, or renal insufficiency develop. Low-risk patients include indolent non-Hodgkin's, ALL with WBC ≤ 50,000, AML/CLL with WBC ≤ 10,000, heme/solid cancers growing slowly. All others = high or intermediate risk.

Source: Howard SC, Trifilio S, Gregory TK, Baxter N, McBride A. Tumor lysis syndrome in the era of novel and targeted agents in patients with hematologic malignancies: a systematic review. *Ann Hematol.* 2016;95(4):563-573.

Table 15-15 Management of Symptomatic, Intermediate, or High-Risk Tumor Lysis Patients

• Hydration with NS to keep urine output 80–100 ml/m^2/hour	• IV Calcium if symptomatic low Ca
• Diuretics may be needed	• Treat K+ ≥ 7 mmol/l
• NaHCO$_3$ is NOT recommended	• Phosphate buffers if high P
• Rasburicase (Elitek): 0.1–0.2 mg/kg IV in 30 minutes (NOT if G6PD deficient)	• Consider dialysis for K+ ≥ 7 mmol/l, uremia, fluid overload, severe hyperphosphatemia
• Allopurinol if Elitek not used	

Modified from Coiffer B, Altman A, Pui CH. Guidelines for the management of pediatric and adult tumor lysis syndrome: an evidence-based review. *J Clin Oncol.* 2008;26:2726-2778.

TRANSFUSION AND BLOOD PRODUCTS

TRANSFUSION AND BLOOD PRODUCTS

Cross-matching and ordering blood products: Type-specific noncross-matched blood causes a fatality in 1 in 30 million transfusions. Non-ABO antibodies occur in 0.04% of nontransfused and 0.3% of previously transfused.

Whole blood has no WBCs and 20% of normal platelets after 24-hour storage. Factors V + VIII decline to 40% after 21 days; 70% of RBCs remain after 21–35 days storage. With storage, K$^+$ and ammonia increase (beware in liver failure) and Ca^{+2} decreases (beware in liver dysfunction as citrate is not effectively metabolized by the liver).

Packed red blood cells (PRBCs): Hematocrit rises 1% for each ml/kg of PRBCs transfused. Fewer antigens are present in PRBCs compared to whole blood. (1) *Leukocyte-poor RBCs* are derived from filtering RBCs and should be used if one (severe), or two (sequential) febrile nonhemolytic transfusion reactions. (2) *Washed RBCs* are useful if prior anaphylaxis due to antibodies to IgA or other proteins. (3) *Frozen deglycerolized RBCs* are the purest RBC product. Use if there is a reaction to washed RBCs or a transfusion reaction due to anti-IgA antibodies. (4) *Irradiated RBCs*— use if immunocompromised.

Fresh frozen plasma (FFP): ABO cross-match prior to transfusion. Indications: (1) coagulation protein deficiency when specific factor concentrates are undesirable or unavailable, (2) warfarin reversal, (3) diffuse bleeding + documented coagulopathy, or (4) active bleeding with liver disease and a secondary coagulopathy.

Factor VIII preparations: (1) cryoprecipitate is made from single donor and contains fibrinogen, VWF, and factors VIII and XIII. (2) Factor VIII concentrate is pooled from multiple donors. (3) Several recombinant factor VIII products are available.

Table 15-16 Blood Products

Component	Indication	Dose	Adverse effects	Special features
Albumin 5%[1]	Shock	10–20 ml/kg	Rare volume overload, fever, urticaria	Stable storage, no filter, no disease transmission
Plasmanate[1]	Shock	See above	Rare volume overload, fever, urticaria, hypotension	Stable storage, no filter, no disease transmission
Hetastarch 6% (Hespan)[1]	Volume expansion	10–20 ml/kg	Pruritus, coagulopathy	Stable leukopheresis, no disease transmission
Dextran[1]	Volume expansion	10 ml/kg	Allergy, bleed, renal failure	Same as hetastarch
Whole blood[2]	Hemorrhagic shock	10 ml/kg will ↑ Hb 1 g/dl	Transfusion reactions, hemolysis, disease transmission	Thrombocytopenia, coagulopathy, leukopenia
Packed RBCs[2]	↑ O_2 carrying capacity and shock	3 ml/kg will ↑ Hb 1 g/dl	Less allergic and febrile reactions than whole blood	Administer 10–15 ml/kg
Washed RBCs	↓ allergic reactions	3 ml/kg will ↑ Hb 1 g/dl	Rare	Takes 1 hour to wash and > 70% of RBCs lost
Leukocyte poor RBCs	99.9% of WBCs are removed	3 ml/kg will ↑ Hb 1 g/dl	Rare	Use if 2 febrile nonhemolytic reactions to washed RBCs
Apheresis platelets	Poorly functioning or decreased platelets	5–10 ml/kg	Transfusion reactions are rare	No cross-matching, ABO compatibility is preferred
FFP	Coagulopathy with bleeding	10–25 ml/kg	Transfusion reactions are rare	No cross-matching, ABO group compatibility preferred

[1]No cross-match needed. [2]For acute hemorrhage, initiate transfusion with 20 ml/kg of whole blood or 10 ml/kg of PRBCs. Request sickle prep negative. Blood if sickle cell disease. Avoid mixing blood + D_5W or Ringer's lactate due to hemolysis and clotting, respectively.

Data from AABB Center for Cellular Therapies (2018), Circular of Information for the Use of Cellular Therapy Products. Retrieved from http://www.aabb.org/aabbcct/coi/Documents/CT-Circular-of-Information.pdf

Factor IX concentrate: Prothrombin complex contains factors II, VII, IX, and X. One unit raises a recipient's activity 1.5%. Factors IX and X are thrombogenic and can cause DIC; therefore, use cautiously in hepatic and vascular disease.

Platelet concentrate: One unit = 5 to 10 thousand platelets. Platelets are not refrigerated and only survive 7 days. Platelet counts > 50,000/ml are desirable prior to surgery. ABO cross-matching is not necessary. ITP dose 0.1–0.4 units/kg.

Albumin and plasma protein fraction (PPF): 25% salt-poor albumin contains excess sodium (160 mEq Na^+/l) and is hyperoncotic compared to plasma. 5% buffered albumin solution is iso-oncotic compared to plasma. PPF contains 88% albumin and 12% globulins and is iso-oncotic compared to plasma.

TESTING BLOOD PRIOR TO ADMINISTRATION

Complete cross-match—Three phases: (1) Immediate spin phase detects ABO incompatibility from IgM and takes 5–10 minutes. (2) Albumin phase takes 15–30 minutes. (3) Antihuman globulin phase takes 15–30 minutes. Albumin and antihuman globulin phases detect IgM, IgG, + other antibodies causing hemolytic transfusion reactions.

Unexpected antibody screen: Uncovers non-ABO antibodies (e.g., Kell, Duffy) in recipient's serum. 0.04% of recipients will have an unexpected positive antibody screen if no prior transfusion, and 1% will have a positive screen if prior transfusion. This test is important if prior transfusion or pregnancy.

Abbreviated cross-match: (1) Immediate spin alone or (2) stat cross-match—omit immediate spin and shorten antihuman globulin and albumin phase to 15 minutes.

TRANSFUSION REACTIONS

Hemolytic transfusion reactions occur in 1/40,000 transfusions and are usually due to ABO incompatibility. Symptoms: Palpitations, abdominal and back pain, syncope, and a sensation of doom. Consider if temperature rises ≥ 2°C. Immediately stop transfusion and look for hemoglobinemia and hemoglobinuria. Notify blood bank and perform direct antiglobulin (Coombs test), haptoglobin, peripheral smear, serum bilirubin, and repeat antibody screen and cross-match. Keep urine output ≥ 1–2 ml/kg/hour and consider alkalization of urine to limit renal failure. Mannitol is not useful. It increases urine flow by decreasing tubular reabsorption without improving renal perfusion.

Anaphylactic reaction almost exclusively occurs with anti-IgA antibodies (1/70 people). It usually begins after the first few ml of blood with afebrile flushing, wheezing, cramps, vomiting, diarrhea, and hypotension. Discontinue the transfusion and treat with diphenhydramine, epinephrine, and steroids.

Febrile nonhemolytic reactions occur during or soon after initiation of 3 to 4% of all transfusions, most frequently in multiply transfused or multiparous patients with antileukocyte antibodies. Stop transfusion and treat as transfusion reaction.

Urticarial reactions cause local erythema, hives, and itching. Further evaluation unnecessary unless fever, chills, or other adverse effects are present. This is the only type of transfusion reaction in which the infusion can continue.

Infections: AIDS, CMV, or hepatitis may be transmitted with blood products.

Modified from Vossoughi S, Perez G, Whitaker BI, Fung MK, Stotler B. Analysis of pediatric adverse reactions to transfusions. *Transfusion.* 2018;58(1):60-69.

16 ■ HYPERTENSION

Hypertension (HTN) = Mean systolic BP or diastolic BP ≥ 95th percentile or BP ≥ 130/80 (whichever is lower) for age, sex, and height on three occasions. Appropriate blood pressure cuff size: R mid-arm, cuff bladder length 80–100%/width ≥ 40% of the arm circumference.

Elevated BP: BP ≥ 90th percentile to <95th percentile, or 120/80 mm Hg to <95th percentile (whichever is lower). Recommend lifestyle interventions (healthy diet, sleep, and physical activity). Repeat BP in 6 months.

Hypertensive urgency: Defined as significantly elevated BP without evidence of end organ damage. Often develops over days to weeks.

Hypertensive emergency: Defined as elevated BP associated with end organ damage. Often develops over hours.

Hypertensive encephalopathy: Most common presentation of acute hypertension, with headache, confusion, vomiting, visual disturbances, focal neurologic findings.

Stage I HTN: BP ≥ 95th percentile to ≥95th percentile +12mm Hg, or 130/80 to 139/89 (whichever is lower). If asymptomatic, lifestyle counseling and refer for repeat BP in 1 to 2 weeks. If you suspect underlying disease or symptomatic, obtain urine analysis, basic metabolic panel, and a complete blood count. CXR and ECG to screen for cardiac hypertrophy/heart failure; however, echocardiogram has been shown to be far more specific. Consider CT head if concerned for intracranial process resulting in HTN. If patient is stable and asymptomatic, can consider oral medications.

Stage II HTN: BP levels ≥95th percentile +12 mm Hg, or ≥140/90 mm Hg (whichever is lower) for age, sex, and height. This requires evaluation (same as Stage I evaluation) including an echocardiogram to evaluate for LVH and cardiac target organ damage and initiation of antihypertensives. Presence of LVH is an indication to initiate therapy.

Table 16-1 Stage I and Stage II Hypertension Cutoffs

Stage I (95th percentile) and Stage II (95th percentile + 12 mm Hg) BP for Child with Average (50th percentile) Height				
		Males		Females	
Age (years)	BP percentiles	SBP	DBP	SBP	DBP
2	95th	106	59	106	64
	95th + 12mm Hg	118	71	118	76
5	95th	109	69	110	71
	95th + 12mm Hg	121	81	122	83

(Continued)

Table 16-1 Stage I and Stage II Hypertension Cutoffs (Continued)

Age (years)	BP percentiles	SBP	DBP	SBP	DBP
8	95th	114	74	113	74
	95th + 12 mm Hg	126	86	125	86
11	95th	118	78	118	77
	95th + 12 mm Hg	130	90	130	89
14	95th	130	81	125	80
	95th + 12 mm Hg	142	93	137	92
17	95th	135	85	127	81
	95th + 12 mm Hg	147	97	139	93

Data from Flynn, J. T., Kaelber, D. C., Baker-Smith, C. M., Blowey, D., Carroll, A. E., Daniels, S. R., ... & Gidding, S. S. (2017). Clinical practice guideline for screening and management of high blood pressure in children and adolescents. *Pediatrics*, 140(3), e20171904.

ETIOLOGY OF PEDIATRIC HYPERTENSION

- *Primary HTN:* Predominant type of HTN in children in the United States. Often in children older than 6 years old with risk factors (positive family history in immediate family member, overweight/obese).
- *Renal disease:* Most common secondary cause of HTN in children. HTN and encephalopathy (or seizures) may be first presentation of acute post-streptococcal glomerulonephritis. Na retention/fluid overload occur due to ↓ glomerular filtration rate, causing ↑ BP, hematuria, periorbital edema, and RBC casts.
- *CNS disease:* Cushing's triad of bradycardia, bradypnea, and HTN is found with ↑ intracranial pressure (ICP) due to tumors, bleeding, trauma, or infection.
- *Neuroblastomas:* Cause HTN due to catecholamine release, similar to neurofibromatosis and pheochromocytoma. HTN may be episodic with flushing, palpitations, anxiety, sweating, and chest pain.
- *Drug toxicity:* HTN can be due to steroids, oral contraceptives, phenylephrine, pseudoephedrine, albuterol, cyclosporine A, and drugs of abuse. Chronic lead toxicity can cause HTN, as can licorice through its mineralocorticoid effects. NSAIDs may interfere with efficacy of antihypertensives (ACE inhibitors specifically); however, they do not appear to impact BP in those without HTN.
- *Aortic coarctation (CoA):* This is the most common cause of HTN in the first year of life. Associated with R arm BP ≥ 20 mm Hg than lower extremity BP. CoA also causes up to 2% of secondary HTN in children and adolescents.
- *Other:* Burn victims often exhibit HTN due to sympathetic discharge. Forty-three percent of babies with bronchopulmonary dysplasia exhibit HTN.

HYPERTENSIVE ENCEPHALOPATHY

BP autoregulation is lost and vasodilation occurs causing cerebral edema. Vasodilators in children with HTN and ↑ ICP may be detrimental.

TREATMENT OF HYPERTENSIVE ENCEPHALOPATHY

Great caution should be taken when treating hypertensive emergencies. BP should be reduced no more than 25% in the first 8 hours to avoid cerebral hypoperfusion, with a BP goal ~95th percentile.

- *Sodium nitroprusside* is a commonly used drug in hypertensive emergencies, except with a space occupying cranial lesion due to its vasodilatory effect. It has a rapid onset and a short half-life; it is light sensitive. Metabolism produces cyanide, which is converted in the liver and excreted by the kidneys; therefore, caution should be used in patients with renal/hepatic failure. Cerebral vasodilation may increase ICP.
- *Esmolol* is a cardioselective β_1 blocker, has rapid onset, and is ultra-short acting. It is not affected by renal/hepatic function; therefore, it is an excellent choice for multiorgan failure. Side effect of bronchospasm, bradycardia, and congestive heart failure (CHF).
- *Hydralazine* is a vasodilator with a long duration of action, making titration difficult. However, it can be administered IV/PO/IM, making it versatile if no IV is established.
- *Nicardipine* is extremely effective for a controlled reduction of BP in children. It ↓ peripheral vascular resistance, has little effect on heart rate, and can ↑ ICP. If given via peripheral IV, it can cause thrombophlebitis.
- *Labetalol* is an α and β blocker, safe in renal disease, does not ↑ ICP, and has little to no effect on cardiac output. It can cause bronchospasm and worsens congestive heart failure. Difficult to titrate due to long half-life.

Table 16-2 Drugs in Hypertensive Emergencies

Drug	Dose (max), route, preparation	Mechanism	Onset (lasts)	Features
Most common				
Esmolol	100–500 mcg/kg/minute, IV	β_1-blocker	<1 minute	Can cause/worsen bronchospasm and severe bradycardia
Hydralazine	0.2–0.6 mg/kg/dose (0.4 mg/kg/dose), IV/IM	Direct vasodilator	5–30 minutes (4–12 hours)	Causes tachycardia. Administer every 4 hours when given IV bolus
Labetalol	0.2–1.0 mg/kg/dose (40 mg/dose), IV/IM bolus Infusion: 0.25–3 mg/kg/hour	α/β blocker	2–5 minutes (3–5 hours half-life)	Contraindicated in asthma and heart failure

(Continued)

Table 16-2 Drugs in Hypertensive Emergencies (*Continued*)

Most common				
Nicardipine	1–3 mcg/kg/minute, as infusion	Calcium channel blocker	15 minutes (10–15 minutes)	Reflex tachycardia. Increases cyclosporine and tacrolimus level
Sodium nitroprusside	0.53–10 mcg/kg/minute, IV infusion	Direct vasodilator	<1 minute	Can cause cyanide poisoning
Less common				
Clonidine	0.05–1 mg/dose, may be repeated up to 0.8 mg total dose	Alpha agonist		Dry mouth and drowsiness
Fenoldopam	0.2–0.8 mcg/kg/minute, IV infusion	Dopamine receptor agonist		High doses worsen tachycardia
Hydralazine	0.2–0.6 mg/kg/dose (25 mg/dose), IV or IM	Direct vasodilator		
Isradipine	0.05–0.1 mg/kg/dose (5 mg/dose), PO, every 6–8 hours	Calcium channel blocker		Exaggerated decrease in BP if co-ingested with azole antifungals
Minoxidil	0.1–0.2 mg/kg/dose (10 mg/dose), PO, every 8–12 hours	Direct vasodilator		Long acting

Data from Constantine, E., & Linakis, J. (2005). The assessment and management of hypertensive emergencies and urgencies in children. Pediatric emergency care, 21(6), 391-396. Patel, N. H., Romero, S. K., & Kaelber, D. C. (2012). Evaluation and management of pediatric hypertensive crises: hypertensive urgency and hypertensive emergencies. Open access emergency medicine: OAEM, 4, 85.

17 ■ IMMUNIZATIONS

Table 17-1 Immunization Schedule

Age	Birth	1	2	4	6	12	15	18	24	4–6	11–12	16–18
	Month									**Year**		
Hepatitis B	HB	HB			HB							
Rotavirus			RV	RV	RV							
DTP			DTP	DTP	DTP		DTP			DTP	**Tdap**	
H influenza B			Hib	Hib	Hib	Hib						
Pneumococci 13[1]			PCV	PCV	PCV	PCV				PPSV23[2]		
Polio			IPV	IPV	IPV					IPV		
MMR						MMR				MMR		
Varicella						VAR				VAR		
Meningococcal[3]			MCV if high risk (asplenia, complement deficient)								MCV	MCV
Papillomavirus											HPV[4]	
Influenza (IIV)[5]					Influenza							
Hepatitis A[6]						HA		HA				

[1]Do not give PCV13 and PPSV23 during the same visit. [2]Add PPSV23 if underlying disease (immunocompromised, sickle cell, functional asplenia or cerebrospinal fluid leak, cochlear implant). Give first dose at age 2 years and booster at 5 years. [3]Routine vaccination with first dose 11 years and second dose 16 years. Meningococcal serogroup B: Start first dose at 16 years. Menveo recommended for asplenia, sickle cell, immunocompromised, and HIV with first dose at 2 months of age, then 4 months, 6 months, and 12 months. Menactra for complement deficient with first dose at 9 months and second dose 12 weeks later. [4]HPV: First dose at 9 years and second dose 6 months later. If first dose after 15 years, then second dose 1 month later, and third dose 6 months later. [5]Inactivated influenza vaccine (IIV): give first dose 6 months and if never vaccinated for influenza and less than 9 years, give second dose at 4 weeks apart from the first dose. [6]Hepatitis A vaccine: First dose given at 12 months and second dose at 18 months.

See website (www.cdc.gov) for details, especially specialized instructions for anyone with underlying medical disorders.

Table 17-2 Hepatitis B Exposure

Type of exposure/source	Status of source	Treatment if exposed patient is:	
		Unvaccinated	Vaccinated
Percutaneous/Mucosal	HBsAg+	HBIG[1], HBV[2]	HBV and HBIG if exposed HBsAb−
Known source	High risk for HBsAg+	HBV and HBIG if source HBsAg+	HBV and HBIG if source HBsAg+ and exposed HBsAb−
Perinatal[3]	Mother is HBsAg+	HBV and HBIG within 12 hours of birth	HBV
Mucosal/Sex/Perinatal	Unknown	HBV	HBV
Sex	HBsAg+	HBIG, HBV	HBV

[1]HBIG—hepatitis B immune globulin. [2]HBV, repeat in 1 month and 6 months. [3]If mother is HBsAg+, give HBV and HBIG within 12 hours of birth. Check anti-HBs and HBsAg at 9 to 12 months after completion of the HBV vaccination.

Hepatitis A Exposure: If ≤2 weeks since exposure, then give immune globulin (IG) and hepatitis A vaccine if ≤12 months, or hepatitis A vaccine if 12 months to 40 years, and if ≥40 years, give IG or hepatitis A vaccine if IG is not available.

Hepatitis C Exposure: No treatment.

See website (www.cdc.gov) for details.

Table 17-3 Tetanus Immunization

Prior immunization	All other wounds	Clean, minor wounds
Uncertain or <3 doses	Tdap[1], TIG[2]	Tdap, DTap, or Td
3 doses or more	Tdap if >5 years since last dose	Tdap if >10 years since last dose

[1]Tdap if ≥7 years old for those who have not received Tdap or then can use Td, and DTaP if <7 years. [2]TIG—tetanus immune globulin.

See website (www.cdc.gov) for details.

POSTEXPOSURE RABIES PROPHYLAXIS

If questions arise regarding prophylaxis and local and state health departments are unavailable, call the CDC at 404-639-1050 (days), 404-639-2888 (nights and weekends).

- Human diploid cell vaccine (HDCV): 1 ml IM, on days 0, 3, 7, and 14.
- RIG (rabies immune globulin)—20 units/kg: *Full dose* SC around wound (if possible) and remainder IM distal to RIG site. Do not give near site of first HDCV.

See website (www.cdc.gov) for details.

Table 17-4 Postexposure Rabies Prophylaxis

Animal			Treatment
Dogs, cats, ferrets	Healthy and can observe for 10 days		Prophylaxis if animal shows signs of rabies
	Rabid or suspected		RIG and HDCV
	Unknown		If high risk then RIG and HDCV
Bats, skunks, raccoons, coyotes, foxes, mongooses	All regarded as rabid unless geographic area known to be free of rabies		RIG and HDCV
Rodents, rabbits, hares, livestock			Consult public health but rarely require rabies prophylaxis

HIV

- Postexposure prophylaxis for someone potentially exposed to HIV to prevent from being infected. Must start within 72 hours.
- PEP hotline number: 888-448-4911.
- See website (www.cdc.gov) for details.

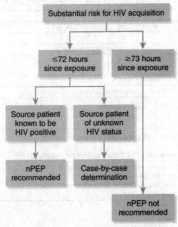

Figure 17-1 Algorithm for Evaluation of HIV Nonoccupational Postexposure Prophylaxis (nPEP)

Substantial risk for HIV acquisition
  • Exposure of: vagina, rectum, eye, mouth, or other mucous membrane, nonintact skin or percutaneous contact.
  • With: blood, serum, vaginal secretions, rectal secretions, breast milk, or any body fluid that is visibly contaminated with blood.
  • When: the source is known to be HIV positive.

Test	Source person	Exposed persons			
	Baseline	Baseline	4–6 weeks after exposure	3 months after exposure	6 months after exposure
For all those considered for or prescribed nPEP for any exposure					
HIV Ag/Ab testing	Yes	Yes	Yes	Yes	Yes
Hepatitis B serology	Yes	Yes	—	—	Yes
Hepatitis C antibody testing	Yes	Yes	—	—	Yes
Syphilis	Yes	Yes	Yes	—	Yes
Gonorrhea	Yes	Yes	—	—	—
Chlamydia	Yes	Yes	—	—	—
Pregnancy	—	Yes	Yes	—	—
For those started on nPEP					
Serum creatinine	Yes	Yes	Yes	—	—
AST and ALT	Yes	Yes	Yes	—	—
For all persons with HIV infection confirmed at any visit					
HIV viral load	Yes	Yes			
HIV genotypic resistance	Yes	Yes			

  • nPEP is not contraindicated for pregnant women.

Table 17-5 Regimens and Drug Choices for Adult and Pediatric HIV PEP

  • Unusual or severe toxicities from antiretroviral drugs should be reported to the manufacturer or the FDA or 1-800-332-1088.
  • Treatment is for 28 days of a three-course antiretroviral regimen.
  • See website (www.cdc.gov) for details.

Table 17-5 Regimens and Drug Choices for Adult and Pediatric HIV PEP (*Continued*)

Adults and adolescents ≥ 13 years with normal renal function	Tenofovir DF 300 mg and emtricitabine 200 mg daily with Raltegravir 400 mg twice daily or dolutegravir 50 mg daily Or Tenofovir DF 300 mg and emtricitabine 200 mg daily with darunavir 800 mg daily and ritonavir 100 mg daily
Children 2–12 years	Tenofovir DF, emtricitabine, and raltegravir with drug dosed to age and weight Or Tenofovir DF, emtricitabine, and lopinavir/ritonavir with drug dosed to age and weight Or Zidovudine and lamivudine with raltegravir or lopinavir/ritonavir
Children 3–12 years	Tenofovir DF, emtricitabine, and darunavir/ritonavir with drug dosed to age and weight
Children 4 weeks to <2 years	Zidovudine oral solution, lamivudine oral solution with raltegravir or lopinavir/ritonavir oral solution with drug dosed to age and weight Or Zidovudine and lamivudine with raltegravir or lopinavir/ritonavir
Children birth to 27 days	Consult a pediatric HIV specialist

Modified from Panlilio AL, Cardo DM, Grohskopf LA, Heneine W, Ross CS. Updated U.S. Public Health Service guidelines for the management of occupational exposures to HIV and recommendations for postexposure prophylaxis. *MMWR*. 2005:54(RR09):1-17.

Table 17-6 Drugs and Dosing for PEP

Drug	Dosing
Tenofovir DF	8 mg/kg max 300 mg every day (2–11 years)
Emtricitabine	6 mg/kg max 200 mg every day (3 months–17 years) 3 mg/kg every day (0–3 months)
Raltegravir	400 mg bid (6–12 years and >25 kg) Chewable tablets: 75 mg bid (2–12 years and 11 to <14 kg) 100 mg bid (2–12 years and 14 to <20 kg) 150 mg bid (2–12 years and 20 to <28 kg) 200 mg bid (2–12 years and 28 to <40 kg) 300 mg bid (2–12 years and ≥40 kg)
Dolutegravir	50 mg every day (≥12 years and ≥40 kg)

Table 17-6 Drugs and Dosing for PEP (*Continued*)

Drug	Dosing
Darunavir/Ritonavir	20 mg/kg darunavir and 3 mg/kg ritonavir (3 to 18 years and 10–15 kg) 375 mg darunavir and 48 mg ritonavir (3–12 years and 15 to <30 kg) 450 mg darunavir and 100 mg ritonavir (3–12 years and ≥40 kg) All dosed twice daily with food
Lopinavir/Ritonavir	Suspension: 16/4 mg/kg bid (14 days–12 months) 12/3 mg/kg bid (>12 months–18 years for <15 kg) 10/2.5 mg/kg bid (>12 months–18 years for 15 kg to 40 kg) 400/100 mg bid (>12 months–18 years for ≥40 kg) Tablets: Two 100/25 mg bid (>12 months–18 years for 15–25 kg) Three 100/25 mg bid (>12 months–18 years for 25–35 kg) Four 100/25 mg bid (>12 months–18 years for >35 kg)
Zidovudine	If ≥ 35 weeks gestational age: 4 mg/kg bid (birth to 41 days) 12 mg/kg bid (at least 4 weeks of age for 4 to <9 kg) 9 mg/kg bid (at least 4 weeks of age for 9 to <30 kg) 300 mg bid (at least 4 weeks of age and ≥30 kg)
Lamivudine	2 mg/kg bid (< 27 days) 4 mg/kg max 150 mg bid (≥4weeks) 75 mg bid (children < 16 years and 14 to <20 kg) 75 mg AM and 150 mg PM (children < 16 years and 20 to <25 kg) 150 mg bid (4 weeks to 18 years and ≥25 kg)

18 ■ INFECTIOUS DISEASE

EMPIRIC ANTIMICROBIAL THERAPY

Table 18-1 Empiric Antimicrobial Therapy

Abscess	• Drainage required, see specific site in text for antibiotics (e.g., brain, parapharyngeal). See methicillin-resistant *Staphylococcus aureus* (MRSA) if skin (page 154)
Acne Retin-A, Epiduo gel, and Tazorac are not approved <12 years old or if pregnant No tetracycline derivatives if ≤8 years old	• *Mild*—Topical benzoyl peroxide (BP) or topical retinoid • *Moderate*—Topical combination therapy (retinoid + BP OR retinoid + BP + antibiotics (abx) • *Severe*—Oral abx + topical retinoid + BP +/− topical abx • *Example product formulations/combinations* ◦ Topical retinoid: tretinoin, adapalene, tazarotene ◦ Topical BP + retinoid: EpiDuo Gel ◦ Topical BP + Abx: Acanya, BenzaClin, Benzamycin, and Duac gel ◦ Topical retinoid + Abx: Veltin or Ziana Gel ◦ Oral abx: Doxycycline 50–150 mg every day, erythromycin 250–500 mg every day, tetracycline 500 mg bid, minocycline IR 50–100 mg every day
Adenitis	• See cellulitis—*face options*; consider cat scratch, mycobacteria
Aeromonas	• Diarrhea—ciprofloxacin or levofloxacin × 3–5 days *Refer to Lexicomp for dosing*
Amebiasis	See *Entamoeba histolytica*
Ancylostoma	*Ancylostoma braziliense*—See cutaneous larval migrans *Ancylostoma duodenale*—See hookworm
Anthrax exposure	See pages 30–32 for exposure prophylaxis and disease treatment
Appendicitis Regimens are for suspected perforation (e.g., pain >36–48 hours, temp >101°F, diffusely tender)	• *First line:* Piperacillin-tazobactam OR ertapenem OR moxifloxacin • *Alternative agents:* Ciprofloxacin or levofloxacin + metronidazole OR cefepime + metronidazole *Refer to Lexicomp for dosing*
Arthritis, septic	See septic arthritis

(Continued)

Table 18-1 Empiric Antimicrobial Therapy (Continued)

Ascaris lumbricoides (roundworm)	• First line: Mebendazole (Vermox) 100 mg PO bid × 3 days OR albendazole 200 mg PO × 1 dose if ≤ 13 kg, or 400 mg PO × 1 dose if > 13 kg • Second line: (≥ 15 kg) ivermectin 150–200 mcg/kg/ dose × 1 dose
Avian "flu"	*See influenzae*
Balanitis	• *Mild*—Topical antibiotic (mupirocin 2% ointment bid) and/or antifungal (clotrimazole 1% cream or miconazole 1% cream four times per day). Addition of 1% hydrocortisone may be beneficial. • *Moderate to severe*— Clindamycin OR Augmentin + Bactrim (see Table 18-2 for dose)
Bell's palsy (Consider otic or mastoid disease)	• *Herpes* is the cause in a large number of cases: prednisone 1–2 mg/kg/day (max 60 mg) × 7–10 days AND (acyclovir 10 mg/kg/day PO 4 × per day OR if ≥ 50 kg, valacyclovir (Valtrex) 1 g PO three times per day × 7–10 days) • Debate exists as to efficacy of antivirals[1]
Bites, animals Oral dosing, see table 18-2 Need to consider tetanus and rabies prophylaxis	• *Dog or Cat*—PO: Augmentin 22.5 mg/kg PO bid OR clindamycin + levofloxacin. *IV*: ampicillin/sulbactam OR clindamycin + levofloxacin • *Rat*—Prophy: penicillin VK or doxycycline (>8 years old); if clinical evidence of infection: IV penicillin, cefuroxime, cefotaxime, or doxycycline • *Reptiles*—First line: Augmentin. Alternatives: cefpodoxime + metronidazole OR levofloxacin + clindamycin
Bite, human Consider MRSA coverage (page 154) If question of joint involvement, consult orthopedic or hand surgeon	• *PO*: Augmentin 22.5 mg/kg PO bid OR clindamycin + (either ciprofloxacin OR TMP-SMX) • *IV*—Ampicillin/Sulbactam, cefoxitin, or piperacillin-tazobactam. PCN allergic: clindamycin + (either ciprofloxacin OR TMP-SMX)
Bordetella pertussis	• Azithromycin (1–5 months: 10 mg/kg/day × 5 days. ≥ 6 months: 10 mg/kg/day PO on day 1, then 5 mg/kg/ day) OR clarithromycin OR TMP-SMX. See dose Table 18-2. Only decreases disease if given in catarrhal stage. Antibiotics can decrease recurrence and transmission.
Botulism	*See Clostridium botulinum*
Bowel perforation	*See appendicitis regimens*
Brain abscess	• Ceftriaxone AND vancomycin AND metronidazole (meningitis doses). Substitute aztreonam for ceftriaxone if penicillin allergy.

Table 18-1 Empiric Antimicrobial Therapy (*Continued*)

Bronchitis	• Antibiotics are not indicated unless cystic fibrosis, bronchopulmonary dysplasia, chronic aspiration, lung hyperplasia, or ciliary dyskinesia. If cough persists > 4 weeks, consider reactive airway disease, foreign body aspiration, cystic fibrosis, sinusitis, pertussis, or tuberculosis.
Bubonic plague	*See plague on page 33 for exposure/disease/treatment and antimicrobials, see Table 18-2*
Campylobacter jejuni	• Diarrhea—Azithromycin 10 mg/kg/day PO × 3 days (max 500 mg/day) OR erythromycin 40 mg/kg/day PO divided four times per day × 5 days (max 2 g/day)
Candida	• Thrush: (neonate)—Nystatin 1 ml/cheek four times per day apply with cotton swab. *(Child)* 400,000–600,000 units swish and swallow four times per day until clear for 48 hours. Suspension: 100,000 units/ml • Pharyngeal candidiasis—Fluconazole 6 mg/kg PO × 1 (max 400 mg/day), then 3 mg/kg/day (max 200 mg/day) × 7–14 days (21 days for *esophageal*) (if <14 days old, dose every 72 hours, otherwise every 24 hours)
Cat scratch disease	• Azithromycin OR TMP-SMX (see dose Table 18-2) • Mild disease resolves without treatment
Cellulitis bite	*See bite recommendations*
Cellulitis—face, periorbital, or orbital	• *Mild, immunized, healthy, no MRSA*—Augmentin or clindamycin • *Ill, unimmunized, sinusitis, or MRSA*—Vancomycin + (either ampicillin/sulbactam OR ceftriaxone OR aztreonam). ADD metronidazole to ceftriaxone or aztreonam containing regimen if dental infection is source.
Cellulitis trunk or extremity *See MRSA page 154*	• *Mild–moderate (and methicillin resistance not suspected)*—Cephalexin OR dicloxacillin OR macrolide (dose Table 18-2) • *Mild–moderate (methicillin resistance possible)*—Linezolid (Zyvox) OR Septra OR clindamycin, see dose Table 18-2 • *Moderate–severe*—Oxacillin OR nafcillin 25–50 mg/kg IV every 6 hours (max 12 g/day) OR ertapenem (Invanz) if > 3 months, 15 mg/kg IV/IM every 12 hours (max 1 g/day) OR cefazolin 25–33 mg/kg IV every 6–8 hours (max 6 g/day) AND *treat* MRSA
Cervical adenitis	*See cellulitis—face options; consider cat scratch, mycobacteria*

(Continued)

Table 18-1 Empiric Antimicrobial Therapy (*Continued*)

Chlamydia trachomatis, urethritis, cervicitis *See PID if needed* also treat empirically for gonorrhea	• Adolescents: Azithromycin 1 g PO × 1 dose OR doxycycline 100 mg PO bid × 7 days • Pregnancy: Azithromycin 1 g PO × 1 dose • Infants/children < 45 kg (anogenital tract): Erythromycin base/ethylsuccinate: 12.5 mg/kg/dose four times per day × 14 days • Dosing is for urethritis, cervicitis, or asymptomatic stage only. *See conjunctivitis for neonatal recommendations*
Cholecystitis	*See Appendicitis choices on Table 18-2*
Cholera	*See Vibrio cholera*
Clostridium botulinum First provide respiratory support.	• *Infant botulism*—age < 1 year: Human botulinum immunoglobulin (BabyBIG). Age > 1 year: Heptavalent equine serum botulinum antitoxin. Contact 770–488-7100 or CDC (1–800-CDC-INFO) via each state's health department for agent. AVOID antibiotics—may lyse *C. botulinum* in gut and increase toxin load. • *Foodborne botulism*—Heptavalent equine serum botulinum antitoxin. See previous contacts
C. difficile	*Clostridium difficile*—See *Pseudomembranous colitis*
Conjunctivitis *Macrolides* (esp. *erythromycin*) may cause pyloric stenosis <6 weeks	• *Neonate*—If gonorrhea, ceftriaxone 25–50 mg/kg IM × 1 dose (max 125 mg) OR cefotaxime 100 mg/kg/day IV divided every 12 hours × 1 day. If severe infection, therapy may need to be continued for > 1 day. ADD azithromycin 20 mg/kg PO × 3 days or erythromycin 7.2–15 mg/kg PO four times per day × 14 days. • *>2 weeks*—Erythromycin (Ilotycin) 0.5% ointment apply every 4 hours until clear × 2 days OR gentamicin (Garamycin) 0.3% ointment/solution—apply every 3–4 hours × 7–10 days OR Polytrim (if > 2 months) 1 drop every 3–6 hours × 7–10 days OR tobramycin (Tobrex) 0.3% solution/ointment—apply every 3–4 hours × 7–10 days • *≥1 year*—Azithromycin (AzaSite) 1 drop twice a day × 2 days, then 1 drop every day × 5 days OR besifloxacin 0.6% (Besivance) 1 drop three times per day × 7 days OR ciprofloxacin (Ciloxan) 0.3% solution 1–2 drops every 2 hours × 2 days, then every 4 hours × 5 days OR moxifloxacin (Vigamox) 0.5% solution 1 drop three times per day × 7 days OR above > 2 weeks old regimen
Corneal ulcer	*See keratitis (bacterial) recommendations* • Do not patch eye if *Pseudomonas* is a concern (e.g., contact lenses); also, consult ophthalmology and ensure *Pseudomonas* coverage if contact lens wearer

Table 18-1 Empiric Antimicrobial Therapy (Continued)

Cryptosporidium parvum	• *If immunocompetent*—Nitazoxanide (Alinia): 100 mg/5 ml or 500 mg tab available. Use 5 ml if 1–3 years old, 10 ml if 4–11 years, 500 mg (or 25 ml) if ≥ 12 years old administered every 12 hours with food × 3 days. Efficacy not established ≥ 12 years old. • *If HIV+*—Treat with antiretrovirals; nitazoxanide may not be effective
Cutaneous larval migrans	• Albendazole (Albenza) 15 mg/kg PO × 1 (max 400 mg; 200 mg tab) OR ivermectin (Stromectol) 200 mcg/kg PO × 1 (if ≥ 15 kg only)
Cyclospora	• TMP-SMX × 7–10 days, see Table 18-2
Dacryocystitis	*See cellulitis—face*
Dental infection	• *Outpatient*—Penicillin VK, amoxicillin-clavulanic acid, or clindamycin (Table 18-2) • *Inpatient*—Ampicillin/sulbactam (Unasyn) 50–100 mg/kg IV every 6 hours (max dose: ampicillin 8 g/day) OR clindamycin 25–40 mg/kg/day IV divide every 8 hours (max 2.7 g/day)
Diarrhea	*See Salmonella, Shigella, Escherichia coli, Campylobacter, Yersinia, traveler's, Vibrio*
Diphtheria *Rare disease, primarily in persons from developing countries*	• *Antitoxin*—(1) Laryngeal-pharyngeal: 20,000–40,000 units IM; (2) nasopharyngeal: 40,000–60,000 units IM; (3) extensive disease > 3 days or neck swelling 80,000–120,000 units IM. Call CDC/state health department: 404-639-8257, 770-488-7100. • *Antibiotics*—Erythromycin OR penicillin G IV × 14 days • *Exposure to infected person (household or habitual contact)*—Erythromycin 40–50 mg/kg/day × 7–10 days (max 2 g/day) OR penicillin G benzathine 600,000 units IM (if <30 kg) or 1,200,000 units IM (if 30 kg) × 1. Culture for *C. diphtheriae* and observe × 7 days with follow-up cultures 2 weeks later.
Discitis	*See osteomyelitis and MRSA*
E. coli diarrhea	• Rifaximin (Xifaxan) if ≥ 12 years old: 200 mg PO three times per day × 3 days OR Septra OR cefixime OR azithromycin (Zithromax) × 5 days (see dosing, Table 18-2) OR STEC Shiga toxin *E. coli* (0157:H7); does not improve with antibiotics
Ehrlichiosis *(disease detail on Table 18-10)*	• Doxycycline 4.4 mg/kg/day PO or IV divided bid (max 200 mg/day) for ≥3 days after defervescence for total of 5–10 days of therapy; rifampin, chloramphenicol, and possibly fluoroquinolones have been recommended as alternatives (consult infectious disease experts for dosing/indications)

(Continued)

Table 18-1 Empiric Antimicrobial Therapy (*Continued*)

Encephalitis	*See herpes simplex*
Endocarditis *(prophylaxis indicated next)*	• *Unknown organism*—Penicillin G 150,000 units/kg/day divided every 4–6 hours (max 24 million units/day) OR ceftriaxone (Rocephin) 100 mg/kg every 24 hours (max 4 g/day) AND gentamicin 2–2.5.5 mg/kg IV every 8 hours AND vancomycin 60 mg/kg/day divided every 8 hours, alter regimen once sensitivity known • *Penicillin allergic*—Daptomycin (Cubicin) 6–8 mg/kg every 24 hours (not FDA approved for peds) OR gentamicin 2–2.5.5 mg/kg every 8 hours AND vancomycin 40–60 mg/kg/day divided every 6 hours (max 2 g/day)
Endocarditis— Prophylaxis *See indications* *Table 8-1*	• Administer PO drugs 1 hour and IV/IM 30 minutes preprocedure: amoxicillin 50 mg/kg PO OR azithromycin 15 mg/kg PO OR clindamycin 20 mg/kg PO/IV OR ceftriaxone (Rocephin) 50 mg/kg IV/IM OR ampicillin 50 mg/kg IV/IM
Entamoeba histolytica	• *Asymptomatic amebiasis*—Iodoquinol 30–40 mg/kg/day PO divided every 8 hours (max 2 g/day) × 20 days OR paromomycin (Humatin) 25–35 mg/kg/day PO divided every 8 hours × 7 days (max 2 g/day) • *Mild to moderate intestinal disease*—Metronidazole (Flagyl) 35–50 mg/kg/day PO/IV divided every 8 hours × 7–10 days OR tinidazole (*Fasigyn/Tindamax*) 50 mg/kg/day (if > 3 years old) PO every 24 hours (max 2 g/day) × 3–5 days AND complete therapy of iodoquinol or paromomycin as per *Asymptomatic amebiasis*. • *Severe intestinal or extraintestinal disease*—(Metronidazole IV regimen above OR tinidazole oral regimen above) PLUS paromomycin as per *Asymptomatic amebiasis*
Enterobius vermicularis (pinworms)	• Primary: Mebendazole 100 mg PO × 1 OR pyrantel pamoate 11 mg/kg base (max of 1 g) • Alternative: albendazole 15 mg/kg PO × 1 (max 400 mg) • Repeat dose in 2 weeks to kill incubating parasites.
Epididymo-orchitis *(consider torsion)*	• *Prepubertal*—Treat as urinary tract infection, see pages 166–167 • *Postpubertal*—Treat as per gonorrhea (*uncomplicated disease* recommendations) AND doxycycline × 10–14 days

Table 18-1 Empiric Antimicrobial Therapy (*Continued*)

Epiglottitis	• Ceftriaxone 75–100 mg/kg IV (max 2 g/day) every 24 hours
Esophagitis	*See Candida—esophageal*
Giardia lamblia	• Primary: Tinidazole (if > 3 years old) 50 mg/kg/day PO × 1 dose (max 2 g/day) • Alternative: Metronidazole 15–30 mg/kg/day divided three times per day × 5–7 days (max 250 mg/dose) OR Nitazoxanide bid for 3 days (100 mg/dose if 1–3 years old; 200 mg/dose if 4–11 years; 500 mg/dose if ≥ 12 years) OR albendazole (if ≥ 2 years old) 10 mg/kg/day once daily × 5 days (max 400 mg/dose)
Gingivitis	*See herpes simplex—gingivostomatitis*
Gonorrhea (*also treat for Chlamydia*)	• *Arthritis, dermatitis*—Ceftriaxone (Rocephin) 50 mg/kg IV/IM (max 1 g/day) every 24 hours × 7 days • *Meningitis or endocarditis*—Ceftriaxone 50 mg/kg IV every 12 hours (max 4 g/day) × 14 days if meningitis OR × 28 days if endocarditis • *Ophthalmia neonatorum or conjunctivitis*—Ceftriaxone 50 mg/kg IM/IV × 1 (max neonatal dose 125 mg, otherwise max dose 1 g) • *PID—see pelvic inflammatory disease* • *Uncomplicated* (cervicitis/urethritis/pharyngitis or proctitis)—Ceftriaxone 125 mg IM OR cefixime (Suprax) 8 mg/kg PO × 1 (max 400 mg)
Helicobacter pylori	• 2 antibiotics (amoxicillin, clarithromycin, or metronidazole) PLUS [(proton pump inhibitor—lansoprazole, esomeprazole, pantoprazole, omeprazole) or bismuth subsalicylate] × 14 days[2]
Herpes simplex *keratitis* (contact ophthalmologist for treatment coordination and recommendation)	• *Encephalitis*[3,4]— (non-HIV-exposed/-positive) 3 months–12 years: Acyclovir 10–15 mg/kg/dose IV every 8 hours × 21 days. ≥ 12 years: 10 mg/kg/dose every 8 hours for 21 days. • *Genitals*—first episode— Acyclovir < 12 years old: 40–80 mg/kg/day PO divided into 3–4 doses/day × 5–10 days (max 1,200 mg/day); ≥ 12 years old: 200 mg five times daily, or 400 mg three times per day × 7–10 days. OR *unapproved options*—(1) famciclovir if ≥ 45 kg or adolescents: 250 mg PO three times per day × 7–10 days OR (2) valacyclovir 20 mg/kg/dose (max 1000 mg/dose) bid × 7–10 days.

(Continued)

Table 18-1 Empiric Antimicrobial Therapy (*Continued*)

	• *Genitalis—recurrence*—Acyclovir < 12 years old: 20 mg/kg/dose (max 400 mg/dose) three times per day. ≥ 12 years old 200 mg five times daily, or 400 mg three times per day, or 800 mg bid × 5 days, or 800 mg three times per day × 2 days OR *unapproved options* (1a) famciclovir (adolescents) 1 g PO bid × 1 day or 500 mg × 1, then 250 mg bid × 2 days total or 125 mg bid × 5 days (1b) 125 mg PO bid × 5 days OR (2) valacyclovir <50 kg: 20 mg/kg/dose (max 1000 mg/dose) bid × 5 days; ≥ 50 kg: 1000 mg once daily × 5 days. • *Genitalis—suppressive therapy*—Use each agent for 1 year; acyclovir 20 mg/kg/dose (max 400 mg/dose) bid, OR *unapproved options* (1) famciclovir (adolescents only) 250 mg PO bid × 1 year OR (2) valacyclovir 20 mg/kg/dose (max 1000 mg) once daily • *Gingivostomatitis and labialis*—Acyclovir 20 mg/kg/dose four times per day × 5–7 days (max 1.2 g/day); for *herpes labialis*— acyclovir 5% cream or ointment, topically 5×/day × 4 days OR penciclovir 1% cream every 2 hours while awake × 4 days OR docosanol 10% 5×/day until healed OR famciclovir 1.5 g PO × 1 dose (adolescents only) • *Keratitis*[3,4,5]—[ganciclovir 0.15% gel 1 drop 5×/day until corneal ulcer heals then 1 drop three times per day × 7 days (only approved ≥ 2 years old) OR trifluridine 1% 1 drop every 2 hours (max 9 drops/day) while awake until re-epithelialization of corneal ulcer occurs, then 1 drop every 4 hours for another 7 days] many experts recommend adding oral therapy (such as acyclovir 80 mg/kg/day (max dose 400 mg) divided 5×/day × 7–14 days). Topical therapy might cause corneal toxicity—close follow up by an ophthalmologist is recommended. Topical steroids are relatively contraindicated; they are sometimes used during stromal (not epithelial) stage to decrease scarring.
Herpes simplex	• *Neonatal disease*[3,4]—Acyclovir 20 mg/kg IV every 8 hours × 14 days for disseminated disease, and for 21 days if CNS/neurologic involvement. *Premie neonates*—20 mg/kg IV every 8–12 hours; ADD topical antiviral if neonate eye disease (*trifluridine* dosing as per keratitis, mentioned previously)

Table 18-1 Empiric Antimicrobial Therapy (*Continued*)

Herpes zoster	• *Immunocompetent/Healthy host and ≥ 12 years old*— Acyclovir 800 mg 5×/day × 5–7 days OR valacyclovir 1 g PO three times per day × 5 days • See *varicella* for chicken pox disease/exposure management • *Disseminated or immunocompromised or severe chicken pox*—Acyclovir 10 mg/kg/dose IV every 8 hours × 7–10 days
HIV exposure	See pages 139–142
Hookworm	• Mebendazole (Vermox) 100 mg PO bid × 3 days or 500 mg PO × 1, OR albendazole (Albenza) 15 mg/kg PO × 1 (max 400 mg) OR pyrantel pamoate 11 mg/kg/day × 3 days (max 1 g/day) • Test for cure in 2 weeks, and if disease still present, repeat treatment.
Impetigo *MRSA, page 154*	• Localized disease or limiting person-to-person spread: topical retapamulin OR mupirocin apply three times per day • More extensive[6] disease or systemic symptoms: Augmentin (90 mg/kg/day in two divided doses for 10 days) OR cefadroxil OR cephalexin OR azithromycin PO for 5 days (dose on Table 18-2); see MRSA if this is a concern
Influenza treatment[7] *Start therapy at any time if any of the following are present: progressive symptomatic illness, <2 years of age, chronic medical condition, immunocompromised, hospitalized, pregnant, within 2 weeks post-partum. Can consider therapy if symptom onset ≤ 2 days for patients not at risk of influenza complications. Peramivir—Not approved, CDC recommended emergency use (see CDC website for updates)*	• *Influenza A or B*—Oseltamivir (Tamiflu) administered bid × 5 days (see dosing on Table 18-2, p. 174) • *Severe disease, not responding, unable to take orals/inhaled medicines*—IV Peramivir: 0–30 days: 6 mg/kg every 24 hours IV; 31–90 days: 8 mg/kg every 24 hours IV; 91–180 days: 10 mg/kg every 24 hours; 181 days–5 years: 12 mg/kg every 24 hours; 6–17 years: 10 mg/kg every 24 hours (max 600 mg/day); do not use if Tamiflu resistant and ↓ dose if renal insufficiency.

(*Continued*)

Table 18-1 Empiric Antimicrobial Therapy (*Continued*)

Influenza prophylaxis	• *Influenza A/B*—Oseltamivir (Tamiflu); use same dose as administered for treatment but only administer every 24 hours
IV catheter-port-central line infection[3,4,5,8,9]	• Vancomycin 15 mg/kg IV every 6 hours AND ceftriaxone 50–100 mg/kg IV every 24 hours OR cefepime 50 mg/kg/dose IV every 8 hours OR piperacillin-tazobactam 240 to 300 mg piperacillin/kg/day divided in 3 to 4 doses; maximum daily dose: 16 g/day. Can add gentamicin 2–2.5 mg/kg IV every 8 hours for severe cases. *Immunodeficient or neutropenic: see neutropenic fever*
Keratitis *Coordinate care with ophthalmologist for most cases*	• *Bacterial*—Bacteria cause 65–90% of all keratitis cases. Consider *Nocardia* and *Mycobacterium* after refractive surgery (LASIK). *Treatment:* (1) Fortified tobramycin (14 mg/ml) AND [fortified cefazolin (50 mg/ml) OR fortified vancomycin (15–50 mg/ml)] OR (2) Fortified cefazolin + third/fourth generation fluoroquinolone topically OR (3) gatifloxacin (Zymar) or moxifloxacin (Vigamox). *Dosing:* One drop is applied every 5–15 minutes × first hour. Then, antibiotic is applied every 30 minutes, but alternated so that a drop is instilled every 15 minutes, for 6–12 hours. Then, administer one 1 drop of each hour while awake × 24–72 hours, then slowly reduce to every 6–8 hours × 10–14 days. Zymar/Vigamox not approved < 1 year old. • *Viral*—See herpes simplex and herpes zoster • *Parasitic*—*Acanthamoeba* can cause infection in contact lens wearer (esp. if wear overnight); specialized treatment
Lice	*See pediculus humanus capitis (pediculosis)*
Ludwig's angina	*See retropharyngeal abscess antibiotics (consult surgeon)*
Lyme disease[3,10] *See Table 18-11 for detail regarding early vs. late disease*	• *Early* (all PO)—Doxycycline 4.4 mg/kg/day divided bid (max 100 mg/dose) × 10 days OR amoxicillin 50 mg/kg/day divided three times per day (max 500 mg/dose) × 14 days OR cefuroxime 30 mg/kg/day divided bid (max 500 mg/dose) × 14 days. If unable to take beta-lactam or doxycycline: Azithromycin 10 mg/kg/day once daily for 7 days. (Administer doxycycline or amoxicillin for 14 days for isolated facial palsy. Administer oral agent for 28 days for arthritis.) • *Early disease with meningitis or carditis or more than mild early arthritis or later stage disease*—Ceftriaxone 75–100 mg/kg/day IV every 24 hours (max 2 g) OR penicillin G 200,000–400,000 units/kg/day IV (max 24 million units/day) divided every 4 hours × 14–28 days.

Table 18-1 Empiric Antimicrobial Therapy (*Continued*)

Mastoiditis[10] CT brain and mastoids	• *Acute*—1st episode: Cefuroxime (Zinacef) 150 mg/kg/day IV/IM divided every 8 hours (max 6 g/day) OR ceftriaxone (Rocephin) 50 mg/kg/day IV/IM administered every 24 hours (max 2 g/day) × 10 days. Consider coverage of MRSA (page 154). • *Acute exacerbation of chronic otitis media*—Vancomycin 15 mg/kg/dose every 6–8 hours + piperacillin-tazobactam 300 mg/kg tazobactam/day divided every 6–8 hours • *Chronic*—Cefepime (Maxipime) 100–150 mg/kg/day divided every 8 hours IV (max 6 g/day) OR meropenem (Merrem) if > 3 months—20 mg/kg IV every 8 hours (max 3 g/day). *If severe infection: 40 mg/kg IV every 8 hours*—max 6 g/day. OR ceftazidime (Fortaz) 100–150 mg/kg/day IV/IM divided every 8 hours (max 6 g/day) PLUS MRSA coverage, page 154, ± surgery.
Measles[3,10]	• *Exposure*—Measles vaccine, if administered within 72 hours of exposures, if *susceptible* and ≥ 6 months. *Susceptible* = all persons unless they had documented measles, born before 1957, lab evidence immunity, or completed appropriate live-virus vaccination. DO NOT give if neomycin allergy, TB, immunosuppressed, steroid use, hematological cancer, pregnant, ≤ 3 months from blood/immunoglobulin use. Use of live vaccine ≤ 72 hours after exposure prevents disease. • Use immunoglobulin (IG) within 6 days of exposure for any of the following: immunosuppressed, pregnant women without evidence of measles immunity, infants < 6 months of age, or infants 6–11 months if unable to receive MMR vaccine. *Infants*: IGIM 0.5 ml/kg (max 15 ml). *Pregnant women without evidence of measles immunity and severely immunocompromised hosts*: IVIG 400 mg/kg. Give measles vaccine 6 months after IGIM, if child is at least 12 months of age. • Treatment: Vitamin A × 2 days, as follows; < 6 months: 50,000 IU once daily; 6–11 months: 100,000 IU once daily; ≥ 12 months: 200,000 IU once daily × 2 days

(Continued)

Table 18-1 Empiric Antimicrobial Therapy (*Continued*)

Meningitis preterm to <1 month old[4,10,11]	• *Empiric Therapy:* Ampicillin + cefotaxime [OR] Ampicillin + gentamicin. Add acyclovir if history or physical exam findings are concerning for HSV encephalitis.
	• Ampicillin dosing: PNA ≤ 7 days 200–300 mg/kg/day every 8 hours. PNA > 7 days 300 mg/kg/day every 6 hours.
	• Cefotaxime: PNA ≤ 7 days and ≥ 2 kg: 100–150 mg/kg/day every 8–12 hours. PNA > 7 days and ≥ 2 kg: 150–200 mg/kg/day every 6–8 hours.
	• Gentamicin dosing:
	  ◦ 0–4 weeks old + birth weight (bw) < 1,200 g, 2.5 mg/kg every 18–24 hours
	  ◦ <1 week old and bw > 1,200 g, use 2.5 mg/kg every 12 hours
	  ◦ 1–4 weeks old and bw 1,200–2,000 g, 2.5 mg/kg every 8–12 hours
	  ◦ 1–4 weeks old and bw > 2,000 g, 2.5 mg/kg every 8 hours

Meningitis[4,10,11] 1 month–50 years *If possible administer dexamethasone before antibiotics*	• *1–2 months old*—Cefotaxime 225–300 mg/kg/day divided every 6–8 hours (max 12 g/day) AND vancomycin 15 mg/kg IV every 6 hours • *2 months–8 years*—Ceftriaxone 100 mg/kg/day IV divided every 12–24 hours (max 4 g/day) AND vancomycin 15 mg/kg IV every 6 hours • Add acyclovir if history or physical exam findings are concerning for HSV encephalitis. • Add dexamethasone 0.4 mg/kg IV every 12 hours × 2 days b if *Haemophilus influenzae* type b or *Streptococcus pneumoniae* suspected (controversial).
Meningococcemia	*See Neisseria meningitidis disease*
Community-acquired MRSA (CA-MRSA)[3,4]	• *Outpatient therapy*—Clindamycin 30–40 mg/kg day PO every 6–8 hours (max single dose: 450 mg) [OR] (if ≥ 2 months) sulfamethoxazole-trimethoprim 8–12 mg trimethoprim/kg/day PO every 12 hours
MRSA *Inpatient treatment*	• *Empiric inpatient therapy*—Vancomycin 15 mg/kg/dose every 6–8 hours
Molluscum contagiosum[3]	• No consensus on management • Most effective and quick cure: physical destruction of lesions (curettage), cryodesiccation with liquid nitrogen, electrodesiccation, and chemical agents (to elicit a local inflammatory response) • Topical cantharidin 0.7% (Cantharone), topical salicylic acid with (lactic acid or acetic acid) (Compound W, Duofilm, Duoplant, Mediplast, Mosco Corn and Callus Remover, Occlusal HP, multiple wart removing products)

Table 18-1 Empiric Antimicrobial Therapy (*Continued*)

Mumps	• Vaccine is NOT effective in preventing disease after exposed
Necator	*Necator americanus—See hookworm*
Necrotizing fasciitis[12] *(surgical consult) See MRSA page 154*	• Vancomycin 15 mg/kg every 6–8 hours PLUS piperacillin-tazobactam 100 mg piperacillin/kg/dose IV every 6 hours (max of 4 g piperacillin/dose) PLUS clindamycin 13 mg/kg/dose IV every 8 hours (max 900 mg/dose).
Neisseria meningitidis[3,4,10]	• *Exposure defined*—Prophylaxis if household contacts, same childcare or nursery, share toothbrush, close social contact, ate or slept in same dwelling in past 7 days or if sat directly next to diseased person on flight > 8 hours. No prophylaxis for healthcare worker unless mouth-to-mouth resuscitation, intubated, or suctioned patient before antibiotic administration. • *Exposure treatment*—Rifampin 10 mg/kg PO every 12 hours × 2 days (max daily dose 600 mg); if < 1 month old, 5 mg/kg PO every 12 hours × 2 days OR ceftriaxone 125 mg if ≤ 15 years old, or 250 mg IM if > 15 years old • *Disease*—See meningitis for empiric coverage. Definitive therapy: Penicillin G IV (300,000 U/kg/day IV; maximum, 12 million units/day, divided every 4–6 hours) OR ceftriaxone 100 mg/kg/day divided every 12–24 hours; maximum daily dose: 4,000 mg/day. Treat for 5–7 days.
Neutropenic fever[3,4,10] *Fever:* Single oral temp. ≥ 38.3°C (101°F) OR ≥ 38°C (100.4°F) for ≥ 1 hour *Neutropenia:* < 500 cells/mm³ OR < 1,000 cells/mm³ and predicted to drop < 500 mm³	• Cefepime 50 mg/kg IV every 8 hours (max 6 g/day) OR meropenem 20 mg/kg IV every 8 hours (max 1 g/dose) OR piperacillin/tazobactam 300–400 mg tazobactam/kg/day divided every 6–8 hours (max 4 g tazobactam/dose) • ADD vancomycin 15 mg/kg IV every 6 hours if: ↓ BP, central catheter, chemotherapy + mucosal damage, quinolone or sulfonamide use before fever onset, known colonization with pneumococci resistant to penicillin, or known gram-positive blood culture, or cellulitis (MRSA). • ADD macrolide if pneumonia (Zithromax, Biaxin); OR antifungal, OR antiparasitic if these infections are a concern.
Omphalitis[13,14]	• ≤ *2 months old*—Vancomycin AND gentamicin (see meningitis dosing) • > *2 months old*—Vancomycin AND ceftriaxone (see meningitis dosing) • ADD metronidazole to above regimens if anaerobic coverage is needed (e.g., foul smelling discharge, born to mothers with amnionitis).

(Continued)

Table 18-1 Empiric Antimicrobial Therapy (Continued)

Onychomycosis	See tinea unguium
Osteomyelitis[10] Consider Pseudomonas if foot/rubber sole puncture or immune deficiency	• Vancomycin 15 mg/kg/dose every 6–8 hours + [ceftazidime or cefepime]. • Cephalosporin dosing: cefepime 50 mg/kg IV every 8 hours (max 6 g/day) OR ceftazidime 50 mg/kg IV every 8 hours (max 6 g/day)
Otitis externa[4,10]	• Ear drops: ciprofloxacin + dexamethasone—4 drops into affected ear twice daily OR ciprofloxacin + hydrocortisone —3 drops into affected ear(s) twice daily OR ofloxacin 5–10 drops into affected ear(s) once daily. Duration: 7 days • If "malignant": chronic, ill or Pseudomonas suspected— See chronic mastoiditis antibiotic choices and doses, page 153
Otitis media	See CDC/AAP/AAFP recommendations, Table 18-15
Papillomavirus[10] If flat anogenital warts test for syphilis (VDRL or RPR) Respiratory papillomatosis—Best treated by ENT with lasers, intralesional interferon, cidofovir, or indole-3-carbinol	• Flat warts on skin—Topical salicylic acid (over the counter), tretinoin (Retin-A) 0.025–0.1% cream applied daily (AVOID these medicines on mucosa), laser surgery. cryotherapy, or laser surgery. • Anogenital warts (condylomata acuminata)—Imiquimod 5% (Aldara; only approved ≥ 12 years) apply every hours 3×/week—wash off in 6–10 hours. UNAPPROVED agents in children (1) podofilox 0.5% (Condylox) apply bid 3 consecutive days/week for up to 4 weeks OR (2) podophyllin 10–25% (Podocon-25, Podofin, Podofilm)— apply initially for 30 minutes to test skin sensitivity, apply one drop at a time and allow to dry until affected area covered. In 1–4 hours wash off. Consider application of petroleum jelly or talcum powder to nonaffected area to avoid skin contact. Repeat once a week for up to 6 weeks. Use lowest dose possible (5–10%), and do not apply to bleeding, friable lesions to decrease systemic toxicity.
Parapharyngeal	Parapharyngeal abscess: See retropharyngeal abscess
Pediculus humanus capitis[4,15,16] (pediculosis or lice)	• First Line: Permethrin 1% lotion/shampoo—Apply sufficient quantity to saturate hair/scalp to shampoo-washed and towel-dried hair/scalp. Also apply behind the ears and at the base of the neck. Leave on × 10 minutes. Repeat in 7–10 days. • Treatment failure with permethrin: Benzyl alcohol (Ulesfia) 5% lotion (use only if ≥ 6 months old)—Saturate dry scalp and hair, rinse off with water after 10 minutes, repeat in 1 week (1 bottle/8 ounces) OR ivermectin 0.8% solution (ivermectin not approved < 15 kg) OR malathion 0.5% shampoo × 10 minutes, reapply in 1 week OR spinosad 0.9% suspension 10 minutes, reapply in 1 week.

Table 18-1 Empiric Antimicrobial Therapy (*Continued*)

	• *Resistance to topical therapy*—Sulfamethoxazole/ trimethoprim (TMP) 5 mg TMP/kg/dose bid PO × 10 days (max 320 TMP/day), best if combined with permethrin OR ivermectin (Stromectol) 200 mcg/kg PO on days 1 and 10 if > 15 kg
Pelvic inflammatory disease[17] (PID) *Age > 12 years* Inpatient (CDC) *treatment* Choose Regimen A, B, or C	• *Regimen A*—[Cefoxitin (Mefoxin) 2 g IV every 6 hours OR cefotetan 2 g IV every 12 hours] AND doxycycline 100 mg PO/IV every 12 hours × 14 days • *Regimen B*—Clindamycin 900 mg IV every 8 hours AND gentamicin 2 mg/kg × 1, then 1.5 mg/kg IV every 8 hours • *Regimen C*—Ampicillin/Sulbactam (Unasyn) 3 g IV every 6 hours AND doxycycline 100 mg IV every 12 hours • *Switch* to oral outpatient medications that follow once clinically improved for 24 hours.
PID, *Outpatient (CDC)[17] treatment* Choose Regimen A or B	• *Regimen A*—Ceftriaxone 250 mg IM × 1 AND doxycycline 100 mg PO bid × 14 days ± ADD metronidazole 500 mg PO bid × 14 days • *Regimen B*—Cefoxitin 2 g IM × 1 AND probenecid 1 g PO × 1 AND doxycycline 100 mg PO bid × 14 days ± ADD metronidazole 500 mg PO bid × 14 days
Perforated bowel	*Or peritonitis; see appendicitis perforation regimens*
Peritonsillar	*Peritonsillar abscess—see retropharyngeal abscess*
Pertussis	*See Bordetella pertussis, pages 144 (antibiotics), 188 (disease)*
Pinworm	*See Enterobius vermicularis*
Pharyngitis[18] *Group A strep. Do not use erythromycin, 48% resistance*	• Penicillin G benzathine (<27 kg: 600,000 units IM × 1; ≥ 27 kg: 1.2 million units IM × 1) OR azithromycin × 3–5 days OR first generation cephalosporin OR amoxicillin 50 mg/kg once daily (max 1000 mg/dose) × 10 days OR penicillin VK (children: 250 mg 2–3 × daily; adolescents 500 mg 2 × daily) × 10 days. • PCN Allergy (nonimmediate hypersensitivity): cephalexin 20 mg/kg/dose bid × 10 days (max 500 mg/dose) or cefadroxil 30 mg/kg/dose once daily (max 1000 mg/ dose) × 10 days • PCN Allergy (immediate hypersensitivity): azithromycin 12 mg/kg/dose once daily (max 500 mg/dose) × 5 days OR clarithromycin 7.5 mg/kg/dose 2×/day (max 250 mg/ dose) × 10 days

(Continued)

Table 18-1 Empiric Antimicrobial Therapy (*Continued*)

Plague (*Yersinia pestis*)[3,19] Side effects vs. disease risk must be considered before drug selection. Streptomycin not widely available.	• *Disease* detail—see page 145. • *Exposure*—(if exposed to known or suspected plague source within the previous 6 days)—Doxycycline or ciprofloxacin × 7 days—dosing Table 18-2 • *Treatment*— (1) streptomycin 15 mg/kg/dose IM twice daily OR (2) gentamicin 2.5 mg/kg/dose every 8 hours. Alternative agents to consider: ciprofloxacin, levofloxacin, moxifloxacin, tetracycline, doxycycline, and chloramphenicol.
Pneumocystis jiroveci[3,4,10,20] (carinii)—Treatment Most require admittance due to high infant/ child mortality rates	• *First line*: Sulfamethoxazole/trimethoprim (15–20 mg TMP/ kg/day PO or IV divided every 6–8 hours × 14–21 days) • *Alternatives*: Pentamidine 4 mg/kg/day × 14–21 days, OR 1 of following (specialized dosing/cautions): (trimethoprim + dapsone) OR atovaquone (Mepron) OR (primaquine + clindamycin) • ADD Solumedrol 1 mg/kg IV every 12 hours OR prednisolone OR prednisone PO 1 mg/kg/day bid if pO₂ < 70 mm Hg
Pneumonia[4,21] Aspiration	• Ampicillin/sulbactam (Unasyn) 150–200 mg ampicillin/ kg/day IV divided every 6 hours (max 2000 mg ampicillin/ dose) OR clindamycin 30–40 mg/kg/day IV divided every 6–8 hours (max dose 2.7 g/day)
Pneumonia 0–3 months old[4,10] If severe, add MRSA coverage, page 154	• *0–4 weeks*—Ampicillin 100–300 mg/kg/day IV divided every 8–12 hours AND (gentamicin—*see meningitis* dosing) OR cefotaxime 50 mg/kg/dose every 12 hours if ≤ 1 week old or every 8 hours if > 1 week old) • *> 4 weeks–3 months*—Ampicillin 100–200 mg/kg/day divided every 6 hours AND cefotaxime 50 mg/kg IV every 6 hours (max 12 g/day) • If *Chlamydia* is cause, use erythromycin 12.5 mg/kg/ dose PO/IV four times daily × 14 days. Beware of pyloric stenosis risk with EM
Pneumonia[22] Community acquired > 3 months old Limited evidence suggests that linezolid has better alveolar penetrance compared to vancomycin	• *Inpatient > 3 months old*—Cefotaxime 100–200 mg/kg/ day divided every 6–8 hours (max 12 g/day) or ceftriaxone 50 mg/kg/day administered every 24 hours (max 2 g/ day) AND azithromycin (Zithromax) or clarithromycin (Biaxin) or erythromycin; see doses on Table 18-2, AND if moderate–severe disease, significant effusion, cavitary lesion, or other MRSA risk, linezolid (Zyvox) 10 mg/kg IV every 8 hours (if full term, >1 week old) or vancomycin 15 mg/kg IV every 6 hours (max 1 g/dose)

Table 18-1 Empiric Antimicrobial Therapy (*Continued*)

	• *Outpatient, < 5 years old* — First line: Amoxicillin 90 mg/kg/day divided every 12 hours (max 4000 mg/day). Alternative: amoxicillin/clavulanate 90 mg/kg/day (amoxicillin component) divided every 12 hours. Amoxicillin allergy: cefpodoxime, cefuroxime or cefprozil; see dosing Table 18-2. NOTE: Mycoplasma *and* Chlamydia *pneumonia can occur ≤ 4 years. If these organisms are suspected (fully immunized infant/child, wheezing, afebrile, interstitial pattern etc.), substitute* azithromycin *as first line OR add* azithromycin *as a second agent. See doses on Table 18-2* • *Outpatient, ≥5 years old:* Amoxicillin 90 mg/kg/day divided every 12 hours (max 4000 mg/day). Add azithromycin if unable to distinguish bacterial from atypical CAP. Alternative: amoxicillin/clavulanate 90 mg/kg/day (amoxicillin component) divided every 12 hours. Amoxicillin allergy: cefpodoxime, cefuroxime or cefprozil; see dosing Table 18-2
Pneumonia *Cystic fibrosis* *If penicillin allergy,* *consider quinolone*	• Ceftazidime (Fortaz) 50 mg/kg IV every 8 hours (max 6 g/day) or ticarcillin clavulanate (Timentin) 200–300 mg/kg/day of ticarcillin IV divided 4–6 hours (max ticarcillin 18 g/day) • AND (gentamicin or tobramycin 2.5 mg/kg IV every 8 hours)
Pneumonia *Hospital acquired*[23] *(cover S. aureus* *(± MRSA),* *Pseudomonas, and* *other gram-negative* *bacilli)*	• Cefepime (Maxipime) 50 mg/kg IV every 8 hours (max 2 g/dose) OR meropenem (Merrem) if > 3 months, 20 mg/kg IV every 8 hours (max 3 g/day; *if severe infection 40 mg/kg IV every 8 hours, max 6 g/day*), OR piperacillin-tazobactam[24] (Zosyn) 240–300 mg/kg/day (piperacillin component) divided every 6–8 hours (max 16 g/day) OR fluoroquinolone • ± *2nd antipseudomonal antimicrobial* (e.g., aminoglycoside: Gentamicin 2–2.5 mg/kg IV every 8 hours) • ± *MRSA coverage (if MRSA risk factors, or >10% of S. aureus isolates in unit are methicillin resistant, or MRSA prevalence unknown, or presence of necrotizing pneumonia, empyema, or lung abscess):* Vancomycin 15 mg/kg IV every 6 hours (max 1 g/dose) OR linezolid (Zyvox) 10 mg/kg/dose IV every 8 hours (max 600 mg/dose)

(Continued)

Table 18-1 Empiric Antimicrobial Therapy (*Continued*)

Pseudomembranous colitis
Only patients with severe disease require treatment with any listed medication
	Children < 5 years old often are asymptomatic carriers of *C. difficile* (most common in infants under 1 year of age) so do not automatically treat positive stool studies < 5 years old.
	• Mild to moderate:
	  ◦ Metronidazole (Flagyl) 30 mg/kg/day PO or IV divided every 6 hours (max 500 mg/dose)
	• Severe:
	  ◦ Vancomycin 40 mg/kg/day PO divided every 6 hours (max 125 mg/dose) × 10 days
	• Severe and complicated:
	  ◦ Vancomycin 40 mg/kg/day PO divided every 6 hours (max 125 mg/dose) PLUS metronidazole 30 mg/kg/day IV every 6 hours (max 500 mg/dose) × 10 days
	  ◦ If complicated with ileus or toxic colitis: vancomycin 40 mg/kg/day PO every 6 hours (max 500 mg/dose) PLUS metronidazole 30 mg/kg/day IV every 6 hours (max 500 mg/dose) PLUS vancomycin 500 mg/100 ml normal saline enema every 8 hours as needed × 10 days

Pterygoid abscess	*See retropharyngeal abscess*
Pyelonephritis	*See urinary tract infection recommendations, pages 166–167.*
Q fever (inhaled biologic with flulike symptoms, fever, endocarditis, hepatitis; 9–40 days incubation)	*Acute Q fever:* • Doxycycline[3] 100 mg orally twice daily (children ≥ 8 years of age) or 4.4 mg/kg/day orally divided twice daily for children <8 years of age (max dose 100 mg) × 14 days • Children younger than 8 years of age with mild illness: doxycycline 4.4 mg/kg/day orally divided twice daily × 5 days[25] • Doxycycline allergic: trimethoprim-sulfamethoxazole 4–20 mg/kg/day (trimethoprim component) orally divided every 12 hours (max 160 mg trimethoprim per dose) *Chronic Q fever:* limited evidence in children; combination doxycycline and hydroxychloroquine (minimum duration of 18 months) • Risk of disease must be weighed against risk of dental staining from the use of doxycycline in children ≤ 8 years old.
Rabies	*See pages 138–139 for exposure recommendations.*

Table 18-1 Empiric Antimicrobial Therapy (*Continued*)

Retropharyngeal abscess	• Clindamycin 40 mg/kg/day divided every 6 hours to every 8 hours[26] OR • Ampicillin-sulbactam 50 mg/kg/dose (ampicillin component) every 6 hours (max 2000 mg ampicillin per dose)[27] OR • Ceftriaxone 50–75 mg/kg every 24 hours (max 2000 mg) PLUS metronidazole 10 mg/kg/dose every 8 hours[28]
Rocky Mountain Spotted Fever *Do not wait for lab confirmation to treat*	• First line: Doxycycline 4.4 mg/kg/day orally or IV divided bid (max 100 mg/dose[29]) OR • *Tetracycline allergy*—Contact infectious disease expert and consider rapid desensitization procedures in an inpatient setting, or chloramphenicol (increased risk of death) 50–100 mg/kg/day IV divided every 6 hours (max 4 g/day). Continue antibiotics until afebrile × 3 days or total duration of 7–10 days.
Roundworm	*See Ascaris lumbricoides*
Salmonella Gastroenteritis (non-typhi)	• *Sepsis or focal infection*—Cefotaxime 100–200 (225–300 if meningitis) mg/kg/day IV divided every 6–8 hours (max dose 12 g/day), OR ceftriaxone 100 mg/kg IV divided every 12 hours to every 24 hours (max 4 g/day) × 7–10 days. • *Diarrhea*—Treat only if septic, age < 3–6 months, immunocompromised, hemoglobinopathy, or bacteremia. Give an initial dose of ceftriaxone 100 mg/kg (max 2000 mg). Step down oral therapy with azithromycin[3,30] 20 mg/kg for the first dose, followed by 10 mg/kg/day × 3 days if immunocompetent (14 days if immunocompromised).
SARS	*See coronavirus, page 193*
Scabies[4]	• Permethrin (drug of choice) 5% cream (Elimite) to entire body (+ scalp in infants) for 8–14 hours then wash off, OR crotamiton 10% lotion or 10% cream (Eurax) apply a thin layer from neck to toes once daily for 3 days followed by a cleansing bath 48 hours after the last application; treatment may be repeated in 7 days, OR ivermectin (Stromectol) 200 mcg/kg per dose PO × 2 doses administered at least 7 days apart (ivermectin not approved < 15 kg), OR 6% sulfur in petroleum ointment massaged into all skin surfaces from neck to toes × 2–3 days with cleansing of each application after 24 hours, OR lindane (not recommended in children <50 kg due to safety concerns, consider alternative agents) 1% lotion to body overnight then wash off

(*Continued*)

Table 18-1 Empiric Antimicrobial Therapy (Continued)

Sepsis	• Treat per meningitis or neutropenia depending on source
	See management algorithm/goal directed therapy, page 175
Septic arthritis *Surgical drainage and orthopedic consult* *Consider* Pseudomonas *if foot puncture or immune deficient*	• Cefazolin 50 mg/kg/dose IV every 8 hours • If community-acquired MRSA represents > 10% of *S. aureus* in geographic area: clindamycin 40 mg/kg/day divided every 6 hours–every 8 hours[31] • If clindamycin resistance is >10% in *S. aureus* isolates: vancomycin[32] • Consider empiric coverage for *Kingella* in children <36 months using a cephalosporin such as cefuroxime (50 mg/kg/dose every 8 hours), or ceftriaxone (100 mg/kg/day)
Shigella diarrhea	• Most infections are self-limited, and rehydration is the mainstay of management. Antimicrobial therapy is indicated in severe disease or immunocompromised patients[3] • Azithromycin (Zithromax) 10 mg/kg PO daily × 3 days OR ciprofloxacin 15 mg/kg/dose (max 500 mg/dose) PO bid × 3 days OR sulfamethoxazole-trimethoprim (use only if susceptible) 10 mg/kg (trimethoprim component, max 160 mg TMP/dose) per day divided bid × 3 days (immunocompetent)
Shunt infection	See ventricular shunt
Sinusitis *Obtain CT of sinus/ orbits, and consult ENT if orbital/periorbital cellulitis*	• First line: Amoxicillin-clavulanate 45–90 mg/kg/day PO divided bid[33] • Ceftriaxone 50 mg/kg IV or IM (if cannot tolerate PO)[34] • Penicillin allergic: Clindamycin 30–40 mg/kg/day divided every 8 hours PLUS cefixime 4 mg/kg/dose bid or cefpodoxime 10 mg/kg/day OR levofloxacin 10–20 mg/kg/day PO divided every 12–24 hours. Continue antibiotics for a total of 10–28 days or until symptom free, then 7 days.
Smallpox	• See page 33 for detail regarding disease. • *Exposure*—(1) Vaccine within 2–3 days of exposure provides some protection. Limited availability through CDC. • Tecovirimat[35] (available only through US Strategic National Stockpile): 13–25 kg: 200 mg PO bid, 25–40 kg: 400 mg PO bid, ≥40 kg: 600 mg PO bid [duration = 14 days]

Table 18-1 Empiric Antimicrobial Therapy (Continued)

Sporotrichosis	Source: Soil/thorny plants (e.g., roses, hay, straw). Typical incubation is 7–30 days (max is 3 months). • *Cutaneous or Lymphocutaneous*[3]—Itraconazole (Sporanox) 6–10 mg/kg/day PO divided bid (max 200 mg/dose) × 3–6 months. *Alternative treatment:* Potassium iodide, initial dose: 50 mg PO three times per day; increase as tolerated to ≤ 50 mg/kg/dose (max 2500 mg/dose) three times per day. Continue at maximum tolerated dosage for several weeks after lesions resolve. • *Disseminated sporotrichosis/severe pulmonary infection*—Amphotericin B 0.7 mg/kg/dose IV once daily followed by a prolonged course of itraconazole
Staphylococcus	*See MRSA, page 154, and specific infection*
Submandibular abscess	*See peritonsillar abscess*
Syphilis[36] *Congenital disease*	• *Possible congenital syphilis (≤ 4 weeks old), possible congenital syphilis, normal physical examination*—(normal CSF, X-rays, CBC/platelets): Aqueous crystalline penicillin G 50,000 units/kg/dose IV every 12 hours for the first 7 days of life followed by 50,000 units/kg/dose IV every 8 hours thereafter for a total of 10 days, OR penicillin G procaine 50,000 units/kg/dose IM × 10 days, OR (if mother received appropriate regimen of penicillin more than 1 month before delivery and there is clinical serologic follow-up) penicillin G benzathine 50,000 units/kg/dose IM × 1 dose. *Proven or probable disease*—Aqueous crystalline penicillin G 50,000 units/kg/dose IV every 12 hours for the first 7 days of life followed by 50,000 units/kg/dose IV every 8 hours thereafter for a total of 10 days OR procaine penicillin G 50,000 units/kg/dose IM once daily × 10 days • *Congenital disease (>4 weeks)*—Aqueous crystalline penicillin G 50,000 units/kg/dose IV every 4–6 hours × 10 days
Syphilis *Early acquired, late, latent, and neurosyphilis*	• *Early acquired [primary, secondary, early latent (acquired in prior 12 months)]*—Penicillin G benzathine 50,000 units/kg IM × 1 (max 2.4 million units). Consult with an infectious disease specialist if penicillin allergic. No pediatric data for use of doxycycline. • *Late (>1 year) or unknown latency*—Penicillin G benzathine 50,000 units/kg (max dose 2.4 million units) IM every week × 3. • *Neurosyphilis*—Aqueous crystalline penicillin G 50,000 units/kg/dose every 4–6 hours × 10–14 days (max dose 24 million units/day)

(Continued)

Table 18-1 Empiric Antimicrobial Therapy (*Continued*)

Tick bite[3]	• **Early localized disease:** ≥8 years: doxycycline 4 mg/kg/day PO divided bid (max 100 mg/dose) × 14 days. < 8 years (or unable to tolerate doxycycline): amoxicillin 50 mg/kg/day PO divided three times per day (max 1.5 g/day) × 14 days OR cefuroxime 30 mg/kg/day divided bid (max 1 g/day) × 14 days • *Disseminated disease:* ∘ Isolated facial palsy: same PO therapy as for early localized disease, × 14–21 days ∘ Arthritis: same PO therapy as for early localized disease, × 28 days ∘ Recurrent arthritis: repeat first oral arthritis regimen OR ceftriaxone 50–75 mg/kg IV once daily (max 2 g/day) × 14 days. *Alternatives to ceftriaxone:* penicillin G 200,000–400,000 units/kg/day IV divided every 4 hours (max 18–24 million units/day) OR cefotaxime 150–200 mg/kg/day IV divided every 8 hours–every 6 hours (max 6 g/day) ∘ AV block or carditis: PO regimen (as per early localized disease) if asymptomatic × 14–21 days, OR ceftriaxone (or alternatives listed above) 50–75 mg/kg/dose IV once daily (followed by PO therapy) × 14 days ∘ Meningitis: ceftriaxone (or alternative regimens listed above) 50–75 mg/kg/dose IV once daily × 14 days OR doxycycline 4–8 mg/kg/day PO divided bid × 14–21 days • Encephalitis/other late neurologic disease: ceftriaxone (or alternative regimens listed above) 50–75 mg/kg/dose once daily × 14–28 days
Tinea capitis or kerion—*Monitor patients closely for liver, hematologic, and electrolyte disorders*	• Griseofulvin microsize (liquid): ∘ *1 month to ≤2 years of age:* 15–25 mg/kg/day PO once daily or divided bid (max 1 g/day) × ≥ 6 weeks ∘ *> 2 years:* 20–25 mg/kg/day PO once daily or divided bid (max 1 g/day) × ≥ 6 weeks • OR Griseofulvin ultramicrosize (tablets): ∘ *> 2 years:* 10–15 mg/kg/day PO once daily (max 750 mg/day) × ≥ 6 weeks • OR terbinafine (tablets may be crushed): 4–6 mg/kg/day PO once daily (max 250 mg) or ∘ *10–20 kg:* 62.5 mg PO once daily ∘ *20–40 kg:* 125 mg PO once daily

Table 18-1 Empiric Antimicrobial Therapy (*Continued*)

	• *>40 kg:* 250 mg PO once daily • Duration: *T tonsurans*—2–6 weeks, *M canis*—8–12 weeks • OR fluconazole (not FDA approved for tinea capitis, lower cure rates) 6 mg/kg/day PO once daily (max 400 mg/day) × 3–6 weeks • Topical treatment with selenium sulfide, ketoconazole, or ciclopirox shampoos may be useful as an adjunct.
Tinea corporis, cruris, pedis	• *Topical options*—Ketoconazole daily, econazole daily • *≥ 2 years:* Miconazole bid, clotrimazole bid, tolnaftate bid, naftifine daily (cream, tinea corporis), sertaconazole daily (tinea corporis) • *≥ 10 years:* Ciclopirox (cream, suspension) bid • *≥ 12 years:* Naftifine daily (cream/gel, tinea pedis and tinea cruris), luliconazole daily, terbinafine (cream-bid for tinea pedis), butenafine (bid for tinea pedis), oxiconazole 1–2 × daily, sertaconazole bid (tinea pedis). *Duration: 2–4 weeks* *Oral (if extensive lesions or failure of topical therapy)*—Griseofulvin, terbinafine, or fluconazole (see Tinea capitis)

Tinea unguium	• *Topical therapies (preferred due to decreased adverse effects)*—Ciclopirox 8% (≥12 years) daily × 4–8 weeks, tavaborole 5% solution (≥6 years) daily × 48 weeks
	• *Oral treatment:*
	  • Terbinafine (tablets):
	    • *10–20 kg:* 62.5 mg PO once daily
	    • *20–40 kg:* 125 mg PO once daily
	    • *> 40 kg:* 250 mg PO once daily
	
	Duration = 6 weeks (fingernails), 12 weeks (toenails)

Tinea versicolor (Pityriasis versicolor)	• *Uncomplicated:* Topical therapy—Selenium sulfide shampoo once daily × 3–7 days OR clotrimazole cream bid × 2–3 weeks. Other topical therapies include ketoconazole, bifinazole, miconazole, econazole, oxiconazole, clotrimazole, terbinafine, ciclopirox, and zinc pyrithione. • *Oral (for extensive lesions or resistant infection)*—Fluconazole 300 mg PO once weekly × 2–4 weeks, OR ketoconazole (Nizoral) if ≥ 2 years old, 3.3–6.6 mg/kg/day PO every 24 hours × 10 days

(Continued)

Table 18-1 Empiric Antimicrobial Therapy (Continued)

Tracheitis, bacterial	• Nafcillin OR oxacillin 100–150 mg/kg/day IV divided every 4–6 hours (max 12 g/day), OR vancomycin 40 mg/kg/day IV divided every 6–8 hours (max 4 g/day) • PLUS a 3rd generation cephalosporin such as ceftriaxone 50–75 mg/kg/day (max 2000 mg) OR if > 2 months old and penicillin allergic, clindamycin 20–40 mg/kg/day IV divided every 6–8 hours (max 2700 mg/day) *If MRSA suspected, see page 154 (rows with MRSA)*
Traveler's diarrhea	*See E. coli antibiotic regimens*

Trichomonas	• Metronidazole (Flagyl):
	  ○ *<45 kg:* 45 mg/kg/day PO divided three times per day × 7 days (max 2 g/day)
	  ○ *≥45 kg:* 2 g PO × 1 OR 500 mg PO bid × 7 days if single dose unsuccessful
	• OR tinidazole:
	  ○ *> 3 years:* 50 mg/kg PO × 1 (max 2 g/dose)
	• *Adolescents:* 2 g PO × 1 OR 2 g PO daily × 5 days if treatment failure

Tularemia	• Gentamicin 5–6 mg/kg/day IV/IM divided every 8 hours to every 12 hours × 7–10 days, OR ciprofloxacin (mild disease) 15 mg/kg/dose (max 400 mg/dose) IV every 12 hours × 10 days *See pages 33–34 for detail presentation and diagnosis*
Urethritis *Adolescent dosing only (≥13 years)*	• *Nongonococcal urethritis:* Azithromycin (Zithromax) 1 g PO × 1, OR doxycycline 100 mg PO bid × 7 days, OR erythromycin base 500 mg PO four times per day × 7 days OR levofloxacin 500 mg PO once daily × 7 days • *M. genitalium:* Azithromycin 1 g PO × 1 OR moxifloxacin 400 mg PO daily × 7–14 days (treatment failure) • Other causes: *N. gonorrhoeae, C. trachomatis, Trichomonas,* HSV, adenovirus
Urinary tract infection[37] *See pages 190–191, for expert guidelines regarding management and Table 18-2 for oral dosing*	• *Inpatient*—Ceftriaxone 50–75 mg/kg/day IV divided every 12–24 hours (do not use < 28 days old), OR gentamicin 2–2.5 mg/kg IV every 8 hours (see meningitis dosing for gentamicin in neonates) + ampicillin 50 mg/kg/dose IV every 6 hours (esp. if gram positive bacteria/*Enterococcus*) OR piperacillin-tazobactam IV 240–300 mg/kg/day (piperacillin component) divided every 6 hours–every 8 hours (max 16 g/day)

Table 18-1 Empiric Antimicrobial Therapy (*Continued*)

	• *Outpatient options*—Cephalexin 50–100 mg/kg/day PO divided every 6 hours–every 8 hours (max 4 g/day), OR cefixime 8 mg/kg/day PO divided every 12 hours–every 24 hours (max 400 mg/day), OR sulfamethoxazole-trimethoprim 6–12 mg/kg/day (trimethoprim component) PO divided every 12 hours (max 160 mg TMP/dose), OR amoxicillin-clavulanate 20–40 mg/kg/day PO divided every 8 hours, OR nitrofurantoin (Furadantin, Macrodantin) 5–7 mg/kg/day PO divided every 6 hours, nitrofurantoin (Macrobid-adolescents) 100 mg PO every 12 hours • Treat 14 days if fever or toxic, 7–14 days if no fever or toxicity. Use of short courses (3–5 days) in pediatrics is controversial and might only be appropriate in adolescents with uncomplicated disease.
Vaginosis (bacterial)[36]	• *Children ≥45 kg or adolescents*—Metronidazole 500 mg PO bid × 7 days, OR metronidazole vaginal gel 0.75% (Metrogel), 1 applicatorful (5 g) intravaginally daily × 5 days, OR clindamycin 2% cream 5 g intravaginally × 7 days, OR tinidazole 2 g PO once daily × 2 days, OR tinidazole 1 g PO once daily × 5 days, OR clindamycin 300 mg PO bid × 7 days.
Varicella disease	Generally, supportive care only. Acetaminophen for fever/ prodromal symptoms and/or antihistamines for relief of pruritis. • *Nonimmunocompromised children ≥2 years (initiate within 24 hours of rash onset)*—Acyclovir 20 mg/kg/ dose PO every 6 hours × 5 days (max 3200 mg/day) OR valacyclovir 60 mg/kg/day PO divided every 8 hours (max 3 g/day) × 5 days; use in preadolescent children is not routinely recommended. Consider use in adolescents (greater risk for more severe disease), or chronic cutaneous/pulmonary disorder, or on chronic salicylates or on steroids ± second household case. • *Immunocompromised or severe disease*—Acyclovir 30 mg/kg/day IV divided every 8 hours × 7–10 days
Varicella exposure	• *Healthy, non-pregnant patients ≥12 months*—Vaccine: Administer vaccine 0.5 ml IM to susceptible children within 3–5 days of exposure if no prior immunization

(*Continued*)

Table 18-1 Empiric Antimicrobial Therapy (*Continued*)

	• *Varicella immune globulin (VZIG or VARIZIG)*—Give to exposed patients if they are (1) immunocompromised, (2) neonates whose mother has varicella (5 days pre to 2 days after delivery), (3) premature infants born ≥ 28 weeks who are exposed during neonatal period whose mothers do not have evidence of immunity, (4) premature infants born < 28 weeks or who weigh ≤ 1,000 g at birth and were exposed during the neonatal period regardless of maternal history of varicella disease or vaccination, (5) pregnant women without evidence of immunity • VZIG/VARIZIG is given within 4–10 days of exposure if above risk factors present. *VZIG dose*—≤ 2 kg: 62.5 units, 2.1–10 kg: 125 units, 10.1–20 kg: 250 units, 20.1–30 kg: 375 units, 30.1–40 kg: 500 units, >40 kg: 625 units (max 625 units) OR • *IVIG (if VZIG unavailable)*: 400 mg/kg IV × 1 (within 4–10 days of exposure) • *Acyclovir*—Acyclovir 20 mg/kg four times per day (max single dose 800 mg) during period of risk (if VZIG or VARZIG contraindicated, mildly immunocompromised without evidence of immunity or patients for whom varicella prevention is desired)
Vascular catheter	*See IV catheter*
Ventricular CSF shunt[38] infection *Consult neurosurgeon*	• Vancomycin 60 mg/kg/day IV divided every 6 hours (max 4 g/day) PLUS an anti-pseudomonal beta-lactam (cefepime 50 mg/kg IV every 8 hours (max 2 g/dose), OR ceftazidime 150 mg/kg/day IV divided every 8 hours (max 6 g/day), OR meropenem 40 mg/kg/dose IV every 8 hours (max 2 g/dose) • *Beta-lactam allergy:* Add aztreonam 90–120 mg/kg/day divided every 6 hours–every 8 hours (max 8 g/day) OR ciprofloxacin 15 mg/kg/dose IV every 12 hours (max 400 mg/dose) • Intrathecal antibiotics and externalization of shunt may be needed and is best guided by a neurosurgeon.
Vibrio species[3,39]	• *Management is typically supportive. Diarrhea is usually mild and self-limited.* • *Sepsis with/without hemorrhagic bullae, wound infections:* 3rd generation cephalosporin (ceftazidime 150 mg/kg/day IV divided every 8 hours, OR ceftriaxone 50–100 mg/kg/day IV divided every 12 hours–every 24 hours) PLUS doxycycline (≥ 8 years) 2.2 mg/kg/dose IV/PO every 12 hours (max 200 mg/day) OR ciprofloxacin 10 mg/kg/dose IV every 12 hours (max 400 mg/dose) OR

Table 18-1 Empiric Antimicrobial Therapy (Continued)

	Sulfamethoxazole-trimethoprim 6–12 mg TMP/kg/day PO divided every 12 hours PLUS gentamicin 2–2.5 mg/kg/dose IV every 8 hours (children whom doxycycline or ciprofloxacin are contraindicated) • *Severe diarrhea:* Doxycycline 2.2 mg/kg/dose PO every 12 hours (max 200 mg/day) OR ciprofloxacin 10–15 mg/kg/dose PO twice a day (max 750 mg/dose)
Warts	*See Papillomavirus*
Yersinia enterocolitica	• Immunocompromised patients, neonates, and those with sepsis or extra intestinal disease require treatment. • 3rd generation cephalosporin (ceftriaxone 50–100 mg/kg/day IV divided every 12 hours–every 24 hours, OR cefotaxime 150–180 mg/kg/day IV divided every 8 hours. Alternatives include sulfamethoxazole-trimethoprim, aminoglycosides, fluoroquinolones, tetracycline, or doxycycline
Yersinia pestis	*See Plague page 33 (disease) and 158 (antimicrobials)*

Sources:

[1]Data from al Almeida JR, Al Khabori M, Guyatt GH, et al. Combined corticosteroid and antiviral treatment for Bell palsy: a systematic review and meta-analysis. *JAMA.* 2009;302:985.

[2]Jones NL, Koletzko S, Goodman K, et al. European Society for Paediatric Gastroenterology, Hepatology, and Nutrition (ESPGHAN)/North American Society for Pediatric Gastroenterology, Hepatology, and Nutrition (NASPGHAN): joint guidelines for the management of Helicobacter pylori in children and adolescents, update 2016. *J Pediatr Gastroenterol Nutr.* 2017;64(6):991-1003.

[3]Redbook.

[4]Lexicomp.

[5]DHHS Panel on Opportunistic Infections in HIV-Exposed and HIV-Infected Children. *Guidelines for the prevention and treatment of opportunistic infections in HIV-exposed and HIV-infected children.* Department of Health and Human Services. November 2013. Available at http://aidsinfo.nih.gov /contentfiles/lvguidelines/oi_guidelines_pediatrics.pdf.

[6]Cole C, Gazewood J. Diagnosis and treatment of impetigo. *Am Fam Physician.* 2007;75(6):859-864.

[7]Uyeki TM, Bernstein HH, Bradley JS. Clinical Practice Guidelines by the Infectious Diseases Society of America: 2018 update on diagnosis, treatment, chemoprophylaxis, and institutional outbreak management of seasonal influenza. *Clin Infect Dis.* 2019;68(6):e1-e47.

[8]Mermel LA, Allon M, Bouza E, et al. Clinical practice guidelines for the diagnosis and management of intravascular catheter-related infection: 2009 update by the Infectious Diseases Society of America. *Clin Infect Dis.* 2009;49(1):1-45.

[9]Flynn PM. Diagnosis and management of central venous catheter-related bloodstream infections in pediatric patients. *Pediatr Infect Dis J.* 2009;28(11):1016-1017.

[10]Gilbert DN, Chambers HF, Eliopoulos GM, Saag MS, Pavia AT, eds. *The Sanford Guide to Antimicrobial Therapy.* Sperryville, VA: Antimicrobial Therapy, Inc.; 2019.

[11]Swanson D. Meningitis. *Pediatr Rev.* 2015;36(12):514-526.

[12]Lee GJ. Skin and soft tissue infections of bacterial and viral etiology. In: Benavides S, Nahata MC, eds. *Pediatric Pharmacotherapy.* Lenexa, KS: American College of Clinical Pharmacy; 2013:606-633; Stevens DL, Bisno AL, Chambers HF, et al.; Infectious Diseases Society of America. Practice guidelines for the diagnosis and

(Continued)

Table 18-1 Empiric Antimicrobial Therapy (*Continued*)

management of skin and soft tissue infections: 2014 update by the Infectious Diseases Society of America. *Clin Infect Dis.* 2014;59(2):e10-e52.

[12]Brook I. Cutaneous and subcutaneous infections in newborns due to anaerobic bacteria. *J Perinat Med.* 2002;30(3):197.

[14]Mason WH, Andrews R, Ross LA, Wright HT Jr. Omphalitis in the newborn infant. *Pediatr Infect Dis J.* 1989;8(8):521.

[15]Gunning K, Kiraly B, Pippitt K. Lice and scabies: treatment update. *Am Fam Phys.* 2019;99(10):635-642.

[16]Hipolito RB, Mallorca FG, Zuniga-Macaraig ZO, et al. Head lice infestation: single drug versus combination therapy with one percent permethrin and trimethoprim/sulfamethoxazole. *Pediatrics.* 2001;107:e30.

[17]Centers for Disease Control and Prevention. 2015 STD treatment guidelines.

[18]Shulman ST, Bisno AL, Clegg HW, et al. Clinical practice guideline for the diagnosis and management of group A streptococcal pharyngitis: 2012 update by the Infectious Diseases Society of America. *Clin Infect Dis.* 2012;55(10):e91.

[19]Centers for Disease Control and Prevention. Plague—Resources for Clinicians. Available at: https://www.cdc.gov/plague/healthcare/clinicians.html.

[20]Kovacs H, Masur H. Evolving health effects of *Pneumocystis* one hundred years of progress in diagnosis and treatment. *JAMA.* 2009;301(24):2578-2585.

[21]Sandora TJ, Harper MB. Pneumonia in hospitalized children. *Pediatr Clin North Am.* 2005;52(4):1059.

[22]Bradley J, Byington C, Shah S, et al. The management of community-acquired pneumonia in infants and children older than 3 months of age: clinical practice guidelines by the Pediatric Infectious Diseases Society and the Infectious Diseases Society of America. *Clin Infect Dis.* 2011;53(7):e25-e76

[23]Kalil A, Metersky M, Klompas M, et al. Management of adults with hospital-acquired and ventilator-associated pneumonia: 2016 Clinical Practice Guidelines by the Infectious Diseases Society of America and the American Thoracic Society. *Clin Infect Dis.* 2016;63(5):e61-e111.

[24]Zar H, Cotton M. Nosocomial pneumonia in pediatric patients. *Pediatr Drugs.* 2002;4(2):73-83.

[25]CDC.gov. Q Fever. https://www.cdc.gov/qfever/healthcare-providers/index.html#treatment.

[26]Al-Sabah B, Bin Salleen H, Hagr A, et al. Retropharyngeal abscess in children: 10-year study. *J Otolaryngol.* 2004;33(6):352-355.

[27]Khudan A, Jugmohansingh G, Islam S, Medford S, Narraynsingh V. The effectiveness of conservative management for retropharyngeal abscesses greater than 2 cm. *Ann Med Surg (Lond).* 2016;11:62-65.

[28]Lalakea ML, Messner AH. Retropharyngeal abscess management in children: current practices. *Otolaryngol Head Neck Surg.* 1999;121(4):398-405.

[29]Biggs H, Behravesh B, Bradley K, et al. Diagnosis and management of tickborne rickettsial diseases: rocky mountain spotted fever and other spotted fever group rickettsioses, ehrlichioses, and anaplasmosis—United States. *MMWR Recomm Rep.* 2016;65(2):1-45.

[30]Wen SC, Best E, Nourse C. Non-typhoidal *Salmonella* infections in children: review of literature and recommendations for management. *J Paediatr Child Health.* 2017;53(10):936-941.

[31]Krogstad P. Septic arthritis. In: Cherry J, Harrison G, Kaplan S, Steinbach W, Hotez P, eds. *Feigin and Cherry's Textbook of Pediatric Infectious Diseases.* 8th ed. Philadelphia, PA: Elsevier; 2019:529-534.

[32]Pääkkönen M. Septic arthritis in children: diagnosis and treatment. *Pediatr Health Med Ther.* 2017;8:65-68. https://www.ncbi.nlm.nih.gov/pmc/articles/PMC5774603/.

[33]Chow A, Benninger M, Brook I, et al. IDSA clinical practice guidelines for acute bacterial rhinosinusitis in children and adults. *Clin Infect Dis.* 2012;54(8):e72-e112.

[34]Wald E, Applegate K, Bordley C, et al. Clinical practice guideline for the diagnosis and management of acute bacterial sinusitis in children aged 1 to 18 years. *Pediatrics.* 2013;132:e262-e280.

[35]Centers for Disease Control and Prevention. Smallpox. https://www.cdc.gov/smallpox/prevention-treatment/index.html.

[36]Centers for Disease Control and Prevention. *2015 Sexually transmitted diseases treatment guidelines.* https://www.cdc.gov/std/tg2015/congenital.htm.

[37]Subcommittee on Urinary Tract Infection, Steering Committee on Quality Improvement and Management. Urinary tract infection: clinical practice guideline for the diagnosis and management of the initial UTI in

Table 18-2 Common Oral Antimicrobial Doses and Mixtures

Antimicrobial	Formulations	Dose (Frequency)[1]
Acyclovir	200, 400, 800, 200 mg/5 ml	See herpes pages 149–151, varicella pages 167–168
Albendazole (Albenza)	200 mg	See infection (max 400 mg/day)
Amoxicillin (Amoxil)	Suspension: 125, 200, 250 and 400 mg/5 ml Caps: 250, 500 mg Tabs: 500, 875 mg	30–50 mg/kg/day (bid to three times per day) 80–90 mg/kg/day DRSP[2]
Amoxicillin/clavulanate (Augmentin)	Suspension*: 125, 200, 250 and 600 mg/5 ml Tabs*: 250, 500, 875 mg Chew tabs*: 200 mg	45 mg/kg/day (bid) 80–90 mg/kg/day if DRSP[2] (*dosing is in mg of amoxicillin)
Ampicillin (Principen)	Suspension: 125 and 250 mg/5 ml Caps: 250, 500 mg	50–100 mg/kg/day (four times per day)
Azithromycin[3] (Zithromax)	Suspension: 100 and 200 mg/5 ml, Tabs: 250, 500 mg	Pneumonia/Otitis media 10 mg/kg × 1 on first day, then 5 mg/kg daily × 4 Pharyngitis 12 mg/kg/day × 5 days 20 mg/kg/day × 3 days Max dose 500 mg
Cefaclor (Ceclor) *Second generation*	Suspension: 125, 250, and 375 mg/5 ml Caps: 250 mg, 500 mg	20–40 mg/kg/day (three times per day) Max 500 mg/dose
Cefadroxil (Duricef) *First generation*	Suspension: 250, 500 mg/5 ml Cap: 500 mg, Tab: 1000 mg	30 mg/kg/day (bid) Max 1,000 mg/dose
Cefdinir (Omnicef) *Third generation*	Suspension: 125 and 250 mg/5 ml Cap: 300 mg	14 mg/kg/day (every 12–24 hours) Max 600 mg/day

(*Continued*)

Table 18-2 Common Oral Antimicrobial Doses and Mixtures (*Continued*)

Antimicrobial	Formulations	Dose (Frequency)[1]
Cefditoren (Spectracef) *Third generation*	Tab: 200, 400 mg (only use ≥ 12 years old)	200–400 mg bid Max 400 mg/dose
Cefixime (Suprax) *Third generation*	Suspension: 100, 200, 500 mg/5 ml Caps: 400 mg Chew tab: 100 and 200 mg	8 mg/kg/day (every 12–24 hours) (UTI: 16 mg/kg on day 1) Max 400 mg/day
Cefpodoxime (Vantin) *Third generation*	Suspension: 50 and 100 mg/5 ml Tabs: 100, 200 mg	10 mg/kg/day (bid) Max 200–400 mg/dose
Cefprozil (Cefzil) *Second generation*	Suspension: 125 and 250 mg/5 ml Tabs: 250 mg, 500 mg	15–30 mg/kg/day (bid) Max 500 mg/dose
Ceftibuten (Cedax) *Third generation*	Suspension: 180 mg/5 ml Caps: 400 mg	9 mg/kg/day (daily) Max 400 mg/dose
Cefuroxime (Ceftin) *Second generation*	Suspension: 125 mg/5 ml Tabs: 250, 500 mg	20–30 mg/kg/day (bid) Max 500 mg/dose
Cephalexin (Keflex) *First generation*	Suspension: 125 and 250 mg/5 ml Caps/Tabs: 250, 500 (750 mg capsule)	25–50 mg/kg/day (four times per day) Max 500 mg/dose
Clarithromycin (Biaxin)	Suspension: 125 and 250 mg/5 ml Tabs: 250, 500 mg	15 mg/kg/day (bid) Max 500 mg/dose
Clindamycin (Cleocin)	Solution: 75 mg/5 ml Caps: 75, 150, 300 mg	8–25 mg/kg/day (three times per day/bid) (30–40 mg/kg/day if DRSP[3]) Max 1800 mg/day
Dicloxacillin (Dynapen)	Caps: 250, 500 mg	12.5–25 mg/kg/day (four times per day), max 250 mg/dose Use 50–100 mg/kg/day if completing osteomyelitis therapy (max dose 500 mg)
Doxycycline(>8 years) (Vibramycin)	Tab/Cap: 50, 75, 100, 150 mg Suspension: 25 mg/5 ml. Syrup: 50 mg/5 ml	4.4 mg/kg/day (bid) Max 200 mg/day
Erythromycin (ERYC, EES, E-mycin)	Suspension: 200 and 400 mg/5 ml Tab: 250, 400, 500 mg	30–50 mg/kg/day (3–4×/day) Max 2000–4000 mg/day

Empiric Antimicrobial Therapy 173

Table 18-2 Common Oral Antimicrobial Doses and Mixtures (*Continued*)

Antimicrobial	Formulations	Dose (Frequency)[1]
Erythromycin/ Sulfisoxazole (Pediazole)	Suspension: 200 mg EM and 600 mg SS per 5 ml	50 mg EM/kg/day (four times per day) Max EM dose 500 mg
Fluconazole (Diflucan)	Suspension: 10 and 40 mg/ml Tabs: 50, 100, 150, 200 mg	6–12 mg/kg/dose × 1, then 3–12 mg/kg/dose once daily Max 600 mg/dose
Griseofulvin Microsize (Grifulvin V) Ultramicrosize tablets (Gris-PEG)	Suspension: 125 mg/5 ml (micro) Tabs: (micro) 500 mg Tabs: (ultra) 125 mg, 250 mg	Micro: 20–25 mg/kg/day (every day to bid) Ultra: 10–15 mg/kg/day (every day) Max dose (micro) 1 g Max dose (ultra) 750 mg
Itraconazole (Sporanox, Tolsura)	Cap: 100 mg, 65 mg Solution: 10 mg/ml	5 mg/kg/dose every 12 hours (see specific infection)
Ivermectin (Stromectol)	Tab: 3 mg	200 mcg/kg/day (see specific infection)
Linezolid (Zyvox)	Tab: 600 mg Suspension: 100 mg/5 ml	30 mg/kg/day (three times per day) if < 12 years Administered bid if ≥ 12 years Max dose 600 mg
Mebendazole (Emverm)	Tabs: 100 mg chewable	Dosing variable—see specific infection
Metronidazole (Flagyl)	Tabs: 250, 500 mg Cap: 375 mg Suspension can be compounded	15–50 mg/kg/day divided three times per day Max 2250 mg/day
Nitrofurantoin (Macrodantin, Macrobid, Furadantin)	Suspension: 25 mg/5 ml Caps: 25, 50, 100 mg	Furadantin, Macrodantin: 5–7 mg/kg/day (four times per day) Macrobid (adolescents): 100 mg bid Max dose 100 mg
Nystatin (Bio-Statin)	Suspension: 100,000 units/ml Tabs: 500,000 units Caps: 500,000 units, 1,000,000 units	Infants: 200,000–400,000 units four times per day or 100,000 units to each side of mouth four times per day Child: 400,000–600,000 units four times per day Max dose 600,000 units

(*Continued*)

Table 18-2 Common Oral Antimicrobial Doses and Mixtures (*Continued*)

Antimicrobial	Formulations	Dose (Frequency)[1]
Oseltamivir (Tamiflu)	Caps: 30, 45, 75 mg Suspension: 6 mg/ml	Treatment: ≤8 months: 3 mg/kg/dose bid Infants ≥ 9 months: 3–3.5 mg/kg/dose bid Children & adolescents: ≤15 kg: 30 mg bid > 15–23 kg: 45 mg bid > 23–40 kg: 60 mg bid >40 kg: 75 mg bid
Penicillin V Potassium	Suspension: 125 and 250 per 5 ml Tab: 250, 500 mg	25–75 mg/kg/day every 6 hours to every 8 hours Max dose 2 g/day
Pyrantel pamoate (Reese's Pinworm Medicine)	Tab: 62.5 mg Suspension: 50 mg/ml	Pinworms, roundworms 11 mg/kg × 1 Hookworm 11 mg/kg × 3 days Max dose 1 g
Rifampin (Rifadin)	Caps: 150, 300 mg Suspension can be compounded	10–20 mg/kg/day (bid) Max dose 600 mg
Terbinafine (Lamisil)	Tab: 250 mg Suspension can be compounded	Tinea capitis: < 25 kg (125 mg/day) 25–35 kg (187.5 mg/day) > 35 kg (250 mg/day)
Trimethoprim/sulfa- methoxazole (Bactrim, Sulfatrim)	Suspension: 40 mg TMP and 200 mg SMX per 5 ml Tabs: 80/400 and 160 /800 mg	6–12 mg TMP/kg/day (bid) Max dose 160 TMP[4]
Vancomycin (Vancocin, Firvanq)	Caps: 125, 250 mg Solution: 25 mg/ml, 50 mg/ml	40 mg/kg/day divided every 6 hours to every 8 hours Max dose 2000 mg/day

[1]Max dose—maximum individual (single) oral dose. [2]DRSP—drug-resistant *S. pneumonia*, for pneumonia and otitis media. [3]20 mg/kg × 1 dose required for *Chlamydia*. [4]Higher doses needed for severe UTI, *Shigella*, and pneumocystis infections.
Source: LexiComp.

NEONATE

Table 18-3 Goal-Directed Therapy for Septic Shock in Infants and Children[1,2]

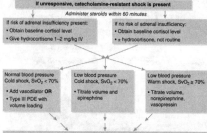

- Recognize altered mental status and decreased perfusion (within minutes of arrival)
- Establish airway and IV, give 20 ml/kg NS or LR up to 60 ml/kg or greater
- Administer broad-spectrum antibiotics depending on source (see page 162, sepsis)
- Correct hypoxia, hypoglycemia, electrolyte disorders (esp. hypocalcemia)

Initiate above within 1st 15 minutes

Fluid-responsive shock
- Observe in pediatric intensive care unit

Fluid-refractory shock
- Place central venous line and arterial line
- Begin dopamine

Fluid refractory, dopamine-resistant shock
- If cold shock, (CR > 2 sec, ↓ pulses, cool/mottled extremities), titrate epinephrine
- If warm shock, (CR < 1–2 sec, ↑ pulses, warm skin) titrate norepinephrine, vasopressin
- Goals (1) SvO₂ > 70% and (2) normal MAP-CVP for age (55 cm H₂O/40 mm Hg term newborn, 60 cm H₂O/44 mm Hg ≤ 1 year old, and 65 cm H₂O/48 mm Hg > 1 year old).

If unresponsive, catecholamine-resistant shock is present

Administer steroids within 60 minutes

If risk of adrenal insufficiency present:
- Obtain baseline cortisol level
- Give hydrocortisone 1–2 mg/kg IV

If no risk of adrenal insufficiency:
- Obtain baseline cortisol level
- ± hydrocortisone is not routine

Normal blood pressure Cold shock, SvO₂ < 70%
- Add vasodilator OR
- Type III PDE with volume loading

Low blood pressure Cold shock, SvO₂ < 70%
- Titrate volume and epinephrine

Low blood pressure Warm shock, SvO₂ ≥ 70%
- Titrate volume, norepinephrine, vasopressin

Persistent catecholamine-resistant shock:
- Measure cardiac output, and direct fluid, inotrope, vasopressor, vasodilator, and hormonal therapies to goals of (1) normal MAP-CVP, (2) CI > 3.3 and < 6.0 l/minute/m²
- If shock still **refractory**, consider ECMO (extracorporeal membrane oxygenation).

[1]Definitions: CR = capillary refill; LR = Lactated Ringers; NS = normal saline; SvO₂ = mixed venous oxygen saturation; PDE = phosphodiesterase inhibitor. **Inotropes:** Dopamine (5 to 10 mcg/kg/minute), dobutamine, milrinone, epinephrine(< 0.3 mcg/kg/minute or > 0.3 mcg/kg/minute with a vasodilator): use to ↑cardiac index (CI/reverse shock if CI < 3.3 l/minute/m² after fluid resuscitation]. **Vasopressors:** Dopamine (≥ 10 mcg/kg/minute), norepinephrine, phenylephrine, epinephrine (> 0.3 mcg/kg/minute), or vasopressin: use to ↑ systemic vascular resistance (SVR) and reverse shock if SVR < 800 dyne-sec/cm⁵/m² after fluid resuscitation]. **Vasodilators:** Nitroprusside or nitroglycerin to SVR if CI < 3.3 l/minute/m² and SVR > 1600 dyne-sec/cm⁵/m² after fluid resuscitation. **[2]**Pulmonary artery catheters are not routine in pediatrics and are generally only placed in ICU setting by experts familiar with their use.

Modified from Carcillo, J. A., & Fields, A. I. Parâmetros de prática clínica para suporte hemodinâmico a pacientes pediátricos e neonatais em choque séptico. Jornal de Pediatria, 2002; 78(6). doi:10.1590/s0021-75572002000600004. Modified from Carcillo JA, Fields AI; American College of Critical Care Medicine Task Force Committee Members. Clinical practice parameters for hemodynamic support of pediatric and neonatal patients in septic shock. *Crit Care Med.* 2002;30(6):1365-1378.

Table 18-4 Management of Febrile Neonates and Young Infants

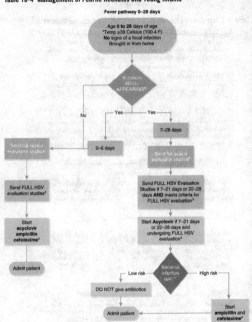

Fever pathway 0–28 days

Age 0 to 28 days of age
*Temp ≥38 Celsius (100.4 F)
No signs of a local infection
Brought in from home

Is patient
WELL-
APPEARING?

No — Yes — Yes

0–6 days   7–28 days

Send full sepsis evaluation studies²

Send FULL HSV evaluation studies³

Start
acyclovir
ampicillin
cefotaxime⁴

Admit patient

Send full sepsis evaluation studies²

Send FULL HSV Evaluation Studies if 7–21 days or 22–28 days **AND** meets criteria for FULL HSV evaluation³

Start **Acyclovir** if 7–21 days or 22–28 days and undergoing FULL HSV evaluation⁴

Bacterial infection risk?

Low risk — High risk

DO NOT give antibiotics

Start ampicillin and cefotaxime⁴

Admit patient

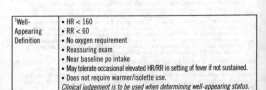

¹Well-Appearing Definition	• HR < 160
	• RR < 60
	• No oxygen requirement
	• Reassuring exam
	• Near baseline po intake
	• May tolerate occasional elevated HR/RR in setting of fever if not sustained.
	• Does not require warmer/isolette use.
	Clinical judgement is to be used when determining well-appearing status.

Table 18-4 Management of Febrile Neonates and Young Infants (*Continued*)

[2]Full Sepsis Evaluation Studies	• Catheterized urinalysis and urine culture • CSF bacterial culture, cell count, protein, glucose, Enterovirus PCR CSF, HSV PCR CSF • Blood Culture x 1 (min. 1.0 ml) • CBC with differential • Procalcitonin (IF 7–28 days) • Enterovirus PCR from plasma during peak season (June – Oct) or if CSF WBC > 13 • Chest x-ray (IF respiratory symptoms) • Respiratory viral testing (RPAN) (IF respiratory symptoms)
[3]Herpes Simplex Virus (HSV) FULL Evaluation Studies	FULL Evaluation Studies on all 0-21 days: • HSV PCR whole blood • HSV PCR CSF • HSV PCR swab of conjunctivae, nasopharynx, mouth, anus, and lesions (if present) • COMP (comprehensive metabolic panel) *If patient < 3 days of age then PCR swab will be changed to culture in the lab.* If 22–28 days old AND 1 of the following criteria: • Ill-appearing • Maternal active HSV lesions at time of delivery • Vesicles on skin exam (including scalp) • Hepatitis (elevated AST or ALT) if otherwise obtained • Abnormal neurologic status, seizure • CSF WBC > 13
[4]Medications	• Acyclovir (20 mg/kg/dose IV Q8) • Ampicillin (50 mg/kg/dose IV/IM Q6) • Cefotaxime (50 mg/kg/dose IV/IM Q8) • Consider cefepime (50 mg/kg/dose IV Q8) instead of cefotaxime if history of prolonged hospitalization (>72 hours). • Consider vancomycin (15 mg/kg/dose IV Q8) if history of MRSA.
[5]Bacterial Infection Checklist	If any Yes then considered High Risk (If lab not obtained then disregard question) • Born at less than 37 weeks gestation? • History of prior hospitalization? • Prolonged (>4 days) newborn nursery course? • Urinalysis positive for nitrites, leukocyte esterase, or WBC >5/HPF? • Is the procalcitonin elevated (>0.5 ng/mL)? • ANC > 4 K/uL? • CSF WBC > 13? • Does the child have a chronic illness? • Received antibiotics prior to this visit? • History of unexplained hyperbilirubinemia?

Pathway adapted from REVISE (Value in Inpatient Pediatrics Network, AAP) and Children s Mercy Hospital Guidelines. *Pathway based on data in febrile infants. Similar considerations may apply to hypothermic (<36C rectal) patients

Table 18-4 Management of Febrile Neonates and Young Infants (*Continued*)

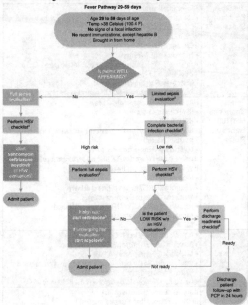

^1 Well-Appearing Definition	• HR < 160
	• RR < 60
	• No oxygen requirement
	• Reassuring exam
	• Near baseline po intake
	• May tolerate occasional elevated HR/RR in setting of fever if not sustained.
	• Does not require warmer/isolette use.
	Clinical judgement is to be used when determining well-appearing status.

Table 18-4 Management of Febrile Neonates and Young Infants (*Continued*)

[2]Sepsis Evaluation Studies	Limited Sepsis Evaluation Studies: • Catheterized urinalysis and urine culture • CBC with differential • Blood Culture x 1 (min 1.0 ml) • Procalcitonin (PCT) • Respiratory viral testing (RPAN) (IF respiratory symptoms) • Chest x-ray (IF respiratory symptoms) For Full Sepsis Evaluation, ADD: • CSF bacterial culture, cell count, protein, glucose, Enterovirus PCR CSF • Enterovirus PCR from plasma during peak season (June–Oct) or if CSF WBC >7
[3]Bacterial Infection Checklist	If any Yes then considered High Risk (If lab not obtained then disregard question) • Born at less than 37 weeks gestation? • History of prior hospitalization? • Prolonged (> 4 days) newborn nursery course? • Urinalysis positive for nitrites, leukocyte esterase, or WBC >5/HPF? • ANC > 4 K/µl? • Is the procalcitonin (PCT) elevated (>0.5 ng/ml)? • Does the child have a chronic illness? • Received antibiotics prior to this visit? • History of unexplained hyperbilirubinemia?
[4]Herpes Simplex Virus (HSV) Checklist	Perform HSV evaluation, see below, if 29–42 days old AND 1 of the following: • Ill-appearing • Maternal active HSV lesions at time of delivery • Vesicles on skin exam (including scalp) • Hepatitis (elevated AST or ALT) if otherwise obtained • Abnormal neurologic status, seizure • CSF WBC > 7 if otherwise obtained HSV Evaluation: • HSV PCR whole blood • HSV PCR CSF • HSV PCR swab of conjunctivae, nasopharynx, mouth, anus, and lesions (if present) • COMP (comprehensive metabolic panel) Up to clinician discretion to send HSV PCR CSF if > 42 days and concern for meningitis/encephalitis.

(*Continued*)

Table 18-4 Management of Febrile Neonates and Young Infants (*Continued*)

[5]Medications	• Ampicillin (50 mg/kg/dose IV/IM Q6) • Ceftriaxone (100 mg/kg x 1 in ED, then 12 hours later, start 50 mg/kg/dose IV/IM Q12) • Acyclovir (20 mg/kg/dose IV Q8) • Vancomycin (15 mg/kg/dose IV Q8) • Cefepime (50 mg/kg/dose IV Q8) Additional considerations: • If UTI is suspected, add ampicillin to cover for Enteroccocus. • If CSF WBC > 7, GP organisms on Gram stain or history of MRSA then add empiric vancomycin. • Consider cefepime instead of cefotaxime/CTX if history of prolonged hospitalization (>72 hours).
[7]Discharge Readiness Checklist	If any No admit the patient • Are the parents comfortable with monitoring their child at home? • Do the parents have reliable means of receiving communication from the hospital ED? • Can bacterial culture results be followed daily by the hospital/ED? • Can the patient follow up with their PCP in 24 hours? • Are they within 30 minutes of an ED?

Courtesy of University of Michigan--C.S. Mott Children's Hospital. Data from REVISE (Value in Inpatient Pediatrics Network, AAP); Kuppermann K, Dayan PS, Levine DA, et. al. A Clinical Prediction Rule to Identify Febrile Infants 60 Days and Younger at Low Risk for Serious Bacterial Infections. JAMA Pediatr. 2019;173(4):342-351.
*Pathway based on data in febrile infants. Similar considerations may apply to hypothermic (<36C rectal) patients.

See viral disease/testing on pages 192–194.

BACTEREMIA

Table 18-5 Fever—Occult Bacteremia (OB)

Overview: Before Hib, pneumococcal vaccine era this was primarily a concern in those aged 3–36 months with fever ≥39°C. In the pre-vaccine era, approximately 3–10% of well-appearing children <3 years old with fever without a source were found to have occult bacteremia. Now, with widespread vaccination this number has fallen to <1%.	*Definition:* Positive blood culture with no infection and well appearance. *Pathogenesis:* Enterococcus spp., *N. meningitidis*, nontype B *H. influenza*, *E. coli*, *Moraxella catarrhalis*, *Salmonella* spp. and *S. aureus* *Testing:* Routine testing and empirical antibiotic administration is not warranted in well-appearing children 3–36 months with fever without a source. New studies suggest that CRP and procalcitonin may be more accurate at identifying serious bacterial infections including bacteremia than previous markers such at WBC and absolute neutrophil count.

Modified from Bressan S, Berlese P, Mion T, et al. Bacteremia in feverish children presenting to the emergency department: a retrospective study and literature review. *Acta Paediatr.* 2012;101(3):271-277; Mahajan P, Grzybowski M, Chen X, et al. Procalcitonin as a marker of serious bacterial infections in febrile children younger than 3 years old. *Acad Emerg Med.* 2014;21(2):171-179; Hsiao AL, Baker MD. Fever in the new millennium: a review of recent studies of markers of serious bacterial infection in febrile children. *Curr Opin Pediatr.* 2005;17(1):56-61.

YALE OBSERVATION SCALE

Table 18-6 Yale Observation Scale (for Infants and Children Age 3–36 Months)[1]

Observation item	Normal (score 1 point)	Moderate impairment (score 3 points)	Severe impairment (score 5 points)
Quality of cry	Strong or none	Whimper or sob	Weak, moans, high pitch, hardly responds
Reaction to parents	Cries briefly, no crying, content	Cries off and on	Persistent cry with little response
State variation	Awake, or if asleep wakens quickly	Eyes close briefly, awake or wakens with prolonged stimulation	No arousal, falls asleep
Color	Pink	Pale extremities, acrocyanosis	Ashen, cyanotic, mottled, or pale
Hydration	Normal skin, eyes, mouth	Normal skin and eyes, mouth slightly dry	Skin doughy/tented, dry mouth, sunken eyes
Response overtures	Alert or smiles (consistently)	Alert or brief smile	No smile, anxious, dull no alerting to overtures

[1]Total ≤ 10 points = 2.7% probability of serious illness (SI); Total 11–15 points = 26% probability of SI; Total ≥ 16 points 92% probability of SI.

NEISSERIA MENINGITIDIS

Occult bacteremia from *N. meningitidis*—Rare cause of occult bacteremia and is found in only 0.03% 3–36 months with fever $\geq$ 39°C. Temperature, WBC, and neutrophil count are useless at discriminating viral syndromes from *N. meningitidis* OB.

Meningococcemia is a symptomatic blood-borne infection; 71% have fever > 38°C, 4% are < 36.8°C, 71% have rash [59% purpura or petechiae, 10% maculopapular (possibly due to misdiagnosis of rash type), pustular/bullae 1%]. The mean WBC count is 14,000 cells/mm^3 while 21% have a WBC count < 5,000; 14% have platelets < 100,000 mm^3; 55% have meningitis, 11% arthritis, 8% pneumonia. If positive culture or suspicion *N. meningitidis*, admit, IV antibiotics spinal tap. See page 155 for antibiotics and treatment of exposed. Because of this disorder, consider adding "return if any new rash" to discharge instructions for febrile patients.

Table 18-7 Evaluation of Petechial Rash[1]

Feature	Possible cause
Ill or toxic	Meningococcemia or Rocky Mountain Spotted Fever
Sick contacts	Meningococcemia, rubella, Epstein-Barr, enterovirus, hepatitis B, gonococcemia, rheumatic fever
Travel or local ticks	Rocky Mountain Spotted Fever, dengue, typhus, rat bite fever
Palpable purpura	Vasculitis and infectious
None of above	Thrombocytopenia (ITP, TTP) or other platelet disorder

[1]Listed disorders are not exhaustive, and features may be absent in many with described possible causes of petechiae.

Table 18-8 Fever and Petechiae Etiology in 190 Children Presenting to a Pediatric ED[1,2]

Organism identified		No organism found—clinical diagnosis	
N. meningitidis	7%	Viral syndrome	45%
With meningitis	4%	Otitis media	13%
Without meningitis	3%	Aseptic meningitis	3%
S. pneumoniae/H. influenzae	1%	Pneumonia	3%
Streptococcus pyogenes pharyngitis	10%	Otitis media with pneumonia	2%
RSV infection	6%	Exudative pharyngitis, partially treated sepsis, or meningitis	1% each
Other hemabsorbing virus	6%		

Table 18-8 Fever and Petechiae Etiology in 190 Children Presenting to a Pediatric ED[1,2] (Continued)

Organism identified		No organism found—clinical diagnosis	
Enterovirus or rotavirus GI tract	2%	Henoch-Schönlein purpura, Rocky Mountain Spotted	0.5% each
Enteroviral meningitis	1%	Fever, ALL	
E. coli urinary tract infection	1%	MMR vaccine reaction	1%

[1]A toxic or ill child with fever and petechiae (or meningeal signs) requires emergent IV antibiotics (see page 154) and IV fluids with blood pressure support if needed. [2]In one study, if fever and petechiae were present, 2% had bacteremia or sepsis. Well-appearing children had a 0% (0–3%, 95% confidence interval [CI]) probability of serious infection (SBI). If they had a WBC of 5–15,000 they had a 0% (0–2%, 95% CI) probability of SBI, and if they had no purpura they had 0% (0–1% 95% CI) probability of SBI. Petechiae limited to face, neck, and chest above the nipples in well-appearing children also may not need further evaluation.

Modified from Baker RC, Seguin JH, Leslie N, Gilchrist MJ, Myers MG. Fever and petechiae in children. Pediatrics. 1989;84:1051; Mandl KD, Stack AM, Fleisher GR. Incidence of bacteremia in infants and children with fever and petechiae. J Pediatr. 1997;131:398

One retrospective study proposes using the irritability, lethargy and low capillary refill (ILL) criteria for identifying children with serious bacterial infections in children who present with fever and petechiae with a sensitivity of 100% (95% CI, 48–100%); specificity 57% (37–76%).

Data from Brogan P, Raffles A. The management of fever and petechiae: making sense of rash decisions. Arch Dis Child. 2000;83(6):506–507.

Table 18-9 Pediatric Bacterial Meningitis Score

Predictors (Points)[1]	Predictive value (PV) of total score[2]	
Bacteria on gram stain (2) CSF protein ≥ 80 mg/dl (1)	Sensitivity (total score ≥ 1)	99.6–100%
Serum WBC count ≥ 10,000 cells/mm³ (1)	Sensitivity (total score ≥ 2)	87%
Seizure at or before presentation (1) CSF neutrophils ≥ 1000 cells/mm³ (1)	Negative PV (total score = 0)	> 99%

[1]CSF—cerebrospinal fluid; WBC—white blood cell. [2]Total score = 2 points for gram stain, and 1 point for each of other listed predictors. Predictive value denotes ability to diagnose bacterial meningitis. If none of the criteria are present in a child with CSF pleocytosis, the risk of bacterial meningitis is 0.1%.

Modified from Nigrovic LE, Kuppermann N, Malley R. Development and validation of a multivariable predictive model to distinguish bacterial from aseptic meningitis in children in the post-Haemophilus influenza era. Pediatrics. 2002;110:712; Dubos F, De la Rocque F, Levy C, et al; Bacterial Meningitis Study Group. Sensitivity of the bacterial meningitis score in 889 children with bacterial meningitis. J Pediatr. 2008;152:378.

TICK-BORNE DISEASE

Table 18-10 Ehrlichiosis

Human monocytic and granulocytic ehrlichiosis (HME and HGE)—a febrile illness due to *Rickettsia* transmitted by Lone Star or wood tick especially in the southeast, south central, and Midwest United States; 90% occur from April to September. Deer, livestock—hosts. Incubation is 12–14 days. Diagnose—Wright stain, antibody titer (*CDC requires compatible Hx + ≥ 1:64 titer or a fourfold change between acute and convalescent titers*). Treatment—See page 147 for disease treatment recommendations.	Features in pediatric HME	
	• Fever	100%
	• Known tick bite	82%
	• Headache/Myalgia	63%
	• ↑ Liver/Spleen	41%
	• Rash trunk + extremity macule/ papule/petechiae	66%
	• ↑ LFT	89%
	• ↓ Platelets	82%
	• ↓ WBC/Lymphocytes	69%/80%
	• ↓ Sodium	65%
	• Anemia	39%

Table 18-11 Lyme Disease

Inflammatory disease vs. multiple organs due to spirochete (*Borrelia burgdorferi*) transmitted by ticks (deer tick). Disease can be (1) *early local* 1–2 weeks (ECM/erythema chronicum migrans), red macule or papule expands to large size (mean 16 cm in adults) resolves over a week. (2) *Early disseminated* 2–12 weeks, carditis, early arthritis (mean 2.4 large joints; knee > ankle; 2 to 100,000 cells/mm³, esp. eosinophils), meningitis, multiple EM lesions. (3) *Chronic* arthritis or neuro deterioration. Diagnose by ELISA or IFA followed by more specific Western immunoblot if equivocal or positive first test. Treatment—see page 152.	Features in children	
	• ECM rash esp. at skin crease (mean adult size 16 cm)	68%
	• Flulike symptoms	64%
	• Arthritis/Arthralgia (40% > 1 joint)	59%
	• Known tick bite	49%
	• ECG changes esp. first-degree AV block	29%
	• Bell's palsy (seventh CN)	14%
	• Aseptic meningitis	4%
	• Myelitis/Neuropathy	1%

Table 18-12 Rocky Mountain Spotted Fever (RMSF)

RMSF—vasculitis due to *R. rickettsii*—most cases occur in the south Atlantic, southeast, and south central United States, although disease is widespread. Wood and dog tick transmit. 90% occur from April to September with 2/3 < 15 years old. Incubation is 2–12 days. Tests are not positive until 7–10 days. The Weil-Felix test is inaccurate and no longer used to diagnose. Instead immunofluorescence assay (IFA) or ELISA testing is often used.	Features in children
	• Headache/Myalgias/Fever
	• + Abdomen pain, diarrhea.
	• Rash (95%)—starts on wrists and ankles and spreads centrally
	• Palm/Sole rash (50–75%)
	• NO tick bite reported (40%)
	• Seizures/Meningismus
	• DIC/Shock

Table 18-12 Rocky Mountain Spotted Fever (RMSF) (*Continued*)

Treatment—Mortality is rare if treated before fifth day of illness; therefore, observe in first 2–4 days if uncertain diagnosis and well appearing. Treat based on clinical picture and not lab tests. Doxycycline is drug of choice with little concern for tooth discoloration if used for < 7–10 days (see Table 18-2 for dose). Fluoroquinolones and chloramphenicol are possible alternatives. In endemic areas, many physicians treat empirically if combination of fever, headache, rash.	• WBC count normal or ↓ Platelets, ↓ Hb • ↓ Sodium, ↑ BUN, ↑ LFTs • Biopsy immunohistology IFA 70% sensitive/100% specific • ELISA/IF antibody tests turn + 7–10 days after onset

Table 18-13 Southern Tick-Associated Rash Illness (STARI)

	Features in children
The exact cause of STARI is unknown, although it may be due to *Borrelia lonestari* with the Lone Star tick serving as a vector centralized to southeast, south central United States. Peak incidence is earlier than Lyme (May to June). Symptoms are similar to Lyme disease although less severe at the time of diagnosis and more rapid clearing of symptoms after treatment. Tests for Lyme disease are usually negative, and there is no definitive diagnostic test. *Treatment*: Many experts recommend doxycycline, amoxicillin, or cefuroxime treatment.	• Erythema chronicum migrans-like rash (smaller) • Rash: Less pruritus, less tender than Lyme • Regional lymph nodes • Flulike symptoms occur • Arthralgias are common • Late complications are uncommon (e.g., arthritis, neurologic deficits)

TICK BITES

Tick bite—In one study, a single doxycycline dose given to those with tick bites in Lyme-endemic areas, decreased erythema migrans from 3.2% to 0.4%. *Dose*: 4 mg/kg PO (maximum 200 mg). Risks, benefits, side effects esp. in those ≤ 8 years must be considered.

Source. Data from Nadelman RB, Nowakowski J, Fish D, et al.; Tick Bite Study Group. Prophylaxis with single-dose doxycycline for the prevention of Lyme disease after and Ixodes scapularis tick bite. *N Engl J Med.* 2001;345(2):79-84.

Tick paralysis—A toxin produced by many different ticks (>60 species identified) inhibits presynaptic acetylcholine release. Exposure to tick occurs 5–10 days prior to symptoms. The most common tick locations are the scalp, behind an ear, neck, and groin. In the United States, 82% are younger than 8 years old, and 64% are females. Rapid ascending paralysis occurs over 12–36 hours. Bulbar (eye muscle) involved early. Focal weakness and pupil dilation are common in Australia (not US ticks). Fifty percent have paresthesias with normal sensory exam, and patients are often misdiagnosed as Guillain-Barré. In one series, all cases occurred from March to June (in the

United States). Removal of tick is curative, although Australian form of disease may worsen more than 48 hours after removal and may be amenable to antitoxin.

Source: Data from Edlow JA, McGillicuddy DC. Tick paralysis. *Infect Dis Clin North Am.* 2008;22(3):397-413.

Table 18-14 Tick Removal—Procedure

- Apply gloves ± inject small wheal of lidocaine + epinephrine directly beneath tick.
- Applying petroleum jelly, alcohol, fingernail polish, or hot match to underside of tick may cause regurgitation (of organisms) and should be avoided.
- Using blunt tweezers, grasp the tick as close as possible to the skin.
- Pull slowly in a firm perpendicular direction, do not squeeze or rotate tick.
- Cleanse area thoroughly after procedure with disinfectant.
- Person performing procedure should thoroughly wash hands afterward.
- Place tick into alcohol or flush down the toilet.

RESPIRATORY TRACT INFECTIONS

Table 18-15 AAP-AAFP Acute Otitis Media (AOM) Guidelines

Certain diagnosis of AOM requires the following:
• Presence of a middle ear effusion (MEE) AND one of the following
• Moderate to severe bulging of the tympanic membrane or otorrhea not due to acute otitis externa OR
• Mild bulging of the tympanic membrane with ≤48 hours otalgia OR intense erythema of the tympanic membrane

Criteria for initial antibiotics or observation in children with AOM		
Age	Severe signs and symptoms[1]	Mild signs and symptoms[2]
<6 months	Antibiotics	Antibiotics
6 months–2 years	Antibiotics	Antibiotics if bilateral; if unilateral antibiotics vs. OBS[3]
≥2 years	Antibiotics	Antibiotics vs. OBS for either bilateral or unilateral disease[3]

Antibiotic recommendations
First line if no antibiotics in the past 30 days and no concurrent purulent conjunctivitis OR if observation failure at 48–72 hours: Amoxicillin 80–90 mg/kg/day, OR if nontype I penicillin (PCN) allergy: Cefdinir 14 mg/kg/day or divided BID, cefuroxime 30 mg/kg/day divided BID, cefpodoxime 10 mg/kg/day divided BID OR if type I PCN allergy[4]: azithromycin, clarithromycin. *If antibiotic failure at 48–72 hours of treatment:* Augmentin 90 mg/kg/day, OR if nontype I PCN allergy, ceftriaxone 50 mg/kg IM × 3 days, OR if type I PCN allergy: clindamycin 10 mg/kg/dose three times per day

Table 18-15 AAP-AAFP Acute Otitis Media (AOM) Guidelines (*Continued*)

If recent antibiotics in the past 30 days or concurrent purulent conjunctivitis: Augmentin 90 mg/kg/day, OR if nontype I PCN allergy, ceftriaxone 50 mg/kg IM × 1 to 3 days. *If antibiotic failure:* Ceftriaxone 50 mg/kg IM × 3 days, OR tympanocentesis plus clindamycin.	

[1]Moderate/severe otalgia ≥ 48 hours; or T ≥ 39°C. [2]Mild otalgia, T < 39°C. [3]Observation based on shared decision making with 48- to 72-hour follow-up. [4]Type I allergy (hypersensitivity) = urticaria or anaphylaxis.

Modified from Lieberthal AS, Carroll AE, Chonmaitree T, et al. The diagnosis and management of acute otitis media. *Pediatrics.* 2013;131:e964; Schilder AG, Marom T, Bhutta MF, et al. Panel 7: Otitis media: treatment and complications. *Otolatyngol Head Neck Surg.* 2017;156:s88–s105.

Table 18-16 CDC/AAP Guidelines for Judicious Use of Antibiotics (Abx) in Pediatric Respiratory Infections

"Cold"	• Mucopurulent rhinitis alone is not indication for Abx. See sinusitis, which follows.
AOM and otitis media with effusion (OME)	• Diagnosis of AOM requires middle ear effusion and signs or symptoms of acute local or systemic illness. • Uncomplicated AOM may treat with 5–7 days of Abx if > 2 years old. • Abx are not indicated for OME unless effusion persists ≥ 3 months. • Abx prophylaxis is reserved for control of recurrent AOM (defined as ≥ 3 distinct/well-documented episodes in 6 months or ≥ 4 in 12 months).
Pharyngitis	• Guidelines recommend group A strep (GAS) testing with treatment decision based on results. • Testing should be performed on patients with ≥ 2 criteria (see table that follows). • Children under the age of 3 should not be routinely tested. • Empiric treatment may be considered for symptomatic children with confirmed GAS exposure.
Sinusitis	• Clinical diagnosis of bacterial sinusitis requires persistent or worsening upper respiratory signs and symptoms (e.g., rhinosinusitis/cough >10–14 days) or more severe features (temp ≥ 39°C, facial swelling or pain, and purulent discharge for ≥3 days). • Radiograph indications: recurrence, suspect complication, diagnosis unclear. CT is reserved if surgery is being considered. • See CDC antibiotic recommendations on Table 18-15.

Modified from Hersh AL; AAP Committee on Infectious Disease. Principles of judicious antibiotic prescribing for upper respiratory tract infections in pediatrics. *Pediatrics.* 2013;132(6):1146-1154.

Table 18-17 Clinical Scoring for Group A Streptococcal Pharyngitis[1]

Individual clinical features	Individual points
Fever > 38.3°C (101°F)	1
Age 5–15 years	1
November–May presentation	1
Cervical adenopathy	1
URI absent (i.e., cough, rhinorrhea, congestion)	1
Pharyngitis (i.e., tonsillar erythema, hypertrophy, or exudate)	1

[1]Total Points: 0–1 (0% group A strep), 2–3 (20% strep), 4 (42%), 5 (63%), 6 (75%). See treatment, page 157.

Modified from Wald ER, Green MD, Schwartz B, et al. A streptococcal score card revisited. *Pediatr Emerg Care.* 1998;14:109.

PNEUMONIA

Bordetella pertussis mimics *Chlamydia pneumonitis*, but has a paroxysmal, inspiratory "whoop" (may be absent in children younger than 6 months). Prolonged coughing attacks may lead to cyanosis, emesis, hypoxia. In one study, the mean age was 55 days, mean WBC count was 20,000/μl while 90% having an absolute lymphocyte count > 9,400.[1] In another study, children with sicker disease had higher mean white blood cell counts (>30,000), higher heart rates and respiratory rates compared to children with less severe illness from pertussis.[2]

Data from [1]Guinto-Ocompo H, Bennett JE, Attia MW. Predicting pertussis in infants. *Pediatr Emerg Care.* 2008;24:16-20. [2]Murray EL, Nieves D, Bradley JS, et al. Characteristics of severe Bordetella pertussis infection among infants ≤90 days of age admitted to Pediatric Intensive Care Units–Southern California, September 2009-June 2011. *J Pediatr Infect Dis Soc.* 2013;2:1-6.

Chlamydia—3–16 weeks. First rhinorrhea, then staccato cough, tachypnea, rales, or wheeze. 95% afebrile, 50% have concurrent/prior conjunctivitis. *Mycoplasma*—low-grade fever, malaise, headache, nonproductive cough lasting weeks. It is responsible for 9–21% of school-aged pneumonia, may occur in epidemics with little seasonal variation. *Pneumococcus* and *H. flu* are typically associated with an abrupt onset of high fever and dyspnea, and may be preceded by a viral URI. *Tuberculosis* is associated with subacute cough, night sweats, and weight loss.

Table 18-18 Most Common Cause of Pneumonia Based on Age[1]

Age	Bacterial	Viral	Other
<3 weeks	Most common • Group B streptococcus • E. coli • Listeria Less common • S. pneumoniae • S. aureus • Anaerobes	• CMV • RSV • hMPV • HSV • Rubella	• B. pertussis • C. trachomatis • Mycobacterium hominis • Treponema pallidum • Ureaplasma urealyticum
3 weeks–3 months	• S. pneumoniae • S. aureus • H. influenzae (nontypable)	• RSV • hMPV • Parainfluenza • Adenovirus • Influenza	• B. pertussis • C. trachomatis
3 months–5 years	• S. pneumoniae • S. pyogenes • S. aureus	• RSV • hMPV • Parainfluenza • Adenovirus • Influenza	• Mycoplasma pneumoniae • Chlamydia pneumoniae • Mycobacterium tuberculosis
>5 years	• S. pneumoniae • S. pyogenes • S. aureus	• hMPV • Influenza • Adenovirus	• M. pneumoniae • C. pneumoniae • M. tuberculosis

[1]CMV–cytomegalovirus; RSV–respiratory syncytial virus; hMPV–human metapneumovirus; HSV–herpes simplex virus.

No single physical exam finding can differentiate pneumonia from other respiratory illnesses. However, hypoxia < 96% and increased work of breathing (grunting, nasal flaring, or retractions) are more suggestive of pneumonia compared to respiratory rate, fever, or auscultatory findings.

Modified from Shah S, Bachur RG, Simel DL. The rational clinical examination. *JAMA.* 2017;318(5): 462-471; Rambaud-Althaus C, Althaus F, Genton B, et al. Clinical features for diagnosis of pneumonia in children younger than 5 years: a systematic review and meta-analysis. *Lancet Infect Dis.* 2015;15:439-450.

Table 18-19 Pneumonia Admission Criteria—British Thoracic Society Guidelines[1,2]

Evaluation	Admit criteria
Pulse oximetry for all admissions	O_2 sat < 93% (some use < 91–92%)
CXR not routine if disease mild, uncomplicated[1]	RR > 60–70/minute (>45–50 child)

(Continued)

Table 18-19 Pneumonia Admission Criteria—British Thoracic Society
Guidelines[1,2] (*Continued*)

Evaluation	Admit criteria
Labs not useful for bacteria vs. viral disease	Dyspnea, apnea, or grunting
Recommend blood culture if suspect bacteria[3]	Poor intake, significant dehydration
Obtain viral antigen studies < 18 months (inpatients)	Family can't observe/supervise
Reevaluate at 48–72 hours if fever persists	Premie infant, or age < 2–3 months

[1]Guidelines for uncomplicated disease in healthy patients (judgment can override this); many US experts
routinely obtain CXR. [2]See pages 158–159 for therapy, also consider admit if failed oral antibiotics. [3]Proven
useless for uncomplicated community acquired disease, consider blood culture if immunocompromised or
ill (e.g., ICU admit).

UTI

Table 18-20 Urinary Tract Infections (UTI) and Pyelonephritis

Organisms in neonates: *E. coli* 74%, *Klebsiella* 7%, *Pseudomonas* 7%, *Proteus* 4%. In older infants/children: *E. coli* is most common. *Proteus* and *Pseudomonas* are more common if hospitalized, recurrent UTI, or male.	Age	UTI risk[1]
	0–2 months	7.5%
	2–24 months	4.1%
	2–5 years	1.7%

[1]If fever present.

Table 18-21 Risk Factors for UTI[1]

- Females < 2 years old
- Fever ≥ 2 days
- No alternate source for fever
- White/Caucasian
- Temperature ≥ 39°C
- Prior urinary infection or anatomic abnormality
- Males < 6 months old (or < 12 months, uncircumcised)

[1]In females, the presence of ≥ 2 of the following five criteria identified 99% (94–100%) with a UTI: white
race, age < 12 months, temperature ≥ 39°C, no other source for fever, or fever ≥ 2 days.

Data from Gorelick MH, Hoberman A, Kearney D, Wald E, Shaw KN. Validation of a decision rule identifying febrile young girls at high risk for urinary tract infection. *Pediatr Emerg Care*. 2003;19:162-164.
doi:10.1097/01.pec.0000081238.98249.40.

Table 18-22 Predictive Value of Urinalysis (UA) in Detecting UTI[1]

Urinalysis feature	Sensitivity	Negative predictive value
Any WBC/high power field (hpf)	77%	97%
≥ 5 WBC/hpf	43–84%	90–98%
Any bacteria	86–93%	99%

Table 18-22 Predictive Value of Urinalysis (UA) in Detecting UTI[1] (*Continued*)

Urinalysis feature	Sensitivity	Negative predictive value
Leukocyte esterase, nitrates, or ≥ 5 WBC/hpf	75–98%	85–99%
Positive gram stain for bacteria	94–99%	99%

[1]93% of culture positive bag urines are false positives; therefore, catheterized urine is preferred for those still in diapers. A UA is insensitive for UTI; therefore, culture all aged < 3 years. Nitrate positive organisms = *E. coli*, *Proteus*, *Klebsiella*, *Enterobacter*, *Salmonella* (not *S. saprophyticus*, *Pseudomonas*, or *Enterococcus*).

Table 18-23 Management Options for Urinary Tract Infections

Admit	• ≤2–3 months old, obstruction, high-grade reflux, dehydration, vomiting, toxicity, nephrolithiasis, or immunocompromised
IV antibiotics	• Ceftriaxone 50–75 mg/kg/dose IV (do not use <28 days old) OR • Cefotaxime (neonates) 50 mg/kg/dose IV every 8 hours–every 12 hours OR • Gentamicin 2–2.5 mg/kg/dose IV every 8 hours + ampicillin 50 mg/kg/dose IV every 6 hours (esp. if gram-positive bacteria) OR piperacillin-tazobactam IV 240–300 mg/kg/day (piperacillin component) divided every 6 hours–every 8 hours (max 16 g/day)
Oral antibiotics	• Cephalexin 50–100 mg/kg/day PO divided every 6 hours – every 8 hours (max 4 g/day), OR cefixime 8 mg/kg/day PO divided every 12 hours–every 24 hours (max 400 mg/day), OR sulfamethoxazole-trimethoprim 6–12 mg/kg/day (trimethoprim component) PO divided every 12 hours (max 160 mg TMP/dose), OR amoxicillin-clavulanate 20–40 mg/kg/day PO divided every 8 hours, OR nitrofurantoin (Furadantin, Macrodantin) 5–7 mg/kg/day PO divided every 6 hours, nitrofurantoin (Macrobid-adolescents) 100 mg PO every 12 hours. Treat for 14 days if fever/toxic, 7–14 days if no fever and no toxicity; see Table 18-2
Urinary tract evaluation	• No clinical response in first 48 hours: urinary tract US/CT (to exclude abscess/obstruction) + voiding cystourethrogram (VCUG) or radionuclide cystography (RNC) at earliest convenience. VCUG preferred in males to assesses urethra for posterior valves. If nontoxic or doing well, VCUG or RNC at earliest convenience. • Continue antibiotics while awaiting the previously mentioned study. Radionuclide renal scans/DMSA and CT will identify acute changes from pyelonephritis or renal scarring. Their exact role in aiding management of a child with UTI is still undefined.

VIRAL RESPIRATORY DISEASE AND TESTING

Table 18-24 Cause of Acute Viral Respiratory Infections ≤ 5–7 Years

Virus	%	Virus	%
Rhinovirus (Picornavirus)	9–52	Influenza	2–7
Respiratory syncytial virus	7–60	Adenovirus	2–9
Human metapneumovirus	3–19	Coronavirus	3–16
Parainfluenza	3–11	Bocavirus	2–19
Multiple viruses	7–22		

Modified from Fillatre A, Francois C, Segard C, et al. Epidemiology and seasonality of acute respiratory infections in hospitalized children over four consecutive years (2012–2016). *J Clin Virol.* 2018;102:27-31; Arbefeuille S, Ferrieri P. Epidemiologic analysis of respiratory viral infections mainly in hospitalized children and adults in a Midwest university medical center after the implementation of a 14-virus multiplex nucleic acid amplification test. *Am J Clin Pathol.* 2017;147:43-49; Wishaupt JO, van der Ploeg T, de Groot R, et al. Single and multiple viral respiratory infections in children: disease and management cannot be related to a specific pathogen. *BMC Infect Dis.* 2017;17:62; Berry M, Gamieldien J, Fielding BC. Identification of new respiratory viruses in the new millennium. *Viruses.* 2015;7:996-1019.

Table 18-25 Comprehensive Respiratory Viral Panel[1] (6–78 hours turnaround time)

Virus	Sensitivity[2] (%)	Specificity (%)
Adenovirus	96.4	99.7
Coronavirus (299E)	82.4	100
Coronavirus (HKU1)	100	100
Coronavirus (NL63)	100	99.7
Coronavirus (OC43)	100	99.4
Influenza A	96.8	100
Influenza A (H1N1)	100	100
Influenza A (H1)	100	100
Influenza A (H3)	100	99.4
Influenza B	41	100
Metapneumovirus	93.3	100
Parainfluenza 1	93.3	100
Parainfluenza 2	63.6	100
Parainfluenza 3	100	100
Parainfluenza 4	100	100
Rhinovirus/Enterovirus	100	98
RSV A	100	99.7
RSV B	95.5	100

[1]Data for the Luminex Molecular Diagnostics xTAG RVP Fast Assay. [2]Rapid tests for these viruses (esp. influenza and RSV) are < 50–90% sensitive.

Modified from Pabbaraju K, Wong S, Tokaryk KL, et al. Comparison of the Luminex xTAG Respiratory Viral Panel with xTAG Respiratory Viral Panel Fast for diagnosis of respiratory virus infections. *J Clin Microbiol.* 2011;49(5):1738-1744.

Table 18-26 Seasonal Variation in Respiratory Viruses (North America, Excluding Tropics)

Jan	Feb	Mar	Apr	May	Jun	Jul	Aug	Sep	Oct	Nov	Dec
RSV											RSV
Influenza											Influenza
Corona virus (SARS)											SARS
Human metapneumovirus (year-round, slightly more common in winter)											
Adenovirus (year-round, more common later winter to June)											
		Parainfluenza [1]					Parainfluenza [2,3]				
		Rhinovirus									

CORONAVIRUS (AND SEVERE ACUTE RESPIRATORY SYNDROME/SARS)

This is the second leading cause of the common cold after the rhinoviruses. Subtype caused 2002 outbreak of SARS. SARS incubation period is 2–7 days (max reported 14 days). In SARS, severe illness can occur with fever, hypoxia, cough, dyspnea, and pneumonia. Serum WBC often <3,500 cells/ml and lymphocytes <1,000 cell/ml. Diagnose via antibody testing, PCR, and viral culture. Low Na, K, and high CK, LDH, ALT, AST may occur. CXR = interstitial infiltrate or diffuse patchy consolidation; effusions, nodes are rare.

Treatment: Anecdotal reports indicate that steroids plus ribavirin, or Tamiflu, or lopinavir/ritonavir may be useful. Interferon may also have an anti-SARS effect.

INFLUENZA (FLU)

Influenza is a highly contagious viral infection. The prior season's subtypes of A: H1N1, H3N2, and influenza B are used to make the seasonal vaccine. Vaccination is 79–90% protective (within 2 weeks). One H1N1 subtype (formerly "swine" flu) caused most cases in 2009 with high mortality in the very young and unhealthy. H5N1 (bird flu) sporadically causes serious illness (esp. Asia).

Clinical: Compared to the common cold, flu has more abrupt onset, headaches, higher temps, severe cough, myalgias, chest pain, fatigue with less rhinorrhea, and sneezing. The triad of headache, cough, and pharyngitis in children predicts flu with 80% sensitivity, 81% specificity. If high-risk medical condition, pneumonia, respiratory distress, history of influenza B, admission is usually warranted. Vomiting and diarrhea are more common with H1N1 than seasonal influenza.

Table 18-27 Accuracy of Antigen-Based Rapid Diagnostic Assays—Influenza

Tests	Sensitivity[1]	Specificity
Direct fluorescent antibody	62%	98%
Indirect immunofluorescent antibody	50–75%	95–97%
Optical immunoassay	71%	82%

[1]Sensitivity of rapid tests for H1N1 was only 10–70% in 2009.

Modified from Uyeki TM. Influenza diagnosis and treatment in children: a review on clinically useful tests and antiviral treatment for influenza. *Pediatr Infect Dis J.* 2003;22(2):164-177.

Diagnosis: CDC recommends diagnostic testing if hospitalized, or if results will aid in making decisions regarding clinical care, infection control, or managing close contacts. The most accurate is a real-time reverse transcription polymerase chain reaction (rRT-PCR), which can take days to receive results.

Complications: Severe viral pneumonia with hypoxia or bacterial superinfection 3–7 days after developing influenza can occur. Important bacterial pathogens are *S. pneumonia* (common in the 2009 season) and *S. aureus*. Meningitis and encephalitis can also occur. Myositis (esp. influenza B) causes severe calf pain and high CK levels. Rhabdomyolysis occurs in < 5% of myositis cases.

Source: Data from Agyeman P, Duppenthaler A, Heininger U, Aebi C. Influenza-associated myositis in children. *Infection.* 2004;32:199.

Treatment: See pages 151–152 for oral and IV antivirals and www.cdc.gov for updates. The CDC does NOT recommend relying on results of a rapid flu test for treating ill or high-risk patients. Treatment is generally indicated if the child is younger than 2 years (CDC states age younger than 5 years is high risk with the highest risk being in children under 2 years), adults 65 years and older, pregnant women up to 2 weeks before delivery, the chronically ill (asthma, heart failure, chronic lung disease), those with weak immune systems (diabetes, HIV, immunosuppressants), or those on long-term aspirin therapy (if younger than 19 years old). Also treat those who are admitted to the hospital.

RESPIRATORY SYNCYTIAL VIRUS (RSV)

The most common cause of bronchiolitis. See pages 267–268 for details regarding bronchiolitis management. Test high-risk patients (e.g., congenital heart disease, chronic lung disease, prematurity).

Table 18-28 Accuracy of Antigen-Based Rapid Diagnostic Assays in RSV[1]

Test	Sensitivity	Specificity
Direct/indirect fluorescent antibody	93–98%	92–97%
Enzyme linked immunoassay	59–97%	75–100%
Direct immunoassay	93%	91%
Optical immunoassay	88–95%	97–100%

[1]Admitted ill patients might benefit from ribavirin (controversial). Prophylactic palivizumab (Synagis), if high risk during RSV season.

Modified from Henrickson K, Hall C. Diagnostic assays for respiratory syncytial virus disease. *Pediatr Infect Dis J.* 2007;26:S36.

19 ■ KAWASAKI DISEASE

Overview: Kawasaki disease (KD) is an acute vasculitis of unknown origin. It leads to cardiac complications in 25% of untreated cases and is the most common cause of acquired heart disease in children. The earliest sign is high fever (often $\geq 40°C$) for up to 10 days. KD is characterized by an initial necrotizing arteritis, followed by subacute/chronic vasculitis, and finally luminal fibroblastic proliferation.

PHASES OF KAWASAKI DISEASE

- *Acute phase* (0–2 weeks from onset): Fever, rash, conjunctivitis, nodes, mucosal edema, ± myocarditis
- *Subacute phase* (2–8 weeks): Arthritis, epidermal desquamation (usually begins in periungual region), possibility of cardiac thrombi/aneurysm forming
- *Convalescent phase* (up to 2 years): Risk of coronary aneurysm

Table 19-1 Diagnostic Criteria[1,2]

Fever lasting at least 5 days without other source, and at least four of the following:
• Bilateral bulbar, nonexudative conjunctival injection (often spares limbus)
• Mucous membrane changes (e.g., injected pharynx, strawberry tongue or redness, fissuring, and crusting of lips)
• Edema or erythema of palms or soles (desquamation in subacute phase)
• Rash (polymorphous and truncal)
• Cervical adenopathy, with at least one node > 1.5 cm (least common feature)

[1]Other *nondiagnostic* features: sleep disturbances (90%), urethritis and sterile pyuria (75%), uveitis/iritis (80%), arthralgias/arthritis (~30%), or hemolytic uremic syndrome (rare). [2]*Incomplete or atypical KD*: If 2 or 3 criteria with fever ≥ 5 days OR infants with unexplained fever ≥ 7 days. Measure CRP and ESR, if CRP ≥ 3.0 mg/dl or ESR ≥ 40 mm/hour, then obtain serum albumin, CBC, serum transaminase and urine. If ≥ 3 of following labs are present, diagnose KD plus treat and perform echocardiogram: albumin ≤ 3 g/dl, anemia (for age), WBC > 15,000/mm^3, high ALT, urinalysis ≥ 10 WBCs/hpf, platelets $\geq 450,000/$ mm^3 (> 7 days from onset); if < 3 labs are present, obtain echo. If echo+, treat as KD. If echo negative, consider serial examination and labs, repeat echo, or consult KD expert.
Modified from McCrindle BW, Rowley AH, Newburger JW, et al. Diagnosis, treatment, and long-term management of kawasaki disease: a scientific statement for health professionals from the American Heart Association. *Circulation.* 2017;135(17):e927-e999.

DIAGNOSTIC TESTS

- Elevated platelet count during (subacute) thrombosis stage, normal acutely
- Leukocytosis, with left shift, normochromic/normocytic anemia, CRP and ESR elevation
- Urine—Moderate sterile pyuria (avoid catheterization, can be urethral in origin), occasional bilirubinuria due to gallbladder hydrops
- CXR—Cardiomegaly in up to 30%, electrocardiogram (ECG) in first week: low voltage, ST depression; second to third week: PR and QT prolongation, ST elevation

TREATMENT

- *Gamma globulin*: Administer 2 g/kg IV over 10–12 hours as a single infusion (10–20% will be refractory to IVIG).
- *Aspirin*: 80–100 mg/kg/day PO or PR divided four times per day until 14th day of illness, then 3–5 mg/kg PO daily until 6–8 weeks after onset. If coronary artery aneurysm present on echocardiogram, continuation of aspirin > 8 weeks may be indicated.
- *Obtain echocardiogram and ECG* on presentation. Repeat in 14, 21, and 60 days.

20 ■ INBORN ERRORS OF METABOLISM

Table 20-1 Specific Inborn Errors of Metabolism (IEM), by Biochemical Features[1]

Metabolic acidosis	Serum NH₃	Glucose	IEM type
↔	↔	↔	Nonketotic hyperglycinemia
↔	↑	↔	*Citrulline normal* (transient hyperammonemia of newborn or hyperornithinemia, hyperammonemia, and homocitrullinuria [HHH]). **Urea cycle disorders** *low citrulline* (↓ ornithine trans-carbamylase or ↓ carbamyl phosphate synthetase), *mild ↑ citrulline* (↓ argininosuccinate lyase), ↑ *citrulline* (citrullinemia)
↑	↑	↓	**Fatty acid oxidation:** Carnitine transferase deficiencies (NK), medium/very long chain acyl CoA dehydrogenase deficiencies (NK). **Organic acidemia:** Glutaric acidemia type II (K), methylmalonic acidemia (K,L), propionic acidemia (K,L), congenital lactic acidosis (K,L)
↑	↑	↔	**Organic acidemia:** beta-ketothiolase deficiency (K)
↑	↑	↑	**Organic acidemias:** Isovaleric acidemia (K,L), methylmalonic acidemia (K,L), propionic acidemia (K,L)
↑	↔	↔	**Organic acidemia:** Isovaleric acidemia (K,L)
↑	↔	↓	**Carbohydrate metabolism:** Fructose 1,6 diphosphatase deficiency (K,L). **Glycogen storage type:** I (L), III (K). **Amino aciduria:** Maple syrup urine disease (early onset), glutaric aciduria type I

[1] *MA:* ↑ metabolic acidosis with anion gap vs. ↔ no metabolic acidosis; NH₃: ↑ hyperammonemia vs. ↔ normal ammonia; Glu: ↑ hyperglycemia vs. ↔ normoglycemia vs. ↓ hypoglycemia; K—ketotic; NK—nonketotic; L—lactic acidosis.

TYPICAL PRESENTATIONS

Hyperammonemic disorders—Neonatal catastrophe, seizures, ↓ feeding, loss of tone, recurrent coma, vomiting, lethargy after high-protein food, FTT, ataxia, clinical improvement with IV fluids, developmental delay, growth failure
Organic acidemias—Neonatal catastrophe, recurrent coma, developmental delay, growth failure, liver failure after virus, distinctive odors (e.g., maple syrup, sweaty sock, musty)

Table 20-2 Management

Evaluation	• Blood—Glucose, CBC, electrolytes, Ca, LFTs, bilirubin, NH_3, quantitative amino acids, lactate, pyruvate, carnitine, fatty acids • Urine—Ketone bodies, reducing substances, protein, organic acids, galactose • CSF (undiagnosed neonates)—Glucose, protein, cell count, microscopy, lactate, amino acids
Catabolism	• Reverse catabolism with IV fluids (10% dextrose plus age appropriate electrolytes at $1.5\times$ maintenance); intralipids for severe presentations
Precipitant	• Search for/treat precipitant (e.g., infection) and coexisting hypoglycemia
Acidosis	• Liberal $NaHCO_3$ due to ongoing acid production + dialysis • For specific organic acidemias: B_{12} 1 mg IM (methylmalonic acidemia) + biotin 10 mg PO or NG (multiple carboxylase deficiency), thiamine 25–100 mg PO (MSUD), folic acid 1–5 mg PO (methylmalonic acidemia with homocystinuria), vitamins C and K (primary lactic acidosis due to electron transport defect), glycine (isovaleric acidemia), and carnitine ($\downarrow$ carnitine)
Hyperammonemia	• If urea cycle defect (NH_3 with no acids): (1) arginine HCl 6 ml/kg of 10% solution IV over 90 minutes (citrullinemia, argininosuccinic aciduria), (2) sodium benzoate and sodium phenylacetate (Ammonul) for OTC/CPS deficiency) • Dialysis for severe/recalcitrant cases

RENAL DISORDERS

Key history: Unexplained fever, vomiting, and diarrhea (pre-renal), preceding history of streptococcal infection (pharyngitis, impetigo), strenuous exercise, bloody diarrhea (HUS), joint/rash (HSP), edema, medications, and foods.
Urinalysis: False + dipstick for blood occur with betadine and ascorbic acid. RBC casts or dysmorphic RBCs suggest *glomerular disease*. Infants younger than 3 months old cannot concentrate urine well; therefore, specific gravity is unreliable at this age.

CAUSES OF RED URINE

Hematuria, alcaptonuria, bilirubinemia, phenazopyridine, phenothiazines, ibuprofen, L-dopa, phenolphthalein, methyldopa, adriamycin, deferoxamine, phenytoin, quinine, sulfa, chloroform, naphthalene, oxalic acid, anilines, food color, beets, blueberries, rhubarb, fava beans, hemoglobinuria or myoglobinuria (heme + dipstick with no RBCs), porphyrins, red diaper syndrome (*Serratia*), tyrosinosis

DIFFERENTIAL DIAGNOSIS OF HEMATURIA

- **Extrarenal disorders:** Coagulation disorders, salicylates, sickle cell disease/trait
- **Renal**
  - **Extraglomerular:** Hemorrhagic cystitis, trauma, nephrolithiasis, familial hypercalciuria, nephritis, hydronephrosis, polycystic kidneys, renal vein thrombosis, papillary necrosis, hemangiomas, tumor (e.g., Wilm's), foreign body, posterior urethral valves, ureteropelvic junction obstruction, renal tuberculosis
  - **Glomerular:** Glomerulonephritis (acute, rapidly progressive, recurrent macroscopic, chronic and post-streptococcal), IgA nephropathy, Alport's syndrome, exercise, familial benign hematuria, focal glomerulosclerosis
- **Systemic:** Allergy, hepatitis B antigenemia, endocarditis, cardiac shunt or valve, HSP, HUS, polyarteritis

Table 21-1 Normal Bladder Volume and Normal Plasma Creatinine (PCr)

Bladder volume estimate	• < *1 year old*: Weight (kg) × 10 ml • > *1 year old*: (age in years + 2) × 30 ml
Plasma creatinine estimate	• *Males*: PCr (mg/dl) = 0.35 + (0.025 × age in years) • *Females*: PCr (mg/dl) = 0.35 + (0.018 × age in years)

Table 21-2 Differentiating Between Causes of Renal Failure

Test	Prerenal	Renal	Postrenal
Urine sodium	< 20	> 40	> 40
Fractional excretion of sodium (FE_{Na})[1]	< 1	> 2	> 2
Renal failure index (RFI)[2]	< 1	> 2	> 2
Urine osmolality	> 500	< 300	< 400
Urine/serum creatinine ratio	> 40	< 20	< 20
Serum BUN/creatinine ratio	> 20	< 10–20	< 10–20
Renal size by ultrasound	Normal	Normal	Normal or ↑hydronephrosis or obstruction
Radionuclide renal scan	↓Uptake ↓excretion	Uptake OK ↓excretion	Uptake OK ↓excretion

[1]FE_{Na} = 100 × (urine Na^+/plasma Na^+)/(urine creatinine/plasma creatinine). Normal FE_{Na} is 1–2%, except under 2 months when FE_{Na} up may be to 5%. [2]RFI = (urine Na^+)/(urine creatinine/serum creatinine).

22 ■ NEUROLOGY

Figure 22-1 Neurology

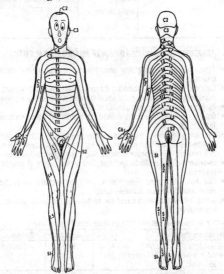

Motor level	Motor function
C4	Spontaneous breathing
C5	Shoulder shrug
C6	Elbow flexion
C7	Elbow extension
C8/T1	Finger flexion
T1–T12	Intercostal and abdominal muscles

Motor level	Motor function
L1/L2	Hip flexion
L3	Hip adduction
L4	Hip abduction
L5	Great toe dorsiflexion
S1/S2	Foot plantar flexion
S2–S4	Rectal tone

Table 22-1 Assessment of Coma and Altered Level of Consciousness

Differential diagnosis of coma and altered LOC, mnemonic TIPS-AEIOU	Trauma or tumor	Abuse or alcohol
	Infection/ intussusception	Encephalopathy, endocrine, or electrolytes
	Poisons	Insulin/hypoglycemia or inborn metabolic error
	Sepsis, seizure, or shock	Opiates
		Uremia

TREATMENT OF INFANT/CHILD WITH AN ALTERED MENTAL STATUS

- Assess airway and breathing (immobilizing cervical spine if possible trauma).
- Consider endotracheal intubation if poor or labored respiratory effort, diminished airway reflexes, suspicion of elevated ICP, or severe hypoxemia.
- Assess pulse oximetry, and administer 100% oxygen.
- Obtain rapid glucose measurement, or administer glucose (dosage, Table 11-3).
- Consider naloxone 0.1 mg/kg/dose; repeat every 2–3 minutes if needed (children younger than 5 years or <20 kg). Dose 2 mg/dose; repeat every 2–3 minutes if no response (children older than 5 years or >20 kg).
- Measure child's length to facilitate dosing and sizing of equipment (pages 5-6).
- Complete vital signs: Temperature (obtained rectally), respirations, pulse, and BP. Perform complete exam.
- Direct further evaluation based on the previous measures, history, and examination.

Table 22-2 Normal Neonatal/Infant Reflexes Appearance/Disappearance

Reflex (description)	Appears	Disappears
Moro—Lift head 30° and let fall to neutral. A positive test = arm extension and abduction, then arm adduction.	Birth	1–3 months
Palmar grasp—Object in hand causes flexion/grasping.	Birth	4 months
Root response—Stroking cheek causes mouth to turn in direction of stimulus.	Birth	3–4 months
Tonic neck—Turn head to side while child is supine, with ipsilateral arm and leg extending and opposite arm/leg flexing. Normal infant tries to break reflex position.	Birth	5–6 months
+*Babinski*—Stroking lateral border of sole, to big toe. A positive reflex causes big toe dorsiflexion, and fanning of other toes.	Birth	1–2 years

Table 22-3 Most Common Etiologies of Headache in Children Presenting to a Pediatric Emergency Department

Viral illness	39%	Brain tumor	2.7%
Migraine	18%	Intracranial hemorrhage	1.3%
Sinusitis	9%	Postconcussive	1.3%
Strep throat	9%	Other[1]	10.3%
Viral meningitis	9%		

[1]Includes VP shunt malfunction (2%), postictal headache (1.3%), and undetermined causes (7%).
Modified from Lewis, D. W. and Qureshi, F. Acute Headache in Children and Adolescents Presenting to the Emergency Department. Headache: *The Journal of Head and Face Pain*, 2000; 40: 200-203.

SEIZURES (FEBRILE AND NONFEBRILE)

Table 22-4 Practice Parameter: Evaluation of First Nonfebrile Seizure > 1 Month Old

Lab tests[1]	• Order labs (CBC, glucose, electrolytes) based on clinical circumstances (e.g., vomiting, diarrhea, dehydration, failure to return to baseline status). ↓Na and ↓Ca (most common unrecognized Δ) are rare—more common if ≤ 6 months. • Consider UA, NH₃, blood gas (arterial or venous), lactate. • Consider toxicology screen if any question of exposure.[3]
Lumbar puncture[1]	• Perform only if suspect CNS infection/subarachnoid bleed.
EEG[2]	• Perform on all first nonfebrile seizures (usually outpatient).
Neuroimaging[1] MRI is preferred to CT for identifying etiology; CT is more available acutely and excludes life threats: bleed or mass effect.	• Perform emergent neuroimaging if postictal focal deficits or altered mental status does not resolve rapidly. • *Nonurgent* MRI should be seriously considered in any child with (1) significant cognitive or motor impairment of unknown etiology, (2) abnormal exam, (3) focal seizure without secondary generalization, (4) EEG that does not represent a benign partial epilepsy of childhood or primary generalized epilepsy, or (5) age ≤ 1 year.

[1]Options: Not necessary in all. [2]Standard: Recommended in all. [3]See Table 31-2 for drugs/toxins causing seizures.
Modified from Hirtz, D., Ashwal, S., Berg, A., Bettis, D., Camfield, C., Camfield, P., Shinnar, S. Practice parameter: Evaluating a first nonfebrile seizure in children: Report of the Quality Standards Subcommittee of the American Academy of Neurology, the Child Neurology Society, and the American Epilepsy Society. *Neurology*, 2000; 55(5): 616-623

Febrile seizures—Seizures between 6 months and 5 years with fever, but without evidence of intracranial infection or cause. Specific infections/agents associated with causing febrile seizures including human herpes virus 6 (HHV-6; roseola infantum), HHV-7, influenza A, adenovirus, enteroviruses, *Shigella*, MMR vaccine (1–2 weeks after vaccination), DTaP vaccination within 24 hours of vaccination.

   Simple febrile seizures are generalized, last > 15 minutes, occur only once in 24 hours, and associated with a normal post-seizure neurologic exam/mental status; 25–33% reoccur especially if first-degree relative with seizure, complex features, age younger than 1 year (50% recurrence) or lower temperature at onset. Manage by identifying and treating the cause of the fever. A lumbar puncture is primarily indicated if there are signs of meningitis, or the exam is unreliable (on antibiotics, very young, persistent irritability).

   Complex febrile seizures last > 15 minutes, are focal, occur more than once in 24 hours, or have an abnormal neurological exam after seizure. Consider CT, LP and labs, EEG. Serious CNS infections (bacterial meningitis, herpes) are rare (without signs of meningitis) in complex febrile seizures, and LP is not mandatory.

Sources: Seltz LB, Cohen E, Weinstein M. Risk of bacterial or herpes simplex virus meningitis/encephalitis in children with complex febrile seizures. *Pediatr Emerg Care.* 2009;25(8):494-497; Callegaro S, Titomanlio L, Donegà S. Implementation of a febrile seizure guideline in two pediatric emergency departments. *Pediatr Neurol.* 2009;40(2):78-83.

   French guideline recommends (1) *antibiotics and lumbar puncture* if altered mental status pre-seizure, GCS < 15 (>1 hour after onset), petechiae, neck stiff, or bulging fontanelle; (2) *2 hours observation* for meningitis if complex features; (3) admit first-time seizures younger than 12 months (US experts DO NOT use age cutoff for admission if within defined age for febrile seizure); (4) low threshold for LP if younger than 12–18 months; (5) *urinalysis* in all (see page 190-191, UA recommendation); (6) short-term observation if no infection focus; (7) no blood tests for a simple febrile seizure if no concern regarding serious infection.

Source: Callegaro S, Titomanlio L, Donegà S. Implementation of a febrile seizure guideline in two pediatric emergency departments. *Pediatr Neurol.* 2009;40(2):78-83.

STATUS EPILEPTICUS

Table 22-5 Most Common Etiologies of Status Epilepticus in Children Younger Than 16 Years Old

Fever/Infection	36%	Anoxia	5%
Med Change	20%	Infection	5%
Unknown	9%	Trauma	4%
Metabolic	8%	Stroke	3%
Congenital	7%	Ethanol/Drugs	2%

Modified from Haafiz A, Kissoon N. Status epilepticus: current concepts. *Pediatr Emerg Care.* 1999;15(2):119-129. Comparable to recent evidence in Singh RK, Stephens S, Berl MM, et al. Prospective study of new-onset seizures presenting as status epilepticus in childhood. *Neurology.* 2010;74(8):636-642.

Table 22-6 Evaluation (Guidelines) and Management of Status Epilepticus

- Protect airway, administer O_2, start IV, cardiac monitor, pulse oximeter.
- Perform stat bedside glucose test and send electrolytes and drug levels.
- IV glucose if hypoglycemia (Table 11-3), and pyridoxine 50–100 mg IV if neonate.
- Intravenous drug therapy (see sequence in table that follows).
- Treat fever/infection and correct sodium, calcium, or magnesium abnormalities.
- Evaluation guidelines (Am Acad Neurol): Obtain antiseizure drug levels for all on antiepileptics. Obtain blood cultures and LP only if clinical suspicion of bacteremia, serious infection, or meningitis. Obtain CT/MRI after stabilization if clinical indication or unknown cause. Consider a toxicology screen, metabolic panel for inborn errors if no cause is found or other clinical indicators present.

Modified from Riviello JJ Jr, Ashwal S, Hirtz D, et al. Practice parameter: diagnostic assessment of the child with status epilepticus (an evidence-based review): report of the Quality Standards Subcommittee of the American Academy of Neurology and the Practice Committee of the Child Neurology Society. *Neurology.* 2006;67(9):1542-1550.

Table 22-7 Drug Therapy for Status Epilepticus (A–E Preferred Order)

	Drug	Dose and route	Maximum rate	Special features
A	Lorazepam	0.05–0.1 mg/kg IV	<0.5–1 mg/minute	May repeat every 5 minutes ×2
	or midazolam	0.2 mg/kg nasal/buccal	*Quicker onset than rectal diazepam*	May repeat every 5 minutes ×2
	or diazepam	0.5 mg/kg PR		May repeat 1/2 dose ×1
B	Fosphenytoin PE[1]	10–20 mg/kg IV	≤3 mg/kg/minute	Monitor closely
	or phenytoin	10–20 mg/kg IV	≤1 mg/kg/minute	Monitor closely
C	Phenobarbital[2]	15–20 mg/kg IV	<1 mg/kg/minute	Monitor closely
D	Midazolam	0.05–2 mg/kg IV/IM	Bolus 0.2 mg/kg (max 10 mg) over 2–5 minutes, with initial infusion at 100 mcg/kg/hour. Titrate as needed by 50–100 mcg/kg/hour (max 400–2,000 mcg/kg/hour).	
E	Pentobarbital (coma)[3]	5 mg/kg IV load 0.5–3 mg/kg/hour	Over 10–30 minutes and <50 mg/minute	Intubation required; vasopressors as needed

Alternates (not all are FDA approved for all ages or for this indication/dose; however, international studies available):

- Levetiracetam (*Keppra*) 60 mg/kg IV load. (Maximum dose 2,500 mg.)
- Valproic acid 40 mg/kg IV load. (No maximum dose.) Do not use valproic acid in patients younger than 2 years, those with hepatic failure or mitochondrial disease.

[1]PE—Phenytoin equivalents: All doses and rates are in phenytoin equivalents. [2]May ↑ to total 40 mg/kg or 1 g max. [3]Attach EEG if possible.

Modified from Kirmani BF, Crisp ED, Kayani S, Rajab H. Role of intravenous levetiracetam in acute seizure management of children. *Pediatr Neurol.* 2009;41(1):37-39; Abend NS, Monk HM, Licht DJ, Dlugos DJ. Intravenous levetiracetam in critically ill children with status epilepticus or acute repetitive seizures. *Pediatr Crit Care Med.* 2009;10(4):505-510.

SHUNTS (CEREBROSPINAL SHUNT INFECTION AND MALFUNCTION)

Table 22-8 Shunt Failure/Shunt Obstruction—Predictive Score[1,2]

Early presenters (within 5 months of surgery)		Late presenters (> 9 months to 2 years since surgery)	
Clinical feature	Points	Clinical feature	Points
Fluid tracking around shunt	1	Nausea and vomiting	1
Headache	1	Loss of developmental milestones	1
Irritability	1		
Fever	1	↑Head circumference	1
Bulging fontanelle	2	Fluid tracking around shunt	1
Erythema at surgery site	3	↓LOC	3
↓LOC	3		

Early shunt score (total points above)	Shunt failure probability	Late shunt score (total points above)	Shunt failure probability
0 points	4%	0 points	8%
1 point	50%	1 point	38%
2 points	75%	≥ 2 points	100%
≥ 3 points	100%		

[1]Features not found to be *independent* predictors of shunt failure included inability to depress or refill CSF reservoir, papilledema, cranial nerve palsy, abdomen pain/mass, meningismus, and peritonitis. [2]A more recent prospective study found that 88% of infants/children older than 2 months old at shunt insertion with failure had irritability, vomiting, or headache. The absence of these features indicated a <7% probability of shunt failure.

Modified from Garton HJ, Kestle JR, Drake JM. Predicting shunt failure on the basis of clinical symptoms and signs in children. *J Neurosurg.* 2001;94(2):202-210; Piatt JH Jr, Garton HJ. Clinical diagnosis of ventriculoperitoneal shunt failure among children with hydrocephalus. *Pediatr Emerg Care.* 2008;24(4):201-210; Boyle TP, Kimia AA, Nigrovic LE. Validating a clinical prediction rule for ventricular shunt malfunction. *Pediatr Emerg Care.* 2018;34(11):751-756.

Table 22-9 CSF Shunt Infections—Presenting Features in Children[1]

Feature	V-P shunt[2]	V-A shunt[2]	Most common organisms	
Fever	95%	100%	*Staphylococcus epidermidis* (SE)	32–57%
Shunt malfunction	57%	14%	*Staphylococcus aureus* (SA)	4–38%
Abdominal pain	48%	0	SA + *Streptococcus viridans*	4–15%
Meningismus	29%	0	Gram negatives ± SE	15% (3%)
Headache	14%	14%	SE + *Enterococcus*	7%
Irritability	19%	43%	SE + *Streptococcus pyogenes*	4%
Nephritis	0	14%	*Enterococcus/Candida*	4%

[1]95% of shunt infections occur <6 months after surgery. [2]V-A→ventriculoatrial; V-P→ventriculoperitoneal. Modified from Kontny U, Höfling B, Gutjahr P, Voth D, Schwarz M, Schmitt HJ. CSF shunt infections in children. *Infection.* 1993;21(2):89-92; Davis SE, Levy ML, McComb JG, Masri-Lavine L. Does age or other factors influence the incidence of ventriculoperitoneal shunt infections? *Pediatr Neurosurg.* 1999;30:253-257; Piatt JH Jr, Garton HJ. Clinical diagnosis of ventriculoperitoneal shunt failure among children with hydrocephalus. *Pediatr Emerg Care.* 2008;24(4):201-210.

MANAGEMENT OF SHUNT MALFUNCTION/INFECTION

- Apply cardiac telemetry and pulse oximeter (risk of apnea, bradycardia).
- Head-to-toe examination with emphasis on shunt tract and neurologic exam.
- AP/lateral films of skull, torso where shunt located, CT scan of the head (up to 24% will have CT read as unchanged/normal/smaller ventricles or negative). Some institutions may have a fast-protocol MRI available.
- Consult neurosurgeon if suspect infection/failure of shunt even if normal CT.
- Shunt tap (by neurosurgeon) for pressure assessment, cell count, culture (do not perform LP in ED due to risk of herniation and ↑rate of missed infection).
- Shunt failure requires surgery. Treat impending herniation as needed. Infection usually requires external ventricular drainage or shunt externalization, and empiric antibiotics until culture results return (see drug dosing Page 168).

WEAKNESS AND ATAXIA

Upper motor neuron (UMN) lesions cause damage to the cortex (e.g., stroke), brain stem, or spinal cord. Lower motor neuron (LMN) lesions damage the anterior horn cells (e.g., poliomyelitis), the neuromuscular junction (e.g., myasthenia gravis, botulism toxin), peripheral nerves (e.g., Guillain-Barre), or muscle (e.g., muscular dystrophies).

Table 22-10 Differentiation of Upper Motor Neuron from Lower Motor Neuron Disease

Category	UMN disease	LMN disease
Muscular deficit	Muscle groups	Individual muscles
Reflexes	Increased	Decreased/Absent
Tone	Increased	Decreased
Fasciculations	Absent	Present
Atrophy	Absent/Minimal	Present

ATAXIA

Ataxia is the incoordination of movement with normal strength. Disorders of the cerebellar hemispheres cause ipsilateral limb ataxia, while disorders of the vermis cause truncal ataxia. Other causes of acute ataxia include cerebral cortex disorders (frontal ataxia), peripheral sensory nerve and spinal cord disorders (sensory ataxia), labyrinth disorders (vestibular ataxia), and metabolic and toxin-induced ataxia.

SPECIFIC DISEASES CAUSING ATAXIA

- *Acute cerebellar ataxia*—The most common cause of acute ataxia in children. This is a post-viral autoimmune ataxia typically occurring in 1- to 3-year-olds 1–3 weeks after viral infection. This disorder causes a sudden onset of ataxia, paroxysmal vertigo, nystagmus in 50%, possibly elevated CSF protein and mild CSF pleocytosis (but commonly CSF normal), and frequently dysarthria. Ataxia may persist for weeks to a year in up to a third of patients. The majority recover within 30 days.
- *Drug ingestion*—Common drugs causing ataxia include phenytoin (and most anticonvulsants), alcohol, tricyclic antidepressants, hypnotics, sedatives, heavy metals (e.g., lead), insecticides, and drugs of abuse (e.g., PCP).
- *Neuroblastomas*—Occult neuroblastomas can cause a classic triad of symptoms with acute ataxia, opsoclonus (jerky, random eye movements), and myoclonus.
- *Posterior fossa tumors*—Direct cerebellar involvement or hydrocephalus.
- *Diseases causing weakness* easily mistaken for ataxia include Guillain-Barre, transverse myelitis, tick paralysis, and myasthenia gravis.
- *Other causes* include head trauma, stroke, acute disseminated encephalomyelitis (ADEM), cerebral vein thrombosis, vasculitis, and congenital disorders such as inborn errors of metabolism.

EVALUATION OF ATAXIA

If unexplained ataxia: CBC, electrolytes, toxin/drug screens (alcohol, drug level for antiseizure medicines), CT, or MRI (MRI more sensitive for brain stem lesions). Consider EEG, lumbar puncture, and more in depth metabolic evaluation (e.g., ammonia, ketones, lactate, amino acids) and neurological consultation.

Sources: Thakkar K, Maricich SM, Alper G. Acute ataxia in childhood: 11-year experience at a major pediatric neurology referral center. *J Child Neurol.* 2016;31(9):1156-1160; Ryan MM, Engle EC. Topical review: acute ataxia in childhood. *J Child Neurol.* 2003;18(5):309-316.

23 ■ NUTRITION AND FEEDING

Energy requirements—A child younger than 12 months of age requires 105–115 kcal/kg/day. Overfeeding exceeds this amount and often provides volumes that can lead to reflux/vomiting. Breast milk or commercially prepared formulas are usually the sole source of energy and nutrients in the first few months of life. Semisolid foods (e.g., cereals and purees) are usually introduced into the diet at 4 to 6 months of age and soft table foods at 9 to 12 months.

Breast milk—The American Academy of Pediatrics (AAP) recommends exclusive breastfeeding until approximately 6 months of age for several reasons. The composition of breast milk changes to meet the changing nutritional needs of the growing infant. In addition, breastfeeding may be protective against some illnesses and diseases. Contraindications to breastfeeding include (1) a diagnosis of classic galactosemia in the infant, (2) untreated brucellosis in the mother, (3) maternal infection with HTLV-1/2 or Ebola virus, (4) certain maternal medications, and (5) maternal use of illicit drugs. In the developed world, mothers who are positive for HIV also should not breastfeed. Furthermore, mothers should temporarily refrain from breastfeeding or provide expressed breast milk, if they have an active, untreated TB infection; an active HSV lesion on the breast; a varicella infection 5 days before or 2 days after delivery; or H1N1 influenza infection with fever. Mastitis is not a contraindication. Breastfed babies should receive supplemental vitamin D 400 IU daily unless they are consuming ~1 l of vitamin D–fortified formula or whole milk daily.

Infant formulas—Most commercially prepared infant formulas supply 19 to 20 calories per ounce. Their nutritional content is established by legislative mandate (the Infant Formula Act of 1980) that prescribes the minimum concentration of 29 nutrients. The AAP strongly recommends iron-fortified formulas to help prevent anemia as iron stores in the body become depleted. Infant formulas are available in powdered, liquid concentrate, or ready-to-feed formulations. As formula powder is now recognized as a potential source of *Cronobacter* infection, the CDC recommends that powered formula for young infants younger than 3 months be prepared with boiled water that has been cooled to no less than 158°F/70°C, and then allowed to cool to a safe drinking temperature. If fluoridated drinking water is not available, fluoride supplementation is recommended for all infants older than 6 months.

Table 23-1 Summary of Different Types of Common Infant Formulas and Uses[1]

Infant Formula Type	Brand Examples	Details
Cow milk protein	Earth's Best Organic Enfamil Infant Similac Advance Similac Non-GMO	Most commonly used and most do well on this type Contains: choline, DHA, ARA May contain: prebiotics (gluco-oligosaccharides)
Partially hydrolyzed protein	Gerber Good Start Similac Sensitive	May be easier to digest
Extensively hydrolyzed protein or hypoallergenic	Enfamil Nutramigen Gerber Extensive HA Similac Alimentum	Proteins broken down into small peptides Lactose free Uses: infants with food protein allergies (cow milk protein, allergic proctocolitis)
Amino acid	Alfamino Elecare Neocate Puramino	Proteins broken down into amino acids Uses: infants with food protein allergies (cow milk protein, allergic proctocolitis)
Soy protein	Enfamil Prosobee Gerber Good Start Soy Similac Isomil	Lactose-free Uses: vegetarians, metabolic disorders (e.g., galactosemia) Contains: soy protein, DHA, ARA
Low-lactose or lactose-free*	Enfamil Gentlease Similac Sensitive	Less casein than whey Whey may be partially broken down
Premature	Enfamil Premature Similac Neosure *Hospital only:* Enfamil Enfacare Similac Special Care	More calories per ounce Higher levels of protein, minerals, and electrolytes

[1]GMO, genetically modified organism; DHA, docosahexaenoic acid; ARA, arachidonic acid; HA, hypoallergenic
*Primary lactose intolerance is rare in children. Most children will be able to tolerate traditional formulas even with transient lactose intolerance following gastroenteritis.

NUTRITIONAL DISORDERS

Failure to thrive (FTT)—Inadequate growth commonly defined as weight $\leq$ third or fifth percentile for age or crossing two or more major percentile lines on an appropriate growth chart. FTT should not be a stand-alone diagnosis as there are a multitude of interrelated causes of FTT that must be investigated.

Bovine milk allergy—Bovine milk allergy is due to sensitivity to the primary protein in cow milk, β-lactoglobulin. Infants with cow milk protein allergy usually present during the first 6 weeks of life with diarrhea, mucous or blood in stools, and occasional respiratory symptoms. Treatment is aimed at eliminating bovine milk protein from the diet and substituting soy-based (e.g., Pregestimil) or hydrolyzed casein formulas (e.g., Nutramigen).

Table 23-2 Approximate Feeding Schedule for the First Year After Birth

Age	Newborn (full-term)	1 month old	2–4 months old	4–6 months old	6–8 months old	8–12 months old	Over 12 months old
Formula amount	2 oz	3–4 oz	3–6 oz	4–6 oz	6–8 oz	7–8 oz	16–24 oz whole milk
Frequency	Every 3–4 hours	Every 3–4 hours	5–8 times per day	4–6 times per day	3–5 times per day	3–4 times per day	Per day
Breastfeeding frequency	Every 2–3 hours (on demand), or 8–12 times per day	Every 2–4 hours (on demand), or 7–8 times per day	5–8 times per day (on demand)	4–6 times per day	3–5 times per day	3–4 times per day	1–2 up to multiple times per day, as long as both mom and baby desire

Data from: DiMaggio DM, Cox A, Porto AF. Updates in infant nutrition. *Pediatr Rev.* 2017;38(10):449–462.

Table 24-1 Diagnosis of Ectopic Pregnancy in Clinically Stable Patients

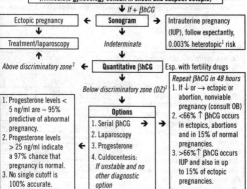

[1][Concurrent IUP + ectopic]. [2]DZ is 1,000–1,500 mIU/ml for transvaginal ultrasound (US) and 6,500 mIU/ml for transabdominal US.

Table 24-2 Ultrasound (US) Findings[1] and Quantitative βhCG in IUP[2,3]

Intrauterine pregnancy (IUP)	Time	mIU/ml
(1) Decidual reaction	<1 week	<5–50
(2) Gestational sac seen at 4.5 weeks with βhCG > 1,000–1,400 via transvaginal US or 6 weeks with βhCG > 6,500 via transabdominal US	1–2 weeks	40–300
	2–3 weeks	100–1000
	3–4 weeks	500–6,000
(3) Yolk sac: Seen at 5.5 weeks (βhCG > 7,200)	1–2 months	5,000–200,000
(4) Fetal pole/heartbeats are seen at 5.5 to 7 weeks (βhCG > 10,800–17,200)	2–3 months	10,000–100,000
	2nd trimester	3,000–50,000
	3rd trimester	1,000–50,000

(Continued)

Table 24-2 Ultrasound (US) Findings[1] and Quantitative βhCG in IUP[2,3] (Continued)

Ectopic pregnancy (% with finding)
(1) Empty uterus, decidual reaction, or pseudosac (10–20%)
(2) Cul-de-sac fluid (24–63%): echogenic = blood
(3) Adnexal mass (60–90%)
(4) Echogenic halo around tube (26–68%)
(5) Fetal heart activity (8–23%)

[1]Transvaginal sonography unless otherwise stated. [2]Time from conception. [3]Median time for βhCG to turn negative after spontaneous abortion is 16 days (30 days for elective).

Table 24-3 Ovarian Torsion

	Clinical features	
Overview: Ovarian torsion is usually due to an enlarged ovary with or without a mass (usually benign) that alters its center of gravity causing it to twist on its axis and compress the venous drainage first, then the arterial flow later. Following venous compression, pressure rises within the ovarian capsule. Eventually, ischemia and necrosis occur. *Evaluation:* A βHCG is mandatory. Diagnose by US (color Doppler best)—abnormalities are usually seen on CT. *Management:* Surgical detorsion may salvage many ovaries even if prolonged symptoms (>3 days).	Mean age (years) peds studies	10–13
	Abdomen pain (≥ sudden)	86–100%
	Mean days pain pre-ED visit	3–6 days
	Vomiting	67–91%
	Fever (late finding)	18–57%
	Abdomen tenderness	88–100%
	Palpable ovarian mass	10–64%
	Peritoneal signs	23%
	Lab/radiologic features	
	WBC count > 12,000 cells/mm^3	32–51%
	Plain radiography mass	26%
	CT ovarian mass	95–100%
	CT enlarged fallopian tube	~75%
	Ultrasonography (see tables that follow)	

Modified from Anders JF, Powell EC. Urgency of evaluation and outcome of acute ovarian torsion in pediatric patients. *Arch Pediatr Adolesc Med.* 2005;159(6):532-535; Rha SE. CT and MR imaging features of adnexal torsion. *Radiographics.* 2002;22:283; Anders JF. Ovarian torsion in the pediatric emergency department: making the diagnosis and the importance of advocacy. *Clin Pediatr Emerg Med.* 2009;10(1):31-37.

Table 24-4 Ultrasonographic Findings in Ovarian Torsion

Ultrasonographic Findings	Frequency
Enlarged ovary or ovarian mass	95–100%
Absent venous flow (earlier than arterial flow obstruction)[1]	67–93%
Absent arterial flow (persistent flow esp. if dual blood supply)[1]	46–73%
Twisted vascular pedicle or whirlpool sign (circular/coiled vessels)	>75%
Ovary with ground glass appearance	26%
Free fluid within abdomen	21%

[1]Use color Doppler.
Modified from Chang HC, Bhatt S, Dogra VS. Pearls and pitfalls in diagnosis of ovarian torsion. *Radiograph-ics.* 2008;28:1355-68; Garel L, Dubois J, Grignon A, Filiatrault D, Van Vliet G. US of the pediatric female pelvis: a clinical perspective. *Radiographics.* 2001;21:1393-407; Shadinger LL, Andreotti RF, Kurian RL. Preoperative sonographic and clinical characteristics as predictors of ovarian torsion. *J Ultrasound Med.* 2008;27:7-13.

Table 24-5 Common Gynecologic Conditions

Vulvovaginitis	*Overview:* Common gynecologic problem in prepubertal girls. Most cases are nonspecific and related to normal vaginal flora. Candidal vulvovaginitis is rare in prepubertal girls. Symptoms include vaginal discharge, irritation, pain, dysuria, and redness. Diagnosis is made by history and physical exam.
	Management: Reassurance, stressing importance of good perineal hygiene, use of hypoallergenic soaps, use of cotton underwear. Avoidance of irritants such as bubble baths, synthetic-fabric underwear, tight clothing.
Labial adhesions	*Overview:* Usually asymptomatic and seen in infants. Occasionally can lead to urinary dribbling and vulvar irritation. Not indicative of sexual abuse.
	Management: Can resolve spontaneously. Topical estrogen cream can also be used, typically once daily applied on the midline for 4–6 weeks.
Imperforate hymen	*Overview:* Abnormality of the vagina leading to hematocolpos. Symptoms can range from asymptomatic amenorrhea to cyclic abdominal/pelvic pain, urinary retention, back pain.
	Management: Diagnosis is made on physical examination or ultrasound demonstrating hematocolpos. Treatment is surgical (hymenectomy).

(Continued)

Table 24.5 Common Gynecologic Conditions (*Continued*)

Urethral prolapse	*Overview:* Occurs in prepubertal girls due to the hypoestrogenic state. Repeated Valsava maneuvers are usually the precipitating cause. Symptoms that prompt evaluation include dysuria, blood in the diaper or underwear, vaginal mass, or concern for sexual abuse. Diagnosis is made by visualization of a circular, red, friable mass around the urethral meatus.
	Management: Conservative measures include sitz baths, topical estrogen, and treating the precipitant (i.e., constipation causing repeat Valsava maneuvers). Surgical excision is a possibility if conservative measures fail.

Modified from Ritchie, Joanne K., et al. The paediatrician and the management of common gynaecological conditions. *Archives of disease in childhood*, 2018; 103(7):314-375. doi:10.1136/archdischild -2017-314375.; Eyk, N. V., Allen, L., Giesbrecht, E., Jamieson, M. A., Kives, S., Morris, M., Fleming, N. Pediatric Vulvovaginal Disorders: A Diagnostic Approach and Review of the Literature. *Journal of Obstetrics and Gynaecology Canada*, 2009; 31(9): 850-862. doi:10.1016/s1701-2163(16)34304-3.

Table 24-6 Causes of Vaginal Bleeding in Specific Patient Populations

Prepubertal females	• Vulvovaginitis • Vaginal foreign body • Urethral prolapse • Straddle injury/genital trauma • Precocious puberty • Dermatoses (lichen sclerosus, atopic dermatitis) • Sexual abuse • Neoplasm
Postpubertal females	• Anovulatory cycles • Infections (e.g., cervicitis) • Foreign body • Laceration/trauma • Sexual abuse • Polyp/Fibroid/Myoma • Hematologic conditions (bleeding disorder like Von Willebrand disease, platelet dysfunction, or coagulation defects; thrombocytopenia) • Thyroid disorders • Ectopic pregnancy • Miscarriage • Medication side effects

Table 24-6 Causes of Vaginal Bleeding in Specific Patient Populations (*Continued*)

Pregnancy	• Ectopic pregnancy • Implantation bleeding • Placental abnormalities (previa, accreta, abruption) • Abortion (threatened, spontaneous, missed) • Infections

Modified from Deligeoroglou, E., Karountzos, V., & Creatsas, G. Abnormal uterine bleeding and dysfunctional uterine bleeding in pediatric and adolescent gynecology. *Gynecological Endocrinology*, 2012; 29(1):74-78. doi:10.3109/09513590.2012.705384; Howell JO, Flowers D. Prepubertal Vaginal Bleeding: Etiology, Diagnostic Approach, and Management. *Obstet Gynecol Surv.* 2016; 71(4):231-42. doi: 10.1097/OGX.0000000000000290.

Table 24-7 Sexually Transmitted Infections

Infection/condition	Recommended treatment	Special considerations
Bacterial vaginosis	Metronidazole 500 mg PO bid for 7 days	
Cervicitis	Azithromycin 1 g PO in a single dose	Consider treatment for both gonorrhea and chlamydia given prevalence of coinfection is high.
Chlamydial infections, adolescents and pregnant patients	Azithromycin 1 g PO in a single dose	
Gonococcal infections (cervix, urethra, rectum, pharynx)	Ceftriaxone 250 mg IM in a single dose PLUS Azithromycin 1 g PO in a single dose	
Genital herpes simplex—first episode	Acyclovir 400 mg PO three times daily for 7–10 days	Alternate regimen: valacyclovir 1 g PO twice daily for 7–10 days.
Genital herpes simplex—recurrent episode	Acyclovir 400 mg PO three times daily for 5 days	Alternate regimen: valacyclovir 1 g PO once daily for 5 days.
Syphilis	Penicillin 2.4 million units IM in a single dose	Latent syphilis, neurosyphilis, and congenital syphilis are treated with different dosing of penicillin.

(Continued)

Table 24-7 Sexually Transmitted Infections (*Continued*)

Infection/condition	Recommended treatment	Special considerations
Trichomoniasis	Metronidazole 2 g PO in a single dose	
Pelvic inflammatory disease	Ceftriaxone 250 mg IM in a single dose PLUS Doxycycline 100 mg twice a day for 14 days WITH OR WITHOUT Metronidazole 500 mg twice a day for 14 days	Multiple treatment regimens exist (oral and parenteral).

Modified from Workowski KA, Bolan GA. Sexually transmitted diseases treatment guidelines, 2015. *MMWR*. 2015;64(3).

25 ■ OPHTHALMOLOGY

Table 25-1 Emergency Department Ophthalmologic Exam

Chemical exposure (known or any suspicion of)	• STOP examination • Irrigate immediately	
Obtain visual acuity • Make sure patient is wearing his or her correction	**Snellen Chart** • 20 feet • Each eye separately—completely occlude but not compress each eye • Record smallest line the patient can read for each eye • Give credit for a line if the patient misses up to one letter **Picture Chart** • 2–4 years and moderately mentally impaired **Tumbling E chart** • 3–5 years and mute, illiterate or mildly mentally impaired • More accurate than picture chart	
External exam	Assess lids, skin, conjunctiva, cornea for obvious foreign body, lacerations, disruption; palpate periorbital area for bony step-offs; assess for proptosis, enophthalmos	
Corneal light reflex (CLR) • Assesses ocular alignment	**Position of reflex**	**Ocular alignment**
	Symmetric	Normal
	Outward displacement	Esotropia
	Inward displacement	Exotropia
	Downward or upward displacement	Hypertropia
Cover, uncover test • Also assesses ocular alignment • More accurate than CLR • Requires greater patient cooperation	• Patient fixates on object 15–20 feet away • Cover right eye quickly with hand and observe left eye for movement • Repeat quickly to other side	
	Eye movement	**Ocular alignment**
	None	Normal
	Outward	Esotropia
	Inward	Exotropia
	Downward or upward	Hypertropia

(Continued)

Table 25-1 Emergency Department Ophthalmologic Exam (*Continued*)

Pupillary response	Exam

Assesses:
 Pupils
 Equal
 Round and Reactive to light and Accommodation
 No relative afferent pupillary defect (RAPD)
	(1) Have patient fix on object 10 feet in distance
	 (2) Lights on: Check that pupils are equal in size
	 (3) Lights off: Check that pupils are still equal in size
	 (4) Lights off: Check that each eye has a direct response to light
	 (5) Lights off: Check swinging light test to assess for RAPD
	 Detailed exam
	 (1) **Assess pupil size in light and dark**
	   ◦ Have patient fixate on object 10 feet away throughout exam to avoid normal constriction with convergence and accommodation (e.g., the "near reflex")
	   ◦ Fixating in distance, in the dark makes the pupils as large as possible and pupil reaction easier to see when you shine the light
	   ◦ Assess that pupils are equal in light and dark
	   ◦ Normal: Pupils symmetric
	   ◦ Abnormal: Pupils asymmetric = anisocoria (see the following)
	 (2) **Assess pupil to direct light**
	   ◦ Shine penlight directly into each eye
	   ◦ Normal: Pupils constrict briskly and completely, relax a little, then dilate again after the light is removed
	   ◦ Abnormal: Pupils constrict slowly and incompletely or not at all
	 (3) **Swinging light test in dimmest light possible**
	   ◦ A comparative test of the 2 optic nerves
	   ◦ Assesses for RAPD
	   ◦ RAPD = Margus Gunn pupil
	     ▪ Patient fixates on object 10 feet away in the dark
	     ▪ Shine a bright light directly into the right eye 2–3 seconds
	     ▪ Note if it constricts, then relaxes just a little
	     ▪ Swing the light quickly back and forth over the bridge of the nose to each eye, holding 2–3 seconds each time, assessing pupil response
	     ▪ Normal: The pupil will have just started to dilate when the light hits, causing a small constriction followed by mild relaxation
	     ▪ Abnormal: If one pupil consistently dilates as the light is shined on it, there is an afferent pupil defect (Marcus Gunn pupil) in the eye that dilates
	       ◦ Sign of unilateral optic nerve damage
	       ◦ Seen in optic neuritis, optic nerve compression
	       ◦ One optic nerve is functioning poorly compared to the other

Table 25-1 Emergency Department Ophthalmologic Exam (*Continued*)

Extraocular movements	
Visual fields	
Red reflex	• Using ophthalmoscope dioptric power 0 • 1 foot in front of the patient • Normal: Symmetric red glow • Abnormal: Beet red, gray, black, asymmetry
Fundoscopic exam	Assess retina, blood vessels, and optic nerve
Fluorescein exam	• Tetracaine (onset of action <1 minute) • Then measure visual acuity • Access cornea with a penlight for uneven light reflection, cloudiness, or foreign body • Stain with fluorescein • Assess with Wood's lamp or cobalt blue light after repeat blinking looking for persistent green stain • Evert lid to assess for the foreign body
Slit lamp exam	To assess the anterior chamber and cornea for cloudiness/foreign body
Dilated eye exam	Facilitates slit lamp exam to view the posterior globe—the retina, optic nerve, blood vessels, and macula
CT scans	Radiologic study of choice in ophthalmologic emergencies

Table 25-2 The Red Eye

Signs and symptoms	Distinguishing features	Condition and pearls	Management/treatment
• Lid swelling • Lacrimal gland swelling OR • Proptosis	• Gritty, burning sensation of lids • Matting of eye when awaken • Redness, swelling, irregular contour to lid margin • Scaly, flaky debris to lid margins • Mild to moderate conjunctival injection • Reduced tear secretion	**Chronic blepharitis** **Anterior blepharitis** • Common in atopy • Usually *Staphylococcus aureus* • Infection of skin, cilia, accessory glands of eye	• Lid margin hygiene bid • Warm, moist washcloth over closed lids 5–10 minutes • Wipe away with soft cloth • Moisten cotton tip in 3 oz water with 3 drops baby shampoo—scrub lids • Rinse • Brush off any dry debris • Apply bacitracin or erythromycin ointment nightly ×2 weeks
		Posterior blepharitis • Common in rosacea or seborrheic dermatitis of scalp and face • Inflammation of meibomian sebaceous glands	• Lid hygiene as above • PO tetracycline 0.5 to 1 g/day four times per day OR • doxycycline 50–100 mg PO bid
	• Painful, tender focal swelling to anterior eyelid margin • "Pimple" • Develops over several days	**Stye = Hordeolum** External stye • Anterior lid margin • Focal inflammation of ciliary follicles or accessory glands Internal stye • Posterior lid margin • Due to plugged meibomian glands from inflammation	• Warm compresses to affected eye bid • Hard-boiled egg or boiled potato cooled to touch holds heat and facilitates reheating • Topical antibiotics are useless

• Lump in eyelid • No to mild tenderness • May have previously	**Chalazion** • Due to scarring in the healing process of stye or internal hordeolum	• Observe for several months for regression • Surgical resection if fails to regress, alters vision, or cosmetically unfavorable
• Tender swelling to medial lower lid overlying the lacrimal sac • Excessive tearing • Discharge from punctum, which increases with pressure to the swollen area • Red conjunctiva	**Dacrocystitis** • Most often seen in infants with nasolacrimal duct obstruction • Due to bacterial infection in area of the obstruction	• Mild cases: Amoxicillin • Severe: IV cefuroxime • If progressive inflammation or not improving in 24 hours → urgent ophthalmology referral for imaging to rule out abscess
• Periocular pain • +/− fever • Violaceous discoloration with tender swelling to upper and lower lids • Mild diffuse conjunctival injection	**Orbital cellulitis** • Diffuse bacterial infection of periocular tissue • Usually from paranasal sinusitis, carried to orbit by emissary veins • Less likely due to skin infection **Preseptal** • Infection is located in the soft tissue anterior to orbital septum (anterior 1/3 of the orbit) Postseptal = orbital cellulitis	• Sino-orbital CT scan to rule out sinusitis, orbital subperiosteal abscess, tumor • Young children younger than 9—gram+ coverage cefuroxime • Older children and adults add clindamycin, or metronidazole for anaerobic coverage • Consult ophthalmology, ENT for concerns, subperiosteal infection, or failure to improve in 24 hours

(Continued)

Table 25-2 The Red Eye *(Continued)*

Signs and symptoms	Distinguishing features	Condition and pearls	Management/Treatment
• Subnormal visual acuity • Foreign body sensation • Severe pain OR • Ciliary flush (red rim around cornea)	• Blurred vision • Photophobia • Periocular pain • "Sand in eye" foreign body sensation • Ciliary flush • Corneal opacification	**Keratitis** • Inflammation of the cornea • Usually due to infection, trauma, dry eye, ultra-violet exposure, contact lens overwear, or autoimmune disorders • Prompt recognition imperative to avoid permanent vision loss • Can start with surface breakdown of epithelium • Can start in deeper layers of cornea, thus fluorescein can be normal	• Do not attempt treatment • Immediate ophthalmology referral
	• Periocular pain • Photophobia • Blurred vision (sometimes) • Ciliary flush • Small or irregular pupil due to adherence of iris to anterior lens or posterior corneal surface	**Anterior uveitis** • Inflammation of the iris and ciliary muscle autoimmune reaction (isolated or part of seronegative spondyloarthropathies, sarcoidosis, herpes simplex, herpes zoster, or Behcet's)	• Index of suspicion • Requires slit lamp exam • Immediate ophthalmology referral
	• Periocular pain • Vision loss • Conjunctiva very red • Swollen eyelids • Hazy cornea • Possible layered pus bottom of anterior chamber	**Endophthalmitis** • Infection inside the eye • Can be introduced from outside by corneal infection, trauma, surgery, or via the blood stream • May be mistaken for severe keratitis, conjunctivitis, uveitis	• Immediate ophthalmology referral • Ophthalmologic emergency

• Focal conjunctival redness	**Subconjunctival hemorrhage** • Due to sudden increase in intrathoracic pressure such as a cough, sneeze, straining with stooling; can occur with rubbing eye, after vaginal delivery	• No treatment • Usually resolves in 1 week
• Purulent drainage	**Bacterial conjunctivitis** • Most common pathogens: *Staphylococcus, Streptococcus, Haemophilus influenzae* • Less likely *Neisseria gonorrhoeae, Pseudomonas aeruginosa* • Contact lens wearer—low index of suspicion for virulent pathogen such as *P. aeruginosa* or *Acanthamoeba*	• If pus is present on exam, refer all of the following to ophthalmology urgently due to concern of virulent pathogen: neonates, extended or inappropriate contact lens wear, immunocompromised hosts, hx of trauma or foreign body • Mild non-neonate and immunocompetent, treat with topical erythromycin or trimethoprim • Refer it worsens after 3 days of txt or not improve in 7 days
• Blotchy bulbar conjunctival redness • Extravascular redness • No pain		
• Ocular pain • Diffuse, marked redness, and swelling purulent discharge		
• Itching	**Allergic conjunctivitis** • Usually seasonal. IgE-mediated immediate hypersensitivity to pollens • Usually accompanied by other allergy symptoms	• Oral antihistamines • OTC topical vasoconstrictor-antihistamine • Topical H1 blocker-mast cell stabilizer
• Prominent itching • Eyelid edema • Diffuse boggy edema (chemosis) especially lower fornix • Diffuse conjunctival redness • Watery discharge • Bilateral but can be asymmetric		

(Continued)

Table 25-2 The Red Eye (Continued)

Signs and symptoms	Distinguishing features	Condition and pearls	Management/treatment
• Topical ocular medication use • Cosmetic use • Environmental pollutants	• Red, leathery thickening, and scaling of the periorbital skin	**Contact dermatoconjunctivitis** • Delayed hypersensitivity reaction to topically applied medications or cosmetics • Most common eye meds are aminoglycosides and cycloplegics	• Discontinue offending agent • Consider topical corticosteroid • Ophthalmology referral if not improved in 14 days
	• Mild but persistent ocular discomfort • Sticky eyelids upon awakening • Mild diffuse redness	**Chemical conjunctivitis** • May be confused with chronic infectious conjunctivitis, uveitis, scleritis, or blepharitis	• Discontinue offending agent • Ophthalmology referral if not improved in 14 days
• Watery discharge	• Watery, thin, mucoid discharge • Diffuse conjunctival redness with follicles • +/– tender preauricular nodes • Monocular or binocular involvement	**Viral conjunctivitis** • Most common cause of acute red eye • Usually self-limited, can be isolated or part of a URI • Most often due to adenovirus	• Do not treat with antimicrobials • Wash hands frequently • Avoid touching eyes • Do not share towels • Avoid work, school, day care until discharge resolves • Refer in 48 hours if worsens or concern for keratitis

Table 25-3 Ocular Trauma

Presentation	Pearls	Management
Chemical exposure		
Alkaline Household cleaners Fertilizers Pesticides Lye Cement cleaner Sparklers Firecracker products **Acid** Car battery fluid	• Vision threatening • Conjunctiva may be normal in face of severe injury due to blood vessel destruction • Immediate irrigation • Do not spend time taking history if known or suspected chemical contact • Acid burns → Coagulation necrosis and denature surface proteins but usually do not penetrate the eye • Alkali burns worse: Cause rapid penetration through cornea and anterior chamber → combine with cell membrane lipids causing liquefaction necrosis	• Remove debris • Topical anesthetic • Immediately irrigate with LR for 30 minutes to pH 7 (inferior fornix) • Evert lids • Inspect for corneal opacification and conjunctival swelling Visual acuity • Fluorescein • Do not patch—increases risk of infecting devitalized tissue Emergent referral • Acid or alkaline burn • ↓Visual acuity • Severe conjunctival swelling • Corneal clouding
Blunt ocular trauma		
• Direct blow to the eye	• Increased risk severe injury if ↓visual acuity, diplopia, severe pain. +LOC, "saw stars" • May not produce significant signs	• Assess for severity of impact with assessment of ocular pain, ↓visual acuity • Diplopia, irregular pupil, hyphema • Eye shield • Do not patch • Emergent ophthalmology referral

(Continued)

Table 25-3 Ocular Trauma (*Continued*)

Presentation	Pearls	Management
Hyphema		
• Blood filling lower part of the anterior chamber • Usually blunt, projectile, or penetrating trauma • Pain • Decreased visual acuity • Injected conjunctiva • Irregular pupil • Usually less than 50% of the chamber is filled	• Increased concern for vision threatening contusion to globe even if not apparent • Rebleeding can occur in up to 30% of cases—likely due to lysis and retraction of clot and fibrin aggregates, usually first 5 days • Increased risk of rebleed in younger ages • Rebleeding can cause severe increase in intraocular pressure leading to blindness	• Elevate head of bed 30–45 degrees • Eye shield • No NSAIDs (antiplatelet effect) • Immediate ophthalmology evaluation • Topical cycloplegic • Topical miotics lower intraocular pressure and increase surface area of iris aiding hyphema resorption • Likely antifibrolytics (aminocaproic acid) • Topical steroids decrease associated iritis and synechiae development • Reduced physical activities • Frequent re-exam over 5 days • Consider admit if child
Open globe		
• Obvious perforation or penetrating FB • Usually pain, decreased vision, diplopia • Teardrop or irregular pupil • Increased or decreased depth anterior chamber • Vitreous extrusion • Intraocular structure prolapse • Corneal or scleral tenting at puncture site	• 5–10% of penetrating injuries at risk for endophthalmitis, which leads to vision loss	• Emergent ophthalmology referral • Visual acuity counting fingers • External ocular movement, assess for entrapment • Place eye shield • Avoid increased intraocular pressure (antiemetics) • NPO • Broad spectrum antibiotics (Cefazolin, Ceftazidime, vancomycin) • Avoid eye manipulation • Tetanus prophylaxis

Table 25-3 Ocular Trauma (*Continued*)

Presentation	Pearls	Management
Protruding FB		
• Orbital or intraocular • High-velocity missiles • Metal bits released by drilling, hammering, shotgun, BB pellets • "Sudden impact" to eyelids or eye	• High index suspicion—PE findings can be mild • Can penetrate globe without severe pain • Vision threatening especially if copper or iron	• Visual acuity • Inspect for small lacerations to eyelids, corneal or scleral lacerations, hyphema, irregular pupil, absent red reflex • Leave FB in place, do not manipulate • Immediate ophthalmology referral
Eyelid laceration		
	• Increased risk severe ocular injury if ↓visual acuity, diplopia. Severe pain. +LOC, "saw stars" • May not produce significant signs • Incorrectly repaired lid lacerations can cause cosmetic deformity, dry cornea with persistent pain or vision loss	• Complex lacerations are deep, long, involve lid margin, levator palpebrae muscle (ptosis) or canalicular system and require emergent repair by ophthalmology • Tetanus prophylaxis • If simple, repair skin with 6–0 suture
Orbital wall fracture		
Blunt trauma to face or eye • Auto accidents • Falls • Combat • Eyelid swelling and ecchymosis • Enophthalmos ("sinking in" of affected eye) • Ptosis • Diplopia • Anesthesia of ipsilateral cheek (infraorbital nerve injury) • Impaired upward gaze	• Increased risk of traumatic brain injury • Most common sites are floor (maxillary roof = "blow out" fracture) and medial wall (lamina papyracea of ethmoid)	• Diplopia? • Numbness of ipsilateral cheek? (infraorbital nerve damage) • Assess for signs of severe contusion, rupture, laceration, irregular pupil, hyphema • Assess for limited upward or downward gaze— suggests entrapment of inferior rectus muscle at fracture site or contusion of the muscle • Upward gaze—nausea

(Continued)

Table 25-3 Ocular Trauma (*Continued*)

Presentation	Pearls	Management
		• Limited lateral gaze suggests medial rectus entrapment • CT • Tetanus prophylaxis • Possible surgical repair required if persistently reduced eye movement after 10–14 days as this may resolve spontaneously • Antibiotics if sino-orbital fracture • No nose blowing
Conjunctival foreign body		
• Bulbar (ocular surface) • Palpebral (Inside surface of lid) • Scratching sensation	• Palpebral conjunctival FB gets stuck on inside upper lid in the tarsal sulcus	• Visual acuity • Evert both lids • Remove FB rolling a moistened cotton tip applicator across the conjunctival surface • Fluorescein • Topical antibiotic • Pain control • Ophthalmology follow up 48 hours to confirm epithelial healing without infection
Corneal abrasion		
• Usually confined to epithelium • Pain, tearing, photophobia • Typically from fingernails, hairbrush bristles, branches/bushes, airborne particles, poor contact lens technique or overwear, sun-lamp treatments	• Sun lamp–associated symptoms typically develop several hours after exposure • Most corneal abrasions heal spontaneously within 48 hours • Infection rare	• Topical anesthetic for exam only • Visual acuity • Inspect cornea with light and magnification for uneven light reflection, cloudiness, or foreign body • Assess depth of anterior chamber (shallow indicates perforation)

Table 25-3 Ocular Trauma (*Continued*)

Presentation	Pearls	Management
	• If no clear history of trauma to the eye, consider infection or dry eye • Repeated topical anesthetic is toxic to the cornea	• Fluorescein • Evert lids • Topical antibiotic • And/or cycloplegic for pain relief • Narcotic prn for 24 hours • No topical anesthetic • No patching in children • Follow up with ophthalmology in 48 hours to ensure healing without infection

Table 25-4 Neonatal Conjunctivitis

Onset: During first month of life

Signs: Conjunctival injection with watery or purulent discharge

Causes: Infection, irritation, or blocked tear duct

Differential	Hx and PE	Dx	Txt	Pearls
Chemical conjunctivitis	Onset: Within 6–8 hours of instillation of topical prophylaxis at birth Presentation: Mildly red eyes and some swelling of the eyelids	• Hx	• No treatment • Resolves spontaneously within 36–96 hours	• Prophylaxis (erythromycin ophthalmic ointment) reduces but does not eliminate risk of gonococcal conjunctivitis. • Does not cover *C. trachomatis*.
Chlamydia trachomatis ~40%	Onset: 5–14 days postpartum • Possibly earlier if premature rupture of membranes Presentation: Variable, minimal to severe • Conjunctival injection • Lid swelling • Watery discharge becoming mucopurulent	• Gold standard: NAAT* • Conjunctival swab with epithelial cells from everted eyelid (is obligate intracellular organism)	• Systemic, due to high rate of nasopharyngeal infection and pneumonia First line: • PO erythromycin ethylsuccinate ×14 days • Effective up to 90% conjunctivitis and 80% pneumonia	Consider if: • <1 month of age with conjunctivitis AND • Fx of untreated maternal *C. trachomatis* infection • If mother had no prenatal care OR • There was a maternal hx of *N. gonorrhoeae* infection

	• Bloody discharge • Possible pseudomembrane formation	• Nasopharynx swab • Test for *N. gonorrhoeae* due to a high rate of coinfection	• May repeat course if needed Alternative: • Azithromycin 3 days • Topical treatment not effective • Treat parents	• Up to 50% of newborns with chlamydial conjunctivitis also develop pneumonia • Conjunctiva usually heals without complications with treatment • Untreated infection can persist and cause conjunctival and corneal scarring • Erythromycin in neonates < 2 weeks associated with HPS,** counsel parents on risks, signs, symptoms
N. gonorrhoeae ~< 1%	Onset: 2–5 days postpartum • Possibly earlier if premature rupture of membranes Presentation: • Acute • Severe eyelid edema • Conjunctival injection • Chemosis • Profuse purulent exudate	• Gram stain for gram-negative diplococci • Culture of conjunctival exudate plus oropharyngeal, and rectal sites on modified Thayer-Martin medium	First line: • Ceftriaxone 50 mg/kg IV or IM to max 125 mg single dose • Treat 14 days if disseminated disease • Do not use if hyperbili or on Ca containing IV fluids	Consider if: • Abrupt onset after day one of life • Apparent severe or persistent chemical conjunctivitis • Hx of untreated maternal *N. gonorrhoeae* infection

(Continued)

Table 25-4 Neonatal Conjunctivitis (*Continued*)

Differential	Hx and PE	Dx	Txt	Pearls
	• Possible indolent and delayed onset due to ophthalmic prophylaxis, size of inoculum, or variation in virulence	• Test for *C. trachomatis* due to a high rate of coinfection	Alternative: • Cefotaxime • OK for hyperbili or if receiving Ca containing fluids • Frequent saline irrigation of eyes prevents secretions from adhering • Topical meds are ineffective • Test and treat mother and sexual partner(s)	• No prenatal care OR • Maternal tx *C. trachomatis* infection • Test and treat asymptomatic neonate if untreated maternal infection • Treat empirically after obtaining cultures before confirmatory tests available • Untreated may result in corneal ulcerations, scarring, and blindness • Can be associated with bacteremia and meningitis • Admit to observe for response to therapy and for disseminated disease

Staphylococcus, _Streptococcus_, Gram-negative bacteria ~30–50%	Onset: • Variable • Usually 4 days up to several weeks postpartum Presentation: • Mucopurulent discharge		Gram-positive and _Haemophilus_: • Erythromycin ointment 6× daily Gram-negative organisms: • Topical gentamicin every 2 hours	• Can be associated with sepsis • Can cause corneal perforation
HSV 1 and 2 ~< 1%	Onset: Usually 5–10 days of life Presentation: • Watery discharge • Lid swelling • Conjunctival injection • Excessive tearing • Painful eye symptoms • Choroiditis • Keratoconjunctivitis	Viral Cx from: • Surface swabs of conjunctiva, mouth, nasopharynx, • Skin scrapings of vesicles or surface lesions • CSF HSV PCR • Whole blood or plasma HSV PCR Additionally: • CBC with differential, LFTs, bilirubin, ammonia, BUN, Cr, CSF studies, blood and CSF cultures, EFG	First line: • Acyclovir × 14–21 days depending on pattern of illness and response to therapy First-line alternative: Ganciclovir If eye disease: Systemic acyclovir plus topical ophthalmic treatment (trifluridine 1%, idoxuridine 0.1%, or ganciclovir 0.15%)	• Suppressive therapy during pregnancy markedly reduces but does not eliminate risk • Can occur as isolated infection, or with disseminated or CNS infection • Do full workup even in apparent isolated diseases because clinical findings may be absent early in course

(Continued)

Table 25-4 Neonatal Conjunctivitis (*Continued*)

Differential	Hx and PE	Dx	Txt	Pearls
		• CXR and brain MRI if HSV infection suspected or identified • Ophthalmology exam: Dendritic keratitis is pathognomonic		• Indications for empiric are not standardized, but most experts agree indicated for any clinical features suggestive of HSV infection • Outcome depends on clinical pattern • HSV infection is lifelong even with appropriate therapy • Recurrence of eye disease and other forms may occur • Those with ocular involvement are at risk for long-term complications including vision loss, requiring close follow-up, and oral suppressive therapy is recommended for up to 1 year

*NAAT—nucleic acid amplification test.
**HPS—hypertrophic pyloric stenosis.

ORTHOPEDICS—ARTHRITIS AND JOINT FLUID AND INFECTIONS

Table 26-1 Analysis of Joint Fluid

	Noninflammatory	Inflammatory	Septic	Hemorrhagic
Clarity	Clear	Cloudy	Purulent/Turbid	Bloody
Color	Yellow	Yellow	Yellow	Red/Brown
WBC/ml	< 200–2000	200–100,000	> 50,000	< 200[2]
PMN (%)	< 25%	> 75%	> 75%	< 25%
Glucose[1]	95–100%	80–100%	< 50%	100%
Culture	Negative	Negative	Positive > 50%	Negative
Disease	Degenerative joint disease, trauma, rheumatic fever, osteochondritis	Crystal, spondylo-arthropathy, Lyme, Reiter's, TB, fungi, viral, RA[3]	Septic arthritis	Trauma, bleeding diathesis, neoplasm

[1]Joint/Serum glucose × 100%. [2]Pure blood, joint = serum WBC. [3]Rheumatoid arthritis.

Table 26-2 Etiology of Arthritis Based on Number of Involved Joints[1]

Monoarthritis (1 joint)	Trauma, tumor, septic, gout, or pseudogout	Lyme disease, avascular necrosis, osteoarthritis (acutely)
Oligoarthritis (2–3 joints)	Lyme, Reiter's, rheumatic fever	Gonococcal, ankylosing spondylitis, gout (polyarticular)
Polyarthritis (> 3 joints)	Rheumatoid, lupus, viral (rubella, hepatitis)	Serum sickness, septic (neonate, immunocompromised)

[1]Migratory arthritis causes: Gonococcal, viral, rheumatic fever, Lyme, lupus, subacute endocarditis, mycoplasma, histoplasmosis, coccidioidomycosis, Henoch-Schönlein purpura, serum sickness (esp. cefaclor), sepsis (*Staphylococcus aureus, Streptococcus, Meningococcus*).

Table 26-3 Septic Arthritis

Overview—Neonatal = Group B strep, *S. aureus*, gram-negative > 2 months *S. aureus*, Strep. gram-negative, *Neisseria*, *Salmonella* (esp. sickle cell), *Pseudomonas* (metal nail puncture through rubberized sole of shoe) 90% in 1 joint (knee > hip > ankle), multiple if neonate. Pseudoparalysis and irritability occur in young, and pain/↓ ROM older. Joint usually held in position max. distention. ↑ resistance to movement. US—effusion in 85% acute hips (also trans. synovitis). Joint culture + in 50–80% *Management*—(1) IV antibiotics (see page 162), (2) repeat aspiration, (3) surgical drainage if (a) hip, (b) ↑ debris, fibrin, loculation in joint space, or (c) no improvement within 3 days of IV antibiotics	*Presenting Features*[1]	
	Average age	4 years
	Age < 2 years	46–69%
	Median duration symptoms	3 days
	Recent URI/*trauma*	53/*31%*
	Associated osteomyelitis	22%
	Temperature > 101°F	~75%
	↑ Sedimentation rate (ESR)	60–90%
	Average ESR (mm/hour)	36–56
	↑ C-reactive protein	82–95%
	↑ Serum WBC	46–60%
	X-ray normal (except neonate, hip subluxation)	~80%
	Abnormal Technetium scan	70–90%
	Abnormal MRI (better than US at telling septic joint vs synovitis)	88%

[1]See Table 26-17 for algorithm discriminating between septic and transient synovitis of hip.
Modified from Luhmann JD, Luhmann SJ. Etiology of septic arthritis in children: an update for the 1990s. *Pediatr Emerg Care*. 1999;15(1):40–42; Bonhoeffer J, Haeberle B, Schaad UB, Heininger U. Diagnosis of acute haematogenous osteomyelitis and septic arthritis: 20 years experience at the University Children's Hospital Basel. *Swiss Med Weekly*. 2001;131(39–40):575–581; Welkon CJ, Long SS, Fisher MC, Alburger PD. Pyogenic arthritis in infants and children: a review of 95 cases. *Pediatr Infect Dis J*. 1986;5(6):669–676; Dagan R. Management of acute hematogenous osteomyelitis and septic arthritis in the pediatric patient. *Pediatr Infect Dis J*. 1993;12(1):88-92. DOI: 10.1097/00006454-199301000-00018; Kallio MJT, Unkila-Kallio L, Aalto K, Peltola H. Serum C-reactive protein, erythrocyte sedimentation rate and white blood cell count in septic arthritis of children. *Pediatr Infect Dis J*. 1997;16:411–413; Barton LL, Dunkle LM, Habib FH. Septic arthritis in childhood. A 13-year review. *Am J Dis Child*. 1987;141(8):898–900; Del Beccaro MA, Champoux AN, Bockers T, Mendelman PM. Septic arthritis versus transient synovitis of the hip: the value of screening laboratory tests. *Ann Emerg Med*. 1992;21(12):1418–1422; Greenspan A, Tehranzadeh J. Imaging of infectious arthritis. *Radiol Clin North Am*. 2001;39(2):267–276; Sundberg SB, Savage JP, Foster BK. Technetium phosphate bone scan in the diagnosis of septic arthritis in childhood. *J Pediatr Orthop*. 1989;9(5):579-585.

Most common causes of bacterial arthritis in children according to age[1]

Age group	Most common bacteria
<3 months	*Staphylococcus aureus* (MSSA and MRSA)
	Group B *Streptococcus* (*Streptococcus agalactiae*)
	Gram-negative bacilli
	Neisseria gonorrhoeae

239

Most common causes of bacterial arthritis in children according to age[1] (Continued)

3 months–3 years	*S. aureus* (MSSA and MRSA)
	Kingella kingae
	Group A *Streptococcus* (*Streptococcus pyogenes*)
	Streptococcus pneumoniae
	Haemophilus influenzae type b (Hib) (in incompletely immunized children in regions with low Hib immunization rates)
>3 years	*S. aureus* (MSSA and MRSA)
	Group A *Streptococcus*
	S. pneumoniae
	N. gonorrhoeae (in sexually active adolescents)

[1] MSSA—methicillin-susceptible *S. aureus*; MRSA—methicillin-resistant *S. aureus*.

Suggested doses of parenteral antibiotics commonly used in the treatment of osteoarticular infections in infants and children

Intravenous agent	Dose for infants 8–28 days	Dose for children > 28 days
Ampicillin	150 mg/kg per day divided in 2 doses	200–400 mg/kg per day divided in 4 doses Max dose 12 g/day
Cefazolin	100–150 mg/kg per day divided in 3 doses	100–150 mg/kg per day divided in 3 doses Max dose 6 g/day
Cefepime	60–100 mg/kg per day divided in 2 doses	100–150 mg/kg per day divided in 3 doses Max dose 6 g/day
Cefotaxime	150–200 mg/kg per day divided in 3 doses	150–200 mg/kg per day divided in 3–4 doses Max dose 8 g/day
Ceftazidime	150 mg/kg per day divided in 3 doses	125–150 mg/kg per day divided in 3 doses Max dose 6 g/day
Intravenous agent	Dose for infants 8–28 days	Dose for children > 28 days
Ceftriaxone	50–75 mg/kg per day in 1 dose	75–100 mg/kg per day divided in 1–2 doses Max dose 4 g/day
Clindamycin	20–30 mg/kg per day divided in 3 doses	25–40 mg/kg per day divided in 3–4 doses Max dose 2.7 g/day

(Continued)

Suggested doses of parenteral antibiotics commonly used in the treatment of osteoarticular infections in infants and children (*Continued*)

Intravenous agent	Dose for infants 8–28 days	Dose for children > 28 days
Daptomycin	—	1–6 years: 12 mg/kg per day in 1 dose 7–11 years: 9 mg/kg per day in 1 dose 12–17 years: 7 mg/kg per day in 1 dose
Gentamicin	7.5 mg/kg per day divided in 3 doses	7.5 mg/kg per day divided in 3 doses
Linezolid	30 mg/kg per day divided in 3 doses	< 12 years: 30 mg/kg per day in 3 doses ≥ 12 years: 600 mg twice per day
Nafcillin	100 mg/kg per day divided in 4 doses	150–200 mg/kg per day divided in 4 doses Max dose 12 g/day
Oxacillin	100 mg/kg per day divided in 4 doses	150–200 mg/kg per day divided in 4–6 doses Max dose 12 g/day
Penicillin	150,000 units/kg per day divided in 3 doses	250,000–400,000 units/kg per day divided in 4–6 doses Max dose 24 million units per day
Vancomycin	Loading dose of 20 mg/kg followed by maintenance dose according to serum creatinine: • < 0.7 mg/dl: 15 mg/kg every 12 hours • 0.7–0.9 mg/dl: 20 mg/kg every 24 hours • 1.0–1.2 mg/dl: 15 mg/kg every 24 hours • 1.3–1.6 mg/dl: 10 mg/kg every 24 hours • > 1.6 mg/dl: 15 mg/kg every 48 hours	45–60 mg/kg per day divided in 3–4 doses Max dose 4 g/day

Data from: American Academy of Pediatrics. Antibacterial drugs for newborn infants: Dose and frequency of administration. In: *Red Book: 2009 Report of the Committee on Infectious Diseases*, 28th ed, Pickering LK (Ed), American Academy of Pediatrics, Elk Grove Village, IL 2009. p.745. American Academy of Pediatrics. Tables of antibacterial drug dosages. In: *Red Book: 2018 Report of the Committee on Infectious Diseases*, 31st ed, Kimberlin DW, Brady MT, Jackson MA, Long SS (Eds), American Academy of Pediatrics, Itasca, IL 2018. p.914. Cubicin (daptomycin for injection). United States Prescribing Information. Revised September, 2017. US Food and Drug Administration. Available online at http://www.accessdata.fda.gov/scripts/cder/drugsatfda/index.cfm (accessed August 3, 2018).

Table 26-4 Osteomyelitis (see Table 26-8 for Vertebral Osteomyelitis)

Overview—In neonate, Group B strep, S. aureus, gram-negative	

Presenting features (exclude neonate)	
Average age	5.9 years
Age < 5 years	50%
Complaint of pain/*swelling*	65/*54%*
Local tender/warmth/red	1/3 each
Fever by hx or exam	75–85%
↑ Sedimentation rate (ESR)	89–92%
Average ESR (mm/hour)	42–61
↑ C-reactive protein	98%
↑ Serum WBC	31–43%
Normal WBC and ESR	< 5%
X-ray normal (esp. first 10 days)	42%
Abnormal Technetium scan	82–95%
Abnormal MRI	88–100%

Overview—In neonate, Group B strep, S. aureus, gram-negative

In neonate, most common features are pseudoparalysis (64%), tenderness (55%), fever (32%), red (32%), and irritability (36%). Infants may have paradoxical irritability (pain ↑ with holding).

If older, S. aureus > Strep > gram-negative

Most common sites: femur > tibia > foot > humerus > pelvis.

Management—(1) IV antibiotics (see page 156), (2) Surgery may be indicated for (a) abscess formation, (b) bacteremia beyond 72 hours of IV antibiotics, (c) sinus tract, or (d) sequestra presence.

Modified from Faden H, Grossi M. Acute osteomyelitis in children. Reassessment of etiologic agents and their clinical characteristics. *Am J Dis Child.* 1991;145(1):65–69; Unkila-Kallio L, Kallio MJ, Eskola J, Peltola H. Serum C-reactive protein, erythrocyte sedimentation rate, and white blood cell count in acute hematogenous osteomyelitis of children. *Pediatrics.* 1994;93(1):59–62; Brook I. Microbiology of human and animal bite wounds in children. *Pediatr Infect Dis J.* 1987;6(1):29–32; Mustafa MM, Sáez-Llorens X, McCracken GH Jr, Nelson JD. Acute hematogenous pelvic osteomyelitis in infants and children. *Pediatr Infect Dis J.* 1990;9(6):416–421; Dagan R. Management of acute hematogenous osteomyelitis and septic arthritis in the pediatric patient. *Pediatr Infect Dis J.* 1993;12(1):88–92. DOI: 10.1097/00006454-199301000-00018; Oudjhane K, Azouz EM. Imaging of osteomyelitis in children. *Radiol Clin North Am.* 2001;39(2):251–266; Scott RJ, Christofersen MR, Robertson WW Jr, Davidson RS, Rankin L, Drummond DS. Acute osteomyelitis in children: a review of 116 cases. *J Pediatr Orthop.* 1990;10(5):649–652; Schneeweiss S, Lalani A. Chapter 42: Osteomyelitis and septic arthritis. In *The Hospital for Sick Children Handbook of Pediatric Emergency Medicine.* Jones and Bartlett; 2008:331–338.

Clinical features associated with bacterial pathogens that cause acute hematogenous osteomyelitis in children

Features	
Gram-negative bacteria	
Bartonella henselae	• Exposure to cats • Bones affected: vertebral column, pelvic girdle • Multifocal infection possible
Brucella	• Endemic areas • Consumption of unpasteurized dairy

(Continued)

Clinical features associated with bacterial pathogens that cause acute hematogenous osteomyelitis in children (*Continued*)

Haemophilus influenzae type b (Hib)	• Children who are incompletely immunized in area with low Hib immunization coverage
Kingella kingae	• Children 6–36 months old • Slow onset with oral ulcers prior to musculoskeletal findings • May affect nontubular bones
Mycobacterium tuberculosis	• Contact with endemic area
Nonsalmonella gram-negative bacilli (Escherichia coli, Serratia)	• Ages birth–3 months old • Children with sickle cell disease or immunocompromised • History of instrumentation of gastrointestinal or urinary tract
Nontuberculous mycobacteria	• Associated with: underlying immunodeficiency (HIV infection, chronic granulomatous disease), surgery or penetrating injury
Pseudomonas aeruginosa	• Injection drug use
Salmonella species	• Exposure to reptiles or amphibians • Children with gastrointestinal symptoms, sickle cell disease or similar hemoglobinopathies, or in developing countries
Gram-positive bacteria	
Actinomyces	• Bones affected: face, pelvis, vertebral bodies
Coagulase-negative staphylococci	• Affects: children with indwelling vascular catheters; neonates in intensive care
Group A Streptococcus	• Children younger than 4 years old • Potential complication of varicella-zoster virus infection
Group B Streptococcus	• Typically ages 2-4 weeks old, up to 3 months old
Staphylococcus aureus	• Any age • Skin or soft tissue infection possible • Venous thromboembolism and pulmonary disease possible with methicillin-resistant *Staphylococcus aureus*
Streptococcus pneumoniae	• Children who are incompletely immunized (younger than 2 years old) or with underlying medical conditions (older than 2 years old)

Clinical features associated with bacterial pathogens that cause acute hematogenous osteomyelitis in children[1] (*Continued*)

Polymicrobial infection	• Likely resultant from direct inoculation (e.g., penetrating trauma) or spread of infection from adjacent tissue

Data from Krogstad P. Hematogenous osteomyelitis in children: Evaluation and management. UpToDate. https://www.uptodate.com/contents/hematogenous-osteomyelitis-in-children-evaluation-and-diagnosis. Accessed February 22, 2019.

Table 26-5 Etiology of Back Pain

Etiology[1,2] (n = 225)	<12 years	≥12 years
Musculoskeletal (trauma, strain)	57%	43%
Infection [viral, pneumonia, UTI (5%)][1]	13%	17%
Idiopathic	12%	13%
Sickle cell disease	14%	13%
Psychogenic	2%	2%
Other (gallstones, pancreas, renal)	2%	13%

[1]If fever, 36% had source (meningitis, lung, pharyngitis, PID, UTI), 32% virus, 18% sickle crisis. See the following text and pages 243-245 for discitis, vertebral osteomyelitis, epidural abscess. [2]If fever with bilateral radicular pain, weakness, bowel/bladder dysfunction, or perineal anesthesia, MRI spine or consult neurosurgery.
Data from Selbst SM, Lavelle JM, Soyupak SK, Markowitz RI. Back pain in children who present to the emergency department. *Clin Pediatr (Phila).* 1999;38(7):401-6. DOI: 10.1177/000992289903800704

Table 26-6 Discitis

Overview—Intervertebral disc infection due to hematogenous spread to vascular channels in cartilage of intervertebral disc space that disappear later in life. 1/3 of patients have + cultures (blood or disc) for *S. aureus*. Most are culture negative. X-rays are abnormal in 76%.[1] MRI is diagnostic procedure of choice. Management—(1) Exclude more serious disease (osteomyelitis, abscess, tumor, or other peritoneal, retroperitoneal abscess). (2) Antibiotic use debatable; if used, treat MRSA (page 147).	*Presenting features*	
	Age ≤ 2.5 years	75%
	Refuse/Difficult walking	56%
	Back/Neck pain (100% > 3 years)	25–42%
	Abdominal pain	3–22%
	Average symptom duration	5–22 days
	Hx fever or T > 100.3°F	28–47%
	Tender back	50%
	Lumbosacral involvement	78–82%
	Serum WBC > 10,500	50%
	Average ESR (mm/hour)	39–42
	Abnormal bone scan	72–90%
	Abnormal MRI	90–100%

[1]↓ Disc space, eroded vertebral end plates.
Modified from Fernandez M, Carrol CL, Baker CJ. Discitis and vertebral osteomyelitis in children: an 18-year review. *Pediatrics.* 2000;105(6):1299-1304; Crawford AH, Kucharzyk DW, Ruda R, et al. Diskitis in children. *Clin Orthop Relat Res.* 1991;266:70-79.

Table 26-7 Epidural Abscess (Spinal)

Overview—Abscess in spinal epidural	*Presenting features*	
space usually involves posterior aspect of	Average age	8 years
epidural space (86%), especially lumbar	Average symptom duration	8–9 days
region extending to 7 vertebral levels.	Limb weakness	78%
S. aureus is cause in 79%, Strep. in 8%,	Fever	63%
followed by gram-negatives/mixed flora.	Back pain	54%
Occasionally, *Mycobacterium tuberculosis*	Complete paralysis	45%
is cause.	Partial paralysis	33%
Source is hematogenous in 1/2, seeded	Sphincter disturbance	38%
by skin or soft tissue site. 1/4 had spine	Spine tenderness	27%
trauma precipitant.	Sensory level	24%
Management—(1) IV antibiotics (see	Abnormal plain films[1]	14–50%
osteomyelitis treatment on page 156).	Cerebrospinal fluid WBC	37%
Ensure that MRSA is covered, AND	count elevated	
(2) neurosurgical consult with surgical	Elevated serum WBC	85%
drainage.	Abnormal myelogram	100%
	Abnormal MRI	92–100%

[1]Most commonly loss of intervertebral disc height.
Modified from Kaufman DM, Kaplan JG, Litman N. Infectious agents in spinal epidural abscesses. *Neurology.* 1980;30(8); Auletta JJ, John CC. Spinal epidural abscesses in children: a 15-year experience and review of the literature. *Clin Infect Dis.* 2001;32(1):9-16. DOI: 10.1086/317527; Rubin G, Michowiz SD, Ashkenasi A, Tadmor R, Rappaport ZH. Spinal epidural abscess in the pediatric age group: case report and review of literature. *Pediatr Infect Dis J.* 1993;12:1007-1011; Sexton DJ, Sampson JH. Spinal epidural abscess. UpToDate. July 18, 2018.

Table 26-8 Vertebral Osteomyelitis

Etiology—*S. aureus* > *S. epidermidis*,	*Presenting features*	
gram-negatives, *Bartonella*.	Median age	6–8 years
Infection occurs when organisms settle in	Age ≤ 2.5 years	14%
low-flow vasculature near subchondral	Average symptom duration	33 days
plate. Patients are generally older and	History fever	54–79%
more ill-appearing than those with disci-	Back/Neck pain (all ages)	64%
tis. Recent trauma is noted in 14%.	Prior infection (lung, skin)	29%
Management—Diagnose by MRI, although	Back trauma	21%
technetium scanning may be more useful	Limp	14%
in very young with nonlocalized pain. IV	Abdominal, shoulder, rib	7% each
antibiotics (see osteomyelitis, page 156).	pain, or incontinence	
Surgery may be indicated for (a) abscess	Hip or flank pain	8%
formation, (b) bacteremia or systemic	Temperature > 102°F	79%
illness beyond 48–72 hours on IV antibiot-	Paraspinal mass	11%
ics, (c) sinus tract, (d) sequestra pres-	Average WBC (cells/mm³)	12,600
ence, (e) progressive neurologic deficit,		
(f) progressive vertebral body collapse		
or kyphosis.		

Table 26-8 Vertebral Osteomyelitis (*Continued*)

	Presenting features	
	WBC > 11,000 (cells/mm³)	64%
	Average ESR (mm/hour)	46
	Abnormal X-ray	46%
	Abnormal bone scan	85–95%
	Abnormal MRI	96–100%

Modified from Fernandez M, Carrol CL, Baker CJ. Discitis and vertebral osteomyelitis in children: an 18-year review. *Pediatrics.* 2000;105(6):1299-304. DOI: 10.1542/peds.105.6.1299; Correa AG, Edwards MS, Baker CJ. Vertebral osteomyelitis in children. *Pediatr Infect Dis J.* 1993;12:228-233. *Pediatr Infect Dis J.* 1993;12:228.

Figure 26-1 Age of Onset of Ossification Centers and Physeal Closure

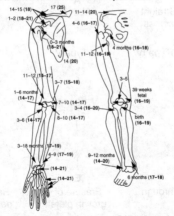

Normal type—Age of onset of secondary ossification centers. **Bold type in parentheses**—Age of physeal closure. All ages are in years unless otherwise specified.
https://www2.aofoundation.org

Figure 26-2 Salter-Harris/Ogden-Harris Physeal Fracture Classification

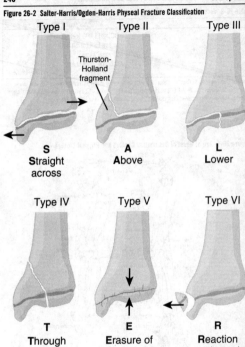

GROWTH PLATES

Salter I	Complete separation of the epiphysis and most of physis from metaphysis due to shearing force. Usually no long-term growth problems (except distal/proximal femur, proximal radius, and proximal tibia—can prematurely close with growth arrest)
Salter II	Fracture line extends along physis into metaphysis. Usually > 10 years. Generally have good prognosis.
Salter III	Fracture line extends from physis through epiphysis to articular surface. Most will require exact reduction and orthopedic consult.
Salter IV	Fracture at articular surface crosses epiphysis to metaphysis. Most will require exact reduction and orthopedic consult.
Salter V	Longitudinal compression of growth plate.
Ogden VI	Peripheral shear to borders of growth plate.
Ogden VII	Intra-articular epiphyseal injury, ligament pulling off distal epiphysis.
Ogden VIII	Fracture through metaphysis with circulation disruption.
Ogden IX	Fracture with loss of periosteum.

EMNote.org. *Ossification Centers of the Elbow*. Retrieved from https://www.emnote.org/emnotes/ossification-centers-of-the-elbow

UPPER EXTREMITY INJURIES

Table 26-9 Management (If Closed, No Neurovascular Injury, No Rotational Deformity)

Shoulder clavicle	
Scapula fracture *Requires high trauma to break (consider chest CT)*	• 75% have other serious injuries with mortality up to 14% • Surgery if body fracture displaced > 10 mm, neck + clavicle fracture, displaced coracoid fracture + distal clavicle or AC joint injury, acromial fracture + subacromial narrowing, glenoid neck fracture + > 10 mm or ≥ 40°, displacement, glenoid rim + shoulder sublux/instability, or glenoid fossa displaced > 3–5 mm • *Splinting*—Sling or shoulder immobilizer
Clavicle fracture	• *Middle 3rd*—Nonoperative. *Medial 3rd*—Usually a Salter-Harris I or II injury and mimics a sternoclavicular dislocation. If posterior-displacement, exclude mediastinal injury. Reduce under general anesthesia. *Distal 3rd*—Immobilize nondisplaced as per middle 3rd. Grossly displaced (types IV–VI) require surgery (esp. > 13 years or if significant tenting of skin). • *Splinting*—Sling arm. A figure of 8 is rarely used.
Humerus/Elbow	
Proximal fracture *(80% of humerus growth occurs here)*	• Proximal humeral ossification cannot be seen on X-ray until 6 months, greater tuberosity at 1–3 years, lesser tuberosity by 4–5 years. • Salter I—Most < 5 years. Salter II occurs in older. III/IV rare. • Majority of severely displaced fractures should be treated by sling and swathe immobilization. Acceptable displacement for closed management (if patient has open physis or is within 1–2 years of physeal closure) is (1) complete displacement, (2) ≤ 3 cm of overriding, and (3) ≤ 60° of angulation. Surgery if (1) open fracture, tenting of skin, displacement greater than (1–3) above, or neurovascular injury. • *Splinting*—Long arm handing cast, coaptation splint, or sling/swathe.
Little League shoulder	• Osteochondrosis/Traction apophysitis proximal humerus. Overuse from throwing. X-ray—Normal or wide physis. Generally treat with rest.

Table 26-9 Management (If Closed, No Neurovascular Injury, No Rotational Deformity) (Continued)

Humeral shaft fracture	• Radial nerve injury most common at distal/mid 3rd. 78–100% recovery. • ≤ 3 years old, accept 45° of angulation. Treat with sling and swathe or Velpeau bandage. • > 3 years old, accept complete displacement and ≤ 2 cm shortening. If proximal shaft, 25–30° of angulation is acceptable. If mid-shaft, 20° of angulation is acceptable. If distal 1/3 shaft, 15–20° of angulation is acceptable. • *Splinting*—Long arm handing cast, coaptation splint, sling/swathe.
Supracondylar fracture *Gartland classification and also denote if extension (95% of cases) or flexion injury*	• Splint undiagnosed/unreduced in 30° of flexion. Posterior-laterally displaced fracture may injure radial nerve. Medially displaced fracture (more common) may injure brachial artery and median nerve. • *Type I*—Nondisplaced + normal Baumann angle (angle physeal line lat. condyle/humeral shaft = 75–80°) = Ia. Ib = comminution, collapse, minimal angulation. Treatment—mobilization. • *Type II*—Displaced, intact posterior cortex. Treatment: Closed reduction with pin fixation for most. • *Type III*—Completely displaced or no cortical contact. 10–20% have absent pulse. Treatment: pinning/surgery. • *Splinting*—Splint undiagnosed elbow injuries with elbow at 20–30° until radiography completed. For type I fractures—Long arm splint with elbow at 90° flexion and forearm/wrist neutral or pronated.
Transphyseal	• Closed reduction and pin fixation required for most.
Lateral condyle fracture	• *Milch I*—Extend to capitellum ossification center. • *Milch II*—Medial to trochlea. • *Stages*—Articular surface: (I) intact, (II) disrupted, (III) displaced/rotated. • *Nondisplaced*—No surgery. • *Displaced* ≥ 2–4 mm—Reduction and surgery. • *Splinting* (for nondisplaced)—Posterior splint with elbow flexed 90°, and neutral or supinated forearm.
Medial epicondyle	• Ulnar nerve injury rate is 10–16%. If associated elbow dislocation, up to 50% may have an ulnar nerve injury. • Displaced < 5 mm—posterior splint, long arm cast or sling. • Displaced ≥ 5 mm, intra-articular fragment, incarcerated fragment, ulnar nerve injury, or late instability may require surgery. • *Splinting*—Posterior splint or long arm cast with elbow at 90°.

(Continued)

Table 26-9 Management (If Closed, No Neurovascular Injury, No Rotational Deformity) (*Continued*)

Medial epicondyle apophysitis	• Little League elbow: Pain/tender medial elbow from repeat valgus stress. Generally, treat with rest, displacement may need surgery.
Radius (R)/Ulna	
Radial head subluxation (Nursemaid's elbow)	• Injury in 6 months to 5 years old from annular ligament slipping over radial head becoming caught between radial head and capitellum. X-ray unnecessary if classic history and exam. • Treat by (1) flex elbow 90° and supinate forearm or (2) hyperpronate wrist/forearm followed by elbow flexion.
Olecranon fracture	• *Nondisplaced*—Immobilization/splinting. • *Displaced*—> 3 mm + extra-articular, closed reduction/ immobilization. If displaced > 3 mm + intra-articular or if comminuted requires surgery. • *Splinting*—Posterior splint with elbow partially extended at 75–80°.
Radial head fractures	• Ossification of radial head epiphysis begins at 5 years. The radial head is largely cartilaginous and rarely injured. 50% have another associated fracture or dislocation involving the elbow. • *Minimally displaced* (< 30°) and no translation—sling/ splint. • *Angulation > 30°*—Closed reduction, flexion-pronation technique. • *Angulation > 45°*—Closed reduction OR percutaneous pin. • *Angulation fixed > 40°, translation > 3 mm with < 60° supinate-pronation, head completely displaced*—Wire or open reduction. • *Splinting*—Sling or posterior splint with elbow 90°/neutral forearm.
Radial neck fractures	• 50% of radial neck fractures have other associated fractures or injury. Most are Salter-Harris I and II injuries. • *If < 10 years old*, accept ≤ 30° of angulation, and < 33% displacement (translation). Up to 45° may be acceptable if able to supinate and pronate 60–70°. *If > 10 years old*, accept ≤ 30° of angulation and ≤ 3 mm displacement (translation). • If they don't meet the previous criteria, closed or open reduction may be needed. • *Splinting*—Posterior splint with elbow 90° and neutral forearm.

Table 26-9 Management (If Closed, No Neurovascular Injury, No Rotational Deformity) (Continued)

Radioulnar (both bones) fracture	• ± Entrapped median, anterior interosseous nerve (FPL, lat. FDPs, pronator quadratus), superficial radial nerve (sensory dorsal web thumb). • *Plastic deformation* (bowing fractures). Treat by reducing plastic deformation under general anesthesia if ≥ 20° (esp. > 4 years), reduction needed to align associated fracture, or unable to fully rotate if > 4 years. • *Greenstick fracture* (complete disruption of only one cortex with plastic deformation of the other cortex; rotation and angular deformity present). Treat by closed reduction by reversing the deforming forces (after appropriate anesthesia). If *apex volar* (distal fragment dorsally angulated), pronate forearm and apply volar surface pressure to fracture apex. If *apex dorsal* (distal fragment is volarly angulated), supinate forearm and apply dorsal surface pressure to fracture apex. Sugar tong or bivalved long arm cast. • *Complete shaft fracture*—Closed reduction. If ≤ 8 years, ≤ 15° of prox/midshaft angulation and 30–45° angulation is acceptable. If ≥ 9 years, ≤ 10° mid and prox. shaft angulation. 9- to 14-year-old female and 9- to 14-year-old male, < 20–30° malrotation acceptable. • *Splinting*—Fractures with the apex of fracture in volar position and distal fragment angulated dorsally: splint in pronation with sugar tong splint encompassing elbow and wrist. Fractures with apex of the fracture in dorsal position and distal fragment angulated volarly splint in supination via sugar tong splint encompassing elbow and wrist. Unstable fractures require splint of elbow in extension.
Monteggia fracture (fracture of proximal ulna with radial head dislocation); *Bado classification*	• 25% posterior interosseous nerve injury (wrist extensors, not ECRL). • *Type I*—Anterior dislocation radial head, fracture ulnar diaphysis. • *Type II* (associated with ulnar nerve injury)—Postdislocation radial head, ulnar diaphyseal or metaphyseal fracture + posterior angulation. • *Type III*—Lat. or anterolat. dislocation radial head, ulnar metaphyseal fracture. • *Type IV*—Anterior dislocation radial head with ulnar/radial fracture at same levels or with radial fracture distal to ulnar fracture.

(Continued)

Table 26-9 Management (If Closed, No Neurovascular Injury, No Rotational Deformity) (*Continued*)

	• Manage primarily based on ulnar fracture. If ulna plastic deformation or incomplete ulnar fracture (greenstick/buckle), closed reduction with up to 10° angle acceptable followed by radial head reduction. Pinning or surgery may be needed if complete transverse, oblique, or comminuted fracture of ulna or unable to reduce radial head. • *Splinting*—Long arm splint with elbow flexed up to 110–120° with forearm mid-supination or neutral.
Proximal and mid-radius fracture	• In general principles of managing both bones (greenstick, plastic, complete), Monteggia, Galeazzi fracture depending on injury. • *Splinting*—Generalities may not always be appropriate depending on associated fractures and initial injury. *Proximal radius*—Long arm cast or sugar tong with forearm supinated. *Middle radius*—Long arm cast or sugar tong with forearm neutral. *Distal radius*—Sugar tong with forearm pronated. For each of these fractures make sure that the distal fragment is immobilized in the degree of rotation so that it is aligned with the bicipital tuberosity.
Distal radius fracture	• *Physeal*—If nondisplaced, immobilization. If displaced or neurovascular compromise, closed reduction and pinning. Open reduction if irreducible, open, displaced Salter-Harris III/IV fracture, compartment syndrome or acute carpal tunnel syndrome. • *Metaphyseal*—If nondisplaced, torus/buckle immobilize. Reduction to following goals is required if displaced fracture. Age 4–9 years, sagittal angulation 20° male, 15° female, frontal 15° (both) Age 9–11 years, sagittal angulation 15° male, 10° female, frontal 5° (both) Age 11–13 years, sagittal angulation 10° male, 10° female, frontal 0° (both) Age > 13 years, sagittal angulation 5° male, 0° female, frontal 0° (both) Open reduction is reserved for fractures that are irreducible/open. • *Splinting*—Sugar tong with forearm pronated.
Galeazzi fractures	• Fracture distal radius with distal radioulnar disruption. • *Type I*—Dorsal displaced distal radius. • *Type II*—Volar displaced distal radius. • *Treat/Splint*: Closed reduction and above elbow cast/full supination.

Table 26-9 Management (If Closed, No Neurovascular Injury, No Rotational Deformity) (*Continued*)

Carpal-metacarpal-phalangeal	
Scaphoid	• *Splint* long arm thumb spica if nondisplaced. If displaced, open reduction and internal fixation.
Metacarpal fractures	• (1) *Epiphyseal/Physeal*—Many are irreducible or unstable requiring pin or surgery. (2) *Neck*—Most can be reduced and splinted in "safe position." (3) *Shaft*—Closed reduction for most. (4) *Base*—Many are high energy with ↑ tissue disruption. Fractures/dislocations usually require surgery. • *Splinting*—*Neck fracture:* "Safe position" is maximum MCP flexion + extend IP joint. *Shaft fracture:* "Beer can" position, wrist extended 10–15°, MCP flexed 70°, IP extended.
Thumb metacarpal fractures	• *Head/shaft*—Closed reduction unless intra-articular or complex. • *Base*—*Type A* (metaphyseal). *Type B* (Salter II + metaphyseal piece on medial side and lateral angulation of shaft). *Type C* (Salter II with metaphyseal piece on lateral side + medial angulation shaft). *Type D* (Salter III – pediatric Bennett fracture). • Type A/B usually can be treated with closed reduction. Many Type C and most (± all) Type D + Salter IV require open reduction. • *Splinting*—Thumb spica.
Proximal and mid-phalanx	• *Physeal fractures*—Most common fractures of the proximal phalangeal base. Surgery indicated if irreducible or open fractures. *Shaft fractures* <10 years, up to 20–25° angulation in the plane of motion is acceptable. If > 10 years, < 10–15° angulation in the plane of motion is acceptable. If above these angles or if spiral, oblique wires/surgery indicated. *Phalangeal neck fractures*—Often unstable and displace due to persistent attached collaterals to the distal fragment. Surgery is usually needed. *Intra-articular fractures*—All displaced intra-articular fractures require pinning or surgery.
Distal phalanx	• (1) *Extraphyseal fractures* usually require splint alone unless very proximal or comminuted. Evacuate subungual hematoma that is > 50% of nail plate ± nail bed repair. (2) *physeal fracture* may cause mallet deformity with DIP in flexed position. An avulsion of insertion of the FDP at the DIP can cause a "jersey finger" or reverse mallet with inability to flex finger at DIP. • *Splinting*—*mallet finger:* Apply volar or dorsal splint to keep finger extended. Unacceptable reduction of mallet or open fracture require surgery. *Jersey finger/reverse mallet* requires surgery.

Modified from Migliaccio D, Ewen Wang N. *Pediatric Emergency Medicine Reports: Common Pediatric Upper Extremity Overuse Injuries.* January 1, 2017, Vol. 22, no. 1; Lalani A, Schneeweiss S. Chapter 9: Orthopedic injuries. In *The Hospital for Sick Children Handbook of Pediatric Emergency Medicine.* Jones and Bartlett; 2008:58-74.

EXTREMITY INJURIES—PELVIS AND LOWER EXTREMITY

Table 26-10 Classification of Pediatric Pelvic Fractures[1]

Torode and Zieg classification[2]		Tile and Pennal classification	
Type I	Avulsion fracture	Type A	Stable fractures
Type II	Iliac wing fracture	A1	Avulsion fractures
IIa	Separated iliac apophysis	A2	Nondisplaced wing/ring fracture
IIb	Fracture bony iliac wing	A3	Transverse fracture of sacrum or coccyx
Type III	Simple ring fractures		
IIIa	Pubis fracture, disrupted symphysis Posterior structures stable	Type B	Partially unstable fracture
		B1	Open book injury
IIIb	Acetabular fracture, no ring fracture	B2	Lat. compress (triradiate)
Type IV	Fracture with unstable segment Ring disruption fracture	B3	Bilateral type B injuries
		Type C	Unstable pelvic ring
IVa	Bilateral sup/inferior rami	C1	Unilateral fractures
IVb	Anterior rami or symphysis + posterior fracture (e.g., sacrum)	C1-1	Ilium fracture
		C1-2	Dislocation ± fracture SI joint
IVc	Fracture—unstable piece between ant. ring pelvis/ acetabulum	C1-3	Sacral fracture
		C2	Bilat fracture (1 type B/1 type C)
		C3	Bilateral type C fractures

Torode class	Mortality	GU injury	Other fractures[3]	Neuro. injury	Abd surgery
II	0%	6%	39%	61%	11%
III	3%	26%	49%	57%	13%
IV	13%	38%	56%	56%	40%

[1]Once triradiate cartilage closed, adult classification (Tile) and treatment is used. [2]Class does not include acetabular fracture. [3]Nonpelvic.

Data from Torode I, Zieg D, Pelvic fractures in children. *J Pediatr Orthop.* 1985;5:76; Silber JS, Flynn JM. Changing patterns of pediatric pelvic fractures with skeletal maturation: implications for classification and management. *J Pediatr Orthop.* 2002;22:22.

Table 26-11 Avulsion Fractures of Pelvis/Proximal Femur[1]

Location (relative frequency)	Mechanism
Ischial tuberosity (38–54%)	Forceful hamstring contraction—jumping
Ant sup. iliac spine (19–32%)	Forceful sartorius contraction—kicking/sprint
Ant inf. iliac spine (18–22%)	Forceful rectus femoris contraction—kicking
Lesser trochanter (9%)	Forceful psoas contraction—sprint, jump, kick, skate
Iliac crest (1–3%)	Contract abdomen/obliques—kicking twisting rotate
Symphysis pubis (0–3%)	Contraction leg adductors—swim, kick, jump, run

[1]*Management*—Rest, no weight bear for ≥ 3–7 days, then gradual weight with crutches, then limited exercise for 2–4 weeks. Surgery if displaced > 2 cm, chronic pain + excess callus (esp. ischial).
Data from el-Khoury GY, Daniel WW, Kathol MH. Acute and chronic avulsive injuries. *Radiol Clin North Am.* 1997;35(3):747-66.

Table 26-12 High-Yield Criteria for Knee, Ankle, and Pelvic Radiographs in the ED

Pelvic criteria[1]	Painful or tender/abraded/contused pelvis, GCS < 15 or distracting injury.
Knee criteria[2]	(1) Unable to flex 90° or (2) unable to bear weight (4 steps) in the ED.
Ankle criteria[3]	(1) Unable to bear weight immediately after injury or (2) unable to take 4 steps in the ED or (3) tender along inferior or posterior edge of malleolus.

[1]Pelvic criteria were 99–100% sensitive. [2]Knee criteria were 92–100% sensitive. [3]Ankle criteria were 100% sensitive.
Data from Junkins EP, Furnival RA, Bolte RG. The clinical presentation of pediatric pelvic fractures. *Pediatr Emerg Care.* 2001;17:15; Cohen DM, Jasser JW, Kean JR, Smith GA. Clinical criteria for using radiography for children with acute knee injuries. *Ped Emerg Care.* 1998;14:185; Khine H, Dorfman DH, Avner JR. Applicability of Ottawa knee rule for knee injury in children. *Ped Emerg Care.* 2001;17:401; Gravel J, Hedrei P, Grimard G, Gouin S. Prospective validation and head-to-head comparison of 3 ankle rules in a pediatric population. *Ann Emerg Med.* 2009;54(4):534-540.e1; Bulloch B, Neto G, Plint A. Validation of the Ottawa Knee Rule in children: a multicenter study. *Ann Emerg Med.* 2003;42(1):48-55; Konan S, Zang TT, Tamimi N, Haddad FS. Can the Ottawa and Pittsburgh rules reduce requests for radiography in patients referred to acute knee clinics? *Ann R Coll Surg Engl.* 2013;95(3):188-191.

Table 26-13 Acetabulum/Femur

Acetabulum	• *Type I*—Small fragments ± hip dislocate; *(II)*—Linear fracture ± pelvic fracture not displaced; *(III)*—Linear fracture, hip unstable; *(IV)*—Central fracture dislocation. • Nondisplaced/minimally displaced/stable (≤ 1 mm): Bed rest, nonweight-bearing. Traction or surgery if unstable or displaced > 1 mm.
Hip fracture *Delbet classification*	• *Type I*—Transepiphyseal ± acetabular dislocation. *Type II*—Transcervical (femoral neck). *Type III*—Cervicotrochanteric (base femoral neck). *Type IV*—Intertrochanteric. Management consists of reduction if needed, spica cast or surgery depending on patient age and specific injury.
Femur shaft	• Classify based on location (prox, mid, distal 3rd), configuration (spiral, oblique, transverse), angle, degree of communication, shortening (unacceptable if > 3 cm), open or closed. • Depending on injury and age, Pavlik harness, spica, traction, surgery.
Distal femur	• Peroneal nerve and rare popliteal artery injury. 23–38% have ligament injuries (usually anterior cruciate). Classify via (1) Salter-Harris (60% type II), (2) displacement [med, lat, ant, post (↑ popliteal artery injury)], and (3) age [infant and juvenile (↑ risk growth disturbance), adolescent]. • If nondisplaced, long leg cast with knee at 15–20° with molding forces opposite to injury mechanism and intact periosteal hinge tightened. • If distal femoral metaphyseal/physeal fracture, closed reduction (general anesthesia) in sagittal plane to < 20° if < 10 years and less if > 10 years. Varus/valgus alignment should be < 5° with no rotation. Irreducible type II and most displaced type III, IV, V fractures require open reduction.

Table 26-14 Knee

Patella and patellar sleeve	• *Patella*—If nondisplaced, intact retinaculum, immobilization. • Surgery indicated if > 4 mm articular displacement, articular step off > 3 mm or comminution. • *Sleeve fracture*—Avulsion distal pole patella with sleeve or articular cartilage, periosteum, and retinaculum (esp. 8–12 years). Often missed on X-ray. Need MRI to diagnose. Treat surgically. • *Splinting*—Long leg splint with knee nearly fully extended.

Table 26-14 Knee (*Continued*)

Tibial tuberosity *Ogden classification*	• *Type I*—Distal to junction of ossification of prox tibia and tuberosity. *Type II*—Junction of ossification of prox tibia and tuberosity. *Type III*—Extend to joint, associated with displaced ant. fragment + discontinuation joint surface. • Surgery is indicated for all except type I with minimal displacement.
Tibial spine *Meyers-McKeever classification*	• *Type I*—Minimally displaced, slight ant. margin elevation. *Type II*—Anterior 3rd to 1/2 of avulsed fragment elevated. *Type III*—Avulsed fragment completely elevated with no bony apposition remaining. • *Type I*—Immobilization, (if tense hemarthrosis, ± needle aspiration). *Type II*—Closed reduction. *Type III*—Open reduction. • *Splinting*—Long leg splint/cast, knee 10–20°.
Osgood-Schlatter	• Tibial tubercle apophysitis—Traction apophysitis of ant. tibial tubercle, in early puberty. Treat with rest, hamstring stretch and quad strengthening.
Jumper's knee	• Sinding-Larsen-Johansson = apophysitis inferior pole patella. Pain if run, jump. Treat—Rest, patellar tendon straps may be tried.
Osteochondritis dissecans of femur	• Medial epincondyle of femur. Occurs in males > females aged 12–16. • Osteochondral bone separates from healthy bone. Progressive, joint pain. Immobilize most, surgery if loose body, or not better after 6 months.

Table 26-15 Tibia/Fibula/Ankle/Foot

Proximal tibial physis	• Popliteal artery injury in 3–7%. Compartment syndrome also occurs. • Nonoperative if non- or minimally displaced. If reduced, general anesthesia. • *Splint*—Long leg splint with knee in full extension.
Tibia and fibula shaft fracture	• Associated—Compartment syndrome of lower extremity. • Proximal metaphyseal/distal tibia fractures can cause anterior tibial artery injury. • Prox tibia fracture—If nondisplaced, long leg splint/cast with knee nearly full extension + varus mold. If displaced, admit + closed reduction in OR. • Diaphyseal—Displaced, closed reduction. Surgery: unstable, shortening uncorrected by closed treatment, displaced fracture in skeletally mature. • *Splinting*—Long leg splint with knee bent 30–40°.

(Continued)

Table 26-15 Tibia/Fibula/Ankle/Foot (Continued)

Toddler's fracture	• History minor trauma, in child <5 years (average age 27 months). • Nondisplaced oblique/spiral distal tibia fracture, may require oblique X-ray to identify. • *Splinting*—Long leg splint with knee bent 30–40°, Jones wrap.
Distal tibia and fibula fractures	• Group I: Low-risk injuries including avulsion fractures, and minor epiphyseal separations (e.g., Salter-Harris I and II). Usually managed by closed reduction and casting. • Group II: High-risk injuries including fractures through the epiphyseal plate (Salter-Harris III, IV, and V), and transitional fractures (occur during time of physeal closure—adolescence). Examples of transitional fracture: (1) *Juvenile Tillaux* (Salter III lateral tibia fracture due to external foot rotation) and (2) triplanar (appears as juvenile Tillaux seen on AP X-ray + Salter II fracture distal tibia primarily seen on lateral X-ray). Group II injuries are usually intra-articular with joint instability. Treat most Group II injuries by open reduction internal fixation to achieve accurate anatomic reduction. • *Splinting*—Initial long leg cast/splint with knee 0–5°, ankle neutral or slightly plantar flexed if recurvatum deformity (backward angle).
Talus fracture	• Neck fracture common. Surgery if ≥ 3 mm dorsal displace or ≥ 5° varus rotate • *Splinting*—Long leg cast knee flexed so no weight-bearing ankle 90°.
Calcaneus fracture	• Immobilize most without reduction of weight-bearing. If severe displacement/intra-articular ± surgery (not needed as often as in adults).
Sever's disease	• Calcaneal apophysitis. Pain at Achilles' insertion. Chronic heel pain. Treat—1 cm heel pad, stretching, resolves as apophysis fuses ~12 years.
Kohler disease	• Avascular necrosis of tarsal navicular from repeated trauma to maturing epiphysis. Most common at 4–7 years. Treat with rest or immobilization.
Metatarsal (MT) fracture	• Compartment syndrome can occur if marked trauma/swelling. • *Shaft/Neck*—Immobilize in short leg walking cast. Wire fixation/surgery may be required if unstable (esp. 1st and 5th MT). *5th MT base*—(1) Avulsion fracture of tuberosity: extra-articular requiring immobilization/NSAIDs. (2) Proximal metaphyseal-diaphyseal (Jones) fracture: nondisplaced immobilize; Ortho follow-up, if displaced ± surgery. (3) Diaphyseal stress fracture.
Freiberg's infraction	• Osteochondrosis of 2nd MT head. 75% female esp. > 13. MT pad, short leg cast. Surgery if persistent pain, MT deformed or MT ↓ ROM.

HIP PAIN

Table 26-16 Differential of Painful Hip

Features	Toxic synovitis	Legg-Calvé-Perthes	Septic arthritis	Slipped capital femoral epiphysis
Age (years)	1.5–12	4–9	< 2, but any age	8–16
Sex (M:F)	3:2	5:1	1:1	2:1
History	Prior URI	Minimally painful	Fever, ± prior URI	Obesity in 88%
Physical exam	↓ Hip abduction and rotation	Limited hip abduction	Hip often held flexed, abducted	Trendelenburg gait, hip external rotation with flexion
X-rays	Enlarged medial joint space	Subchondral lucency femur	↑ Joint space, femur head is laterally subluxed	Line fem. neck crosses < 10% epiphysis
Ultrasound	Effusion ~90%	No effusion	Effusion	No effusion
WBC/ESR	Normal	Normal	Elevated	Normal

Table 26-17 Differentiating Septic Arthritis from Transient Synovitis of Hip

Clinical features	Probability of septic arthritis
• History fever > 101.3°F (38.5°C)	No listed features	0.2%
• No weight bearing	Any one feature	3%
• ESR ≥ 40 mm/hour[1]	Any two features	40%
• Serum WBC > 12,000 cells/mm^3	Any three features	93.1%
	All four features	99.6%

[1]Sedimentation rate.

Modified from Kocher MS, Zurakowski D, Kasser JR. Differentiating between septic arthritis and transient synovitis of the hip in children: an evidence-based clinical prediction algorithm. *J Bone Joint Surg Am.* 1999;81(12):1662-1670; Caird MS, Flynn JM, Leung YL, Millman JE, D'Italia JG, Dormans JP. Factors distinguishing septic arthritis from transient synovitis of the hip in children. A prospective study. *J Bone Joint Surg Am.* 2006;88(6):1251-1257.

NECK PAIN (TORTICOLLIS—"TWISTED NECK")

Table 26-18 Diagnosis in 170 Children Presenting to an ED with Neck Pain or Stiffness[1]

Classification	Diagnosis	Total (%)
Trauma[2]	Neck contusion and "whiplash"	67 (39%)
	False movement	28 (16%)
	Mild traumatic brain injury with neck involved	9 (5%)
	C1–C2 rotary subluxation	1 (< 1%)
Infection	Viral infections of airway and respiratory tract	15 (9%)
	Streptococcal and non-strep. pharyngitis (angina)	13 (8%)
	Retropharyngeal abscess	3 (2%)
	Parotitis and post-tonsillectomy pain (1 case each)	2 (1%)
Unknown	Spontaneous onset with no trauma or infection found	30 (18%)
Other	Congenital and osteoid osteoma (1 case each)	2 (1%)

[1]Excluded cases of obvious meningitis, major trauma (e.g., MVC). [2]See pages 324–325, for discussion regarding cervical spine radiography in trauma.

Modified from Pharisa C, Lutz N, Roback MG, Gehri M. Neck complaints in the pediatric emergency department: a consecutive case series of 170 children. *Pediatr Emerg Care.* 2009;25(12):823-826.

SELECT IMPORTANT CAUSES OF TORTICOLLIS

Atlantoaxial rotary subluxation (AARS)—Subluxation of C1 on C2 can occur after trauma, upper respiratory infections (Grisel's syndrome), or surgery due to laxity of ligaments. Patients with Down syndrome are at risk. The head tilts *away* from the affected sternocleidomastoid muscle (SCM); "cock robin" position). The head rotates opposite to the facet dislocation and laterally flexes in the opposite direction. SCM spasm and neck pain/tenderness occur on the same side as the head rotation. During rotation, C2 spinous process normally is contralateral to head rotate (but same side if AARS). Diagnose via dynamic CT. Need immobilization/surgery.

CNS tumors, bleeding or pressure—Posterior fossa tumors may cause a head tilt (to compensate for diplopia), neck stiffness, or torticollis. Intracranial bleeding, pressure, and cervical tumors may cause neck pain or nuchal rigidity.

Epidural abscess or vertebral osteomyelitis—See details, pages 244–245.

Inflammatory (local) and congenital muscular torticollis The spastic, tender SCM is opposite to the direction of the head rotation (reverse is true for AARS).

Retropharyngeal abscess (RPA)—RPA can occur at any age, but is most common at or younger than 5 years. Most children have a sore throat and many have fever, neck stiffness, neck swelling, and poor oral intake. Stridor is rare (<5%). Nearly 1/2 have limited neck *extension*, 1/3 have torticollis, and 1/10 have limited neck *flexion*. While plain X-rays are usually abnormal (see stridor, page 272), CT is more accurate. *Treat*: IV antibiotics and surgical drainage (not always needed). Modifed from Craig FW, Schunk JE. Retropharyngeal abscess in children: clinical presentation, utility of imaging, and current management. *Pediatrics.* 2003;111(6 Pt 1):1394-1398.

Sandifer syndrome—Gastroesophageal reflux causing abnormal posturing, including torticollis in infants. Torticollis is intermittent, alternates sides, and associated with wheeze, cough, failure to thrive, anorexia. *Treat*: Anti-reflux therapy.

27 ◼ PULMONARY

Table 27-1 Disorders That Alter End Tidal CO₂ (ETCO₂) Concentrations[1]

Increasing ETCO₂	• *Equipment/Mechanical*—Faulty exhalation valve, tourniquet release, reperfusion of an ischemic limb, transient seizure, contamination of sensor or optical bench (↑ baseline and ETCO₂) • *Cardiovascular*—Return of spontaneous circulation, ↑ cardiac output • *Pulmonary*—Hypoventilation, respiratory depression, obstructive disease, rebreathing (increases baseline ETCO₂) • *Metabolic*—Hyperthermia (including malignant), NaHCO₃ (onset within 1 minute, lasts < 2 minutes), shivering
Decreasing ETCO₂	• *Equipment/Mechanical*—Circuit leak, partial airway obstruction, ventilator disconnection • *Cardiovascular*—Cardiac arrest, shock (↓ cardiac output), high-dose epinephrine administration • *Pulmonary*—Hyperventilation, bronchospasm, and upper airway obstruction can ↓ steepness of respiratory upstroke: ↓ slope of waveform, mucous plugging, massive pulmonary embolism • *Metabolic*—Hypothermia, ETCO₂ ≤ 31 is associated with serum bicarbonate ≤ 15 mEq/l (76% sensitive, 96% specific) in children with gastroenteritis

[1]Assuming waveform present (if absent capnographic waveform, assume dislodged ET tube).
Modified from Nagler J, Wright RO, Krauss B. End-tidal carbon dioxide as a measure of acidosis among children with gastroenteritis. *Pediatrics.* 2006;118:260-267.

ASTHMA

Table 27-2 Reference Values (PEFR[1]) for Spirometry

Age		6 years		8 years		10 years		12 years		14 years	
Sex		M[2]	F[3]	M	F	M	F	M	F	M	F
Height (inches)	44	99	149	119	168	139	186	159	205	178	224
	48	146	179	166	197	186	216	206	235	226	254
	52	194	208	214	227	234	246	254	265	274	283
	56	241	235	261	256	281	275	301	295	321	314
	60	289	268	309	287	329	305	349	324	369	343
	64	336	297	356	316	376	335	396	354	416	373
	68	384	327	404	346	424	365	444	384	464	403
	72	431	357	451	376	471	395	491	414	511	432

[1]PEFR—peak expiratory flow rate. [2]M—male. [3]F—female.

Modified from Knudson RJ, Lebowitz MD, Holberg CJ, Burrows B. Changes in the normal maximal expiratory flow-volume curve with growth and aging. *Ann Rev Respir Dis.* 1983;127:725.

Table 27-3 Severity of Acute Asthma Exacerbation[1]

	Features	Initial PEFR or FEV1	Course
Mild	SOB with activity	≥70% of predicted or personal best	Care at home, quick relief with inhaled SABA
Moderate	SOB limits usual activity	40–69% of predicted or personal best	Office or ED visit usual, relief with frequent inhaled SABA with some symptoms for 1–2 days after treatment started; oral steroids often needed
Severe	SOB with rest or with talking	<40% of predicted or personal best	ED visit usual, likely hospital admit, partial relief with frequent inhaled SABA with some symptoms for >3 days after treatment is started; oral steroids in all, other adjuncts may be used
Life threatening	Cannot speak Diaphoresis	<25% of predicted or personal best	Hospitalization in all cases, some require ICU admission, minimal to no relief with frequent inhaled SABA, IV steroids, adjuncts are used

[1]PEFR—peak expiratory flow rate (see Table 27-2); FEV1—forced expiratory volume in 1 second; SOB—dyspnea or shortness of breath; SABA—short-acting β-agonist.

Modified from National Institutes of Health Asthma Guidelines. *Expert Panel Report 3: Guidelines for the Diagnosis and Management of Asthma.* National Heart, Lung, and Blood Institute, 2007.

Table 27-4 Pediatric Asthma Severity Score (PASS) for use ≥ 2 Years Old[1]

Finding	0	1	2
Respiratory rate	Normal rate	Tachypnea	—
Wheezing	None or mild	Moderate	Severe or absent
Work of breathing[2]	None or mild	Moderate	Severe
Prolonged expiration	Normal or mildly prolonged	Moderate prolonged	Severely prolonged

[1]A total PASS ≥ 5 (after treatment) or use of > 3 nebulizer treatments (or > 1 hour continuous) predicted admission with 82% sensitivity/84% specificity. A pretreatment O_2 saturation < 94% was not associated with admission *independent* of PASS and use of > 3 nebulizer treatments. A posttreatment O_2 sat. < 94% is a frequently quoted criterion for admittance (others use < 92%). [2]Use of accessory muscles, retractions, or in-breathing.
Modified from Gorelick MH, Stevens MW, Schultz TR, Scribano PV. Performance of a novel clinical score, the Pediatric Asthma Severity Score (PASS), in the evaluation of acute asthma. *Acad Emerg Med.* 2004;11(1); 10-18; Gorelick M, Scribano PV, Stevens MW, Schultz T, Shults J. Predicting need for hospitalization in acute pediatric asthma. *Pediatr Emerg Care.* 2008;24(11):735-744.

Table 27-5 Risk Factors for Asthma-Related Death

- Prior severe episode (ICU admit, intubation), chest tube
- ≥ 2 admissions, or > 3 ED visits in past year
- Use > 2 canisters of short-acting β-agonist per month
- Difficulty perceiving airway obstruction or the severity of worsening asthma
- Low-socioeconomic status, inner-city residence
- Illicit drug use, major psychiatric/psychosocial problems
- Comorbidity: cardiovascular or chronic lung disease

Modified from National Institutes of Health Asthma Guidelines. *Expert Panel Report 3: Guidelines for the Diagnosis and Management of Asthma.* National Heart, Lung, and Blood Institute, 2007.

Table 27-6 Guidelines for ED Management of Asthma

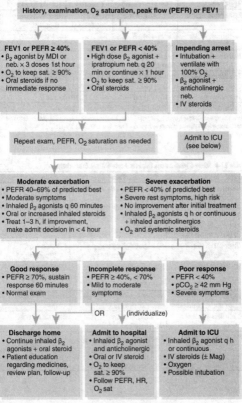

History, examination, O₂ saturation, peak flow (PEFR) or FEV1

FEV1 or PEFR ≥ 40%
- β₂ agonist by MDI or neb. × 3 doses 1st hour
- O₂ to keep sat. ≥ 90%
- Oral steroids if no immediate response

FEV1 or PEFR < 40%
- High dose β₂ agonist + ipratropium neb. q 20 min or continue × 1 hour
- O₂ to keep sat. ≥ 90%
- Oral steroids

Impending arrest
- Intubation + ventilate with 100% O₂
- β₂ agonist + anticholinergic neb.
- IV steroids

↓

Repeat exam, PEFR, O₂ saturation as needed

Admit to ICU (see below)

Moderate exacerbation
- PEFR 40–69% of predicted best
- Moderate symptoms
- Inhaled β₂ agonists q 60 minutes
- Oral or increased inhaled steroids
- Treat 1–3 h, if improvement, make admit decision in < 4 hour

Severe exacerbation
- PEFR < 40% of predicted best
- Severe rest symptoms, high risk
- No improvement after initial treatment
- Inhaled β₂ agonists q h or continuous + inhaled anticholinergics
- O₂ and systemic steroids

Good response
- PEFR ≥ 70%, sustain response 60 minutes
- Normal exam

Incomplete response
- PEFR ≥ 40%, < 70%
- Mild to moderate symptoms

Poor response
- PEFR < 40%
- pCO₂ ≥ 42 mm Hg
- Severe symptoms

OR (individualize)

Discharge home
- Continue inhaled β₂ agonists + oral steroid
- Patient education regarding medicines, review plan, follow-up

Admit to hospital
- Inhaled β₂ agonist and anticholinergic
- Oral or IV steroid
- O₂ to keep sat. ≥ 90%
- Follow PEFR, HR, O₂ sat

Admit to ICU
- Inhaled β₂ agonist q h or continuous
- IV steroids (± Mag)
- Oxygen
- Possible intubation

National Institutes of Health Asthma Guidelines *Nat Heart Lung Blood Inst* 2007

Table 27-7 Parenteral Agents for Treating Acute Asthma

Agent	Dose (max dose)	Frequency	Comments
Epinephrine 1:1,000	0.01 mg/kg IM or SC	every 20 minutes × 3	Nonselective α, β-agonist
Magnesium sulfate	25–50 mg/kg IV (max 2 g)		Administer over 15 minutes
Methylprednisolone	1–2 mg/kg IV (max 125 mg)		
Terbutaline (1 mg/ml)	0.01 mg/kg IM or SC	every 20 minutes × 3	More β selective than epinephrine
Terbutaline	2–10 mcg/kg IV load + 0.1–0.4 mcg/kg/minute IV		
Ketamine	0.2 mg/kg bolus followed by 0.5 mg/kg/hour)		

Data from Howton JC, Rose J, Duffy S, Zoltanski T, Levitt MA. Randomized, double-blind, placebo-controlled trial of intravenous ketamine in acute asthma. *Ann Emerg Med.* 1996;27(2):170-175.

Table 27-8 Inhaled Medications Used for Acute Asthma Exacerbations[1,2]

Agent	Dose[1]	Comments
Albuterol nebulizer solution 20 ml vial (0.5%) OR 3 ml vials (0.021%, 0.042%, or 0.083%)	2.5 mg (min) or 5 mg 3 ml NS every 20 minutes for mod-severe initial with ipratropium then alone continuous or every 1–4 hours	β-agonist (more selective β2 than isoetharine or metaproterenol)
Albuterol HFA MDI (Ventolin HFA)	90 mcg/puff (200/can) Use spacer + mask (<4 years)	4–8 puffs every 4–6 hours prn
Ipratropium (Atrovent)	Neb 250–500 mcg × 3 or 2–3 puffs of 17 mcg/puff via MDI	Anticholinergic, longer onset than most β-agonists
DuoNeb albuterol + ipratropium	Mixed together for 3 doses given every 20 minutes	Moderate or severe asthma
Continuous albuterol	0.5 mg/kg/hour Max 15 mg/hour	Moderate or severe asthma
Heliox (helium/oxygen)	80:20 or 70:30 (Heliox:O_2 mixture)	↓ Airway resistance, ↑ bronchodilator delivery, ↑ CO_2 elimination

Table 27-8 Inhaled Medications Used for Acute Asthma Exacerbations[1,2] (Continued)

Agent	Dose[1]	Comments
Levalbuterol HFA MDI	45 mcg/puff (200/can) Use spacer + mask (< 4 years)	4–8 puffs every 4–6 hours prn
Levalbuterol/Xopenex (0.31, 0.63, 1.25 mg/3 ml or 1.25 mg/0.5 ml)	0.31–1.25 mg in 3 ml NS	

[1]MDI—metered dose inhaler; HFA—hydrofluoroalkane propellant; can—canister. [2]MDI with spacer/holding chamber (e.g., AeroChamber Plus) improves medicine delivery and is equivalent to a nebulizer for mild/moderate asthma.

Modified from National Asthma Education and Prevention Program: Expert Panel Report III: Guidelines for the diagnosis and management of asthma. NIH publication no. 08-4051. Bethesda, MD: National Heart, Lung, and Blood Institute; 2007. www.nhlbi.nih.gov/guidelines/asthma/asthgdln.htm

Table 27-9 Oral Medications for Acute Asthma Exacerbations

Agent	Preparation	Dose	Comment
Dexamethasone (Decadron)	Elixir: 0.5 mg/5 ml Solution: 1 mg/ml	0.6 mg/kg × 1 dose Max 16 mg	Single dose equivalent to 5 days prednisolone
Prednisolone—Pediapred 5/5 Prelone and Orapred 15 mg/5 ml	Solution: 5 and 15 mg/5 ml Tabs: 5 mg	2 mg/kg initial then 1–2 mg/ kg/day	Steroid, if treat 3–7 days No taper needed
Prednisone	Solution: 5 mg/5 ml Tabs: 1, 2.5, 5, 10, 20, 50 mg	2 mg/kg initial then 1–2 mg/ kg/day	Steroid, if treat 3–7 days No taper needed

BRONCHIOLITIS

Table 27-10 Bronchiolitis Respiratory Distress Assessment Instrument (RDAI)[1]

	0	1	2	3	4
Wheezing					
Expiratory	None	End	½ Lung fields	¾ Lung fields	All fields
Inspiratory	None	Part	Throughout	–	–
Location	None	Segmental	Diffuse	–	–
Retractions					
Supraclavicular	None	Mild	Moderate	Marked	–
Intercostal	None	Mild	Moderate	Marked	–
Subcostal	None	Mild	Moderate	Marked	–

[1]Total points 0–4 = mild, 5–8 = moderate, 9–12 = severe, 13–17 = very severe (cutoffs for decision making have not been created).

Modified from Plint AC, Johnson DW, Patel H, et al. Epinephrine and dexamethasone in children with bronchiolitis. N Engl J Med. 2009;360:2079-2089; Lowell DI, Lister G, Von Koss H, McCarthy P. Wheezing in infants: the response to epinephrine. Pediatrics. 1987;79(6):939-945.

Bronchiolitis is a lung infection that commonly occurs in infants at or younger than 8 months old with most cases occurring during the winter. Respiratory syncytial virus (RSV) causes 60–90% followed by other viruses, *Mycoplasma* and *Chlamydia*. The median duration of symptoms is 12 days with 18% ill at 21 days and 9% still ill at 28 days.

Table 27-11 American Academy of Pediatrics Management Guidelines for Bronchiolitis

Diagnosis and risk assessment	• Diagnosis and severity assessment is based on history and exam. Routine labs/X-rays are not recommended. • Routine testing for viruses (RSV) is rarely useful clinically. • High risk: <12 weeks, prematurity, heart or lung disease, or immunocompromised.
Respiratory care	• Nasal suctioning. • Oxygen is indicated if O_2 saturation (sat) falls persistently below 90% (to keep ≥ 90%). • Keep well hydrated with oral feeds or IV fluids. • Bronchodilators are not routinely recommended. • Nebulized epinephrine is not routinely recommended. • Nebulized hypertonic saline is not routinely recommended in ED. • Steroids are not routinely recommended. • Antibiotics are used only if coexisting bacterial infection. • Chest physiotherapy is not routinely recommended.
	• Heliox is not recommended by AAP. It may improve work of breathing and gas exchange while preventing intubation if respiratory distress.
Isolation	• Respiratory/Contact isolation. Alcohol-based hand cleansing is preferred, although antimicrobials soaps are OK to prevent nosocomial spread of RSV.

Modified from American Academy of Pediatrics Subcommittee on Diagnosis and Management of Bronchiolitis. Diagnosis and management of bronchiolitis. *Pediatrics.* 2006;118(4):1774-93. DOI: 10.1542/peds.2006-2223; Yanney M, Vyas H. The treatment of bronchiolitis. *Arch Dis Child.* 2008;93:793; Plint AC, Johnson DW, Patel H, et al. Epinephrine and dexamethasone in children with bronchiolitis. *N Engl J Med.* 2009;360:2079.

COMMUNITY ACQUIRED PNEUMONIA (CAP)

This refers to an infection of the lung in children who acquired the infection in the community as opposed to hospital-acquired pneumonia.

Table 27-12 Antibiotic Treatment > 3 Months of Age

Setting	Type of pneumonia	Pathogen	Antibiotic
Outpatient Immunized	Uncomplicated pneumonia	*Streptococcus pneumoniae*	Amoxicillin PCN allergic: Clindamycin
Outpatient Unimmunized	Uncomplicated pneumonia	*S. pneumoniae* + *Haemophilus influenzae* type B	Augmentin 30 mg/kg dose bid × 7 days PCN Allergic: Levofloxacin 6 months–5 years: 10 mg/kg bid (max 375 mg/dose) > 5 years: 10 mg/kg every day (max 750 mg)
	Atypical features >5 years old	Mycoplasma *Chlamydophila pneumoniae*	Azithromycin 10 mg/kg day 1, 5 mg/kg days 2–5 Levofloxacin will cover atypical
Inpatient Immunized	Uncomplicated	*S. pneumoniae*	Ampicillin IV PCN allergy: Clindamycin IV
Inpatient Underimmunized	Uncomplicated	*S. pneumoniae* + *H. influenzae* type B	Ceftriaxone PCN/Cef allergy: Levofloxacin
Inpatient	Complicated or severe (large effusion, abscess, empyema or ICU)	Strep and Staph Anaerobes if abscess	Ceftriaxone + Vancomycin PCN/Cef allergy Levofloxacin + Vancomycin

Discharge criteria
- Able to take PO
- Pulse ox > 90% in room air
- Baseline mentation
- Improvement of vital signs
- Social environment able to give PO medications and have close follow-up

Modified from Bradley JS, Byington CL, Shah SS, et al. The management of community-acquired pneumonia in infants and children older than 3 months of age: clinical practice guidelines by the Pediatric Infectious Diseases Society and the Infectious Diseases Society of America. *Clin Infect Dis.* 2011;53(7):e25.

Table 27-13 Hospital-Acquired Pneumonia

| *Staphylococcus aureus*, Enterobacteriaceae, *Pseudomonas aeruginosa*, and anaerobes | Aminoglycoside (gentamicin OR amikacin) PLUS
• Piperacillin-tazobactam 300 mg/kg per day in 4 divided doses (max 16 g/day), OR
• Meropenem 60 mg/kg per day in 3 divided doses (max 3 g/day), OR
• Ceftazidime 125 to 150 mg/kg per day in 3 divided doses (max 6 g/day), OR
• Cefepime 150 mg/kg per day in 3 divided doses (max 4 g/day), OR
• Clindamycin 30 to 40 mg/kg per day in 3 or 4 divided doses (max 2.7 g/day) |
| MRSA | Vancomycin (do not use with Piperacillin-tazobactam)* |

*Data from Downes EJ, Cowden C, Laskin BL, et al. Association of acute kidney injury with concomitant vancomycin and piperacillin/tazobactam treatment among hospitalized children. *JAMA Pediatr.* 2017; 171:e173219.

American Academy of Pediatrics. Tables of antibacterial drug dosages. In: Kimberlin DW, Brady MT, Jackson MA, Long SS (Eds.), *Red Book: 2018 Report of the Committee on Infectious Diseases*, 31st ed. Itasca, IL: American Academy of Pediatrics; 2018:914.

CYSTIC FIBROSIS

Inherited defect of exocrine gland secretion characterized by (1) chronic pulmonary disease, (2) malabsorption due to pancreatic insufficiency, and (3) ↑ sweat electrolytes with variable expression and severity of disease manifestations. Suspect based on symptoms and confirm via sweat test, ± newborn immunoreactive trypsinogen, DNA sampling.

Table 27-14 Diseases and Complications Associated with Cystic Fibrosis

Organ	Manifestation and management
GI	• *Cholelithiasis*—Up to 5% have stones, 5% have cholestasis, biliary cirrhosis rare. Ursodeoxycholate slows progression of liver lesions. • *Distal intestinal obstruction syndrome (DIOS)*—Later in childhood, distal small bowel obstruction, pain, ↓ stooling, ± diet/med noncompliance. If incomplete, ± Miralax, GoLYTELY, lactulose. • *Meconium ileus*—15% (obstruct distal small bowel with meconium) in first 48 hours of life. Hyperosmolar enemas 50% relief, others need surgery. • *Meconium plug syndrome*—A more benign blockage of the colon. • *Rectal prolapse*—May be presenting symptom (esp. < 3 years). • *Pancreatic insufficiency*—Leading to malabsorption occurs in 90% by age 1 year. Leads to failure to thrive and later diabetes. Enzyme replacement → adequate fat absorption in up to 80%.

Table 27-14 Diseases and Complications Associated with Cystic Fibrosis (*Continued*)

Lung	• *Airway obstruction*—Inhaled DNase (Pulmozyme) and intermittent inhaled tobramycin will ↓ viscosity sputum, ↑ lung function. Bronchodilators and oral/inhaled steroids may be useful. • *Hemoptysis*—See management (admit if > 30–60 ml). • *Infection*—Use prior cultures to guide antibiotics, obtain new cultures. S. aureus and Pseudomonas are common (may require fluoroquinolones). Antibiotics until baseline symptom status (usually ≥ 14 days). Low admit threshold—pO_2 < 60, infiltrate, atelectasis, distress. • *Pneumothorax* develops in 5–8%, chest tube for all > 10% in size.
Metabolic	• Low K, Na, Cl with alkalosis due to respiratory/sweat loss.

Modified from Orenstein DM, Winnie GB, Altman H. Cystic fibrosis: a 2002 update. *J Pediatr.* 2002;140:156-164.

GRUNTING

Table 27-15 Most Common Etiology of Grunting in Children Presenting to a Pediatric ED

Cardiorespiratory	**57%**
Upper or lower respiratory tract infection	28%
Reactive airway disease	20%
Aspiration foreign body/liquid	4%
Myocarditis, congestive heart failure, congenital heart	4%
Sickle cell—acute chest syndrome	2%
Nonrespiratory infection	**25%**
Bacteremia/sepsis	12%
Fever, viral infection	6%
Meningitis/pyelonephritis (4% each)	4%
Surgical abdomen (intussusception, obstruction) ileus	**8%**
Sickle crisis, VP shunt malfunction, corneal abrasion, skull fracture, hemolytic anemia	**2% each**

Modified from Poole SR, Chetham M, Anderson M. Grunting respirations in infants and children. *Pediatr Emerg Care.* 1995;11(3):158-161.

HEMOPTYSIS

Mild < 150 ml/day; large 150–400 ml/day; massive > 400 ml/day (variable definitions).

Table 27-16 Etiology of Hemoptysis for Children Admitted to Hospital[1]

Cystic fibrosis	65%	Neoplasm	3%	Nasopharyngeal	1%
Congenital heart disease	15%	Pulmonary HTN, bleed,	2%	Sepsis	1%
Pneumonia	6%	embolism		Vasculitides	1%
		Tuberculosis	1%	Other	5%

[1]Overall 13% died, esp. older, ↑ amount, fever, transfusion.
Data from Coss-Bu JA, Sachdeva RC, Bricker JT, Harrison GM, Jefferson LS. Hemoptysis: a 10-year retrospective study. *Pediatrics.* 1997;100(3):E7. DOI: 10.1542/peds.100.3.e7

Management—Intubate if airway compromise, type and cross blood, administer NS, blood as needed for massive bleeding. Reverse bleeding disorder (platelets, FFP). Consult pulmonologist or thoracic surgery/interventional radiologist.

STRIDOR

Table 27-17 Stridorous Upper Airway Diseases in Children

Feature	Croup	Tracheitis[4]	Epiglottitis[4]	Retropharyngeal abscess[4]
Age (years)	0.3–3.0	5–10	2–8	Median 3.5
Prodrome	days	hours to days	minutes to hours	days (prior URI)
Fever	Low grade	Usual	Usual	Usual
X-ray[1]	Steeple sign[1]	Exudate	Ratios[2]	Soft-tissue swelling[3]
Etiology	Viral	*S. aureus*	*H. influenzae*	Streptococcus/ Staphylococcus/anaerobe
Cough	Yes	Yes	No	Uncommon
Drool	No	No	Yes	Yes
Toxic	Usually no	Yes	Yes	Yes

[1]In epiglottitis, films are normal in up to 60%; in croup they are read as normal in 50%. [2]Three calculations reported as 100% sensitive/highly specific for epiglottitis: AEW/C3W > 0.35, EW/C3W > 0.50, and EW/EH > 0.6. EW—epiglottic width; EH—epiglottic height; C3W—C3 vertebral width; AEW—aryepiglottic fold width. [3]Retropharynx soft tissue > 7 mm ant to C2 or > 14 mm ant to C5/6. (CT = more accurate). See retropharyngeal and neck pain due to torticollis detail, pages 260–261. [4]See pages 149 (epiglottitis), 166 (tracheitis), and 161 (retropharyngeal) for antibiotics.
Modified from Keith KD, Bocka JJ, Kobernick MS, Krome RL, Ross MA. Emergency department revisits. *Ann Emerg Med.* 1990;19:978; Shatkiewicz JA, Bowes AK. Croup and epiglottitis: a radiological study. *Laryngoscope.* 1985;95:1159-1160.

Table 27-18 Croup Score (Add the Five Elements Together)[1]

Feature	0	1	2	3
Color	Normal	Dusky	Cyanotic	Cyanotic on O_2
Air movement	Normal	Mild ↓	Moderate ↓	Marked ↓
Retractions	None	Mild	Moderate	Severe
Mentation	Normal	Restless	Lethargic	Obtunded
Stridor	None	Mild	Moderate	Severe/Obstructed
Total score	*Severity*	*Treatment*		
0–4	Mild	Home care		
5–6	Mild/moderate	Consider steroids, admit if < 6 months, unreliable family		
7–8	Moderate	Racemic epinephrine, consider steroids, admit most		
9–14	Severe	Racemic epinephrine, steroids, ICU admission		
15	Life threat	Racemic epinephrine, steroids, intubation		

[1]Any category with score of 3, classify as severe.
Modified from Taussig LM, Castro O, Beaudry PH, Fox WW, Bureau M. Treatment of laryngotracheobronchitis (croup). Use of intermittent positive-pressure breathing and racemic epinephrine. *Am J Dis Child.* 1975;129:790-793.

CROUP MANAGEMENT

- **Oxygen** if respiratory distress (humidity is proven not useful).
- **Dexamethasone** 0.6 mg/kg IM or PO (max 12 mg) or oral prednisolone for 3 days (1–2 mg/kg, max 60 mg)
- **Aerosolized racemic epinephrine** (RE) 0.25–0.50 ml of 2.25% solution diluted 1:8 or standard epinephrine 1 ml of 1:1,000. Observe 2–4 hours after treatment for rebound.
- **Heliox**—When inhaled may be useful at decreasing airway resistance.

Modified from Everard ML. Acute bronchiolitis and croup. *Pediatr Clin North Am*. 2009;56(1):119-133.

VENTILATION—NONINVASIVE

Table 27-19 Contraindications to Noninvasive Mechanical Ventilation

Contraindications	Respiratory arrest, cardiovascular instability, altered mentation, uncooperative, high aspiration risk, viscous or copious secretions, recent face or airway surgery, recent upper GI-esophageal surgery, upper GI tract bleeding, facial trauma, burns, extreme obesity, fixed nasopharyngeal abnormalities limiting use of equipment

Table 27-20 Noninvasive Positive Pressure Ventilation (NPPV) Modes/Parameters[1]

Bilevel positive airway pressure (BiPAP)	(1) Start inspiratory positive airway pressure (IPAP) at 8 cm H_2O. Then, increase to 10–16 cm H_2O (available range 2–25 cm H_2O). (2) The expiratory positive airway pressure (EPAP) is usually set at 5–8 cm H_2O (available range 2–20 cm H_2O). This provides positive end expiratory pressure increasing functional residual capacity and maintaining airway patency at the end of expiration. (3) A backup rate may or may not be provided. (4) Nebulized medications can be delivered via BiPAP. (5) Improvement may be heralded by ↓ respiratory rate, ↑ O_2 saturation, ↓ accessory muscle use, reduction of airway occlusion if upper airway obstruction, and improved lung volumes on chest radiography.
Continuous positive airway pressure (CPAP)	CPAP delivers a constant level of pressure support to the airways during inspiration and expiration. A mask with nasal prongs/adapters or a face mask delivers continuous pressure ranging from 4 to 10 cm H_2O. Nebulized treatments are not routinely administered via CPAP.

[1]NPPV continued on the next page.
Modified from Deis JN, Abramo TJ, Crawley L. Noninvasive respiratory support. *Pediatr Emerg Care*. 2008;24(5):331-338; Hillberg RE, Johnson DC. Noninvasive ventilation. *N Engl J Med*. 1997;337:1746-1752.

Table 27-21 Noninvasive Positive Pressure Ventilation (NPPV) Modes/Parameters

Nasal intermittent positive pressure ventilation (NIPPV)	NIPPV provides periodic increases in positive pressure above a baseline CPAP pressure. NIPPV is delivered via nasal prongs or a tight nasal mask connected to a ventilator or a bilevel nasal CPAP device. If a ventilator is used, the periodic positive pressure can be administered synchronously with an infant's respiratory effort. A low (5 cm H_2O) and a high (8 cm H_2O) CPAP level can be set.
Heated high flow nasal cannula (HFNC)	Heated humidified gas (e.g., ~100% O_2) can be delivered without irritating or drying nasal mucosa. 5 l/minute to 40 l/minute
Weaning parameters for all modes	• Clinically stable for 4–6 hours. • Respiratory rate and heart rate normalize. • Compensated pH > 7.35, SaO$_2$ ≥ 92% on ≤ 2–3 l O$_2$

Modified from Deis JN, Abramo TJ, Crawley L. Noninvasive respiratory support. *Pediatr Emerg Care.* 2008;24(5):331-338; Hillberg RE, Johnson DC. Noninvasive ventilation. *N Engl J Med.* 1997;337(24):1746-1752.

28 ■ PSYCHIATRY, RADIATION RISK

PSYCHIATRY

Table 28-1 Pediatric Suicide Risk Tool

Ask Suicide-Screening Questions (ASQ)
(1) In the past few weeks, have you wished you were dead? Yes/No
(2) In the past few weeks, have you felt that you or your family would be better off if you were dead? Yes/No
(3) In the past week, have you been having thoughts about killing yourself? Yes/No
(4) Have you ever tried to kill yourself? Yes/No
If yes, how? _____
When? _____
If the patient answers Yes to any of the above, ask the following acuity question:
(5) Are you having thoughts of killing yourself right now? Yes/No
If yes, please describe: _____
ASQ is designed to assess suicide risk in youths ages 10–21 in the emergency department. Any question 1 through 4 with a "yes" response or left blank is considered as a positive screen. Anyone with a positive screen must have a safety evaluation prior to leaving the ED. The answer to question 5 determines acuity of risk and urgency of further steps.
ASQ has a sensitivity of 96.9%, specificity of 87.6%, negative predictive value of 99.7% for medical/surgical patients, and 96.9% for psychiatric patients.

Modified from Horowitz LM, Bridge JA, Teach SJ, et al. Ask Suicide-Screening Questions (ASQ): a brief instrument for the pediatric emergency department. *Arch Pediatr Adolesc Med.* 2012;166(12):1170-1176. doi:10.1001/archpediatrics.2012.1276.

EVALUATION AND MANAGEMENT OF THE AGITATED PEDIATRIC PATIENT

Figure 28-1 Clinical Decision Flow Chart for the Agitated Patient

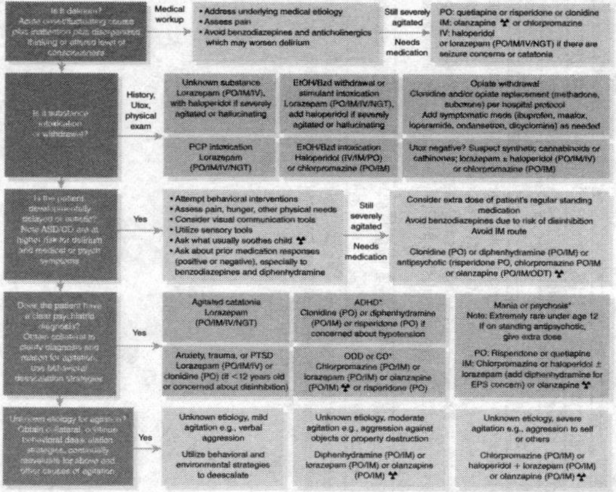

* Medication options are listed alphabetically. NGT—nasogastric tube; EtOH—ethanol; Utox—urine toxicology; PCP—phencyclidine; EPS—extrapyramidal symptoms; ASD—autism spectrum disorder; DD—developmental disability; BZD—benzodiazepines; ODT—orally dissolving tablet; PTSD—post-traumatic stress disorder; AHDH—attention deficit hyperactivity disorder; ODD—oppositional defiant disorder; CD—conduct disorder; ☢—Do not give olanzapine and benzodiazepines within 1 hour of each other.

Reproduced from Gerson R, Malas N, Feuer V, Silver GH, Prasad R, Mroczkowski MM. Best practices for evaluation and treatment of agitated children and adolescents (BETA) in the emergency department: consensus statement of the American Association for Emergency Psychiatry. *West J Emerg Med.* 2019;20(2):409-418.

Expert consensus on the management of agitated pediatric patients in the ED favors an individualized, multidisciplinary approach. The use of medications should be part of a comprehensive strategy, with an emphasis on prevention and de-escalation by treating the root causes of agitation and attempting nonpharmacological interventions first, as well as in conjunction with medication.

The goal of medication management is to provide a calming effect on the patient and should also address the underlying etiology of agitation. Choice of medication is dictated by an assessment of the risk of adverse effects against the potential benefit for an individual patient. Commonly administered medications include diphenhydramine, benzodiazepines, and alpha-2-agonists; neuroleptics should only be used judiciously in cases of severe agitation or delirium. Ketamine, barbiturates, and opioids should be avoided (unless opioids are needed for pain control).

Oral administration is preferred and should be attempted first before using an intramuscular (or intravenous, if access is available) route. In general, if a first dose of medication is ineffective, a second dose of the same medication should be given, rather than adding a new medication. Attention should be paid to the total daily dose and maximum dose of selected medications. Any patient who receives more than one dose of medication requires continuous monitoring for adverse effects. Continual reassessment of the underlying etiology of agitation should be ongoing, along with concomitant application of nonpharmacological treatments for agitation. Table 28-2 Medication Management for the Agitated Patient is found on the following page.

RADIATION RISK

Many medical imaging modalities expose patients to ionizing radiation, which can be associated with higher cancer risks. There is no epidemiological evidence of increased cancer risk with exposures of less than 10 mSv and clear evidence of increased risk with exposures of more than 100 mSv. The risk increases in a dose-dependent fashion, but the exact amount of risk at doses between 10 and 100 mSv remains controversial.

A 10 mSv dose of radiation is estimated to cause a 0.1% increased lifetime risk of cancer and a 0.5% excess risk of death from cancer. The effect of any individual image study on cancer mortality is very small. Natural incidence of cancer mortality is 25%.

Average yearly background radiation exposure is 3 mSv, primarily from radon gas in the home. Some radiation also comes from cosmic rays, so living at higher altitudes causes an increase in background radiation as well. It is useful to think about radiation exposure from imaging modalities in comparison to the amount of time it takes to acquire the same amount of radiation just from daily living.

Young children are about three to four times more sensitive to the effects of radiation than adults. They also have a longer lifetime in which to develop cancer; therefore, it is particularly important to minimize unnecessary radiation exposure in this population.

Table 28-2 Medication Management for the Agitated Patient

Medication	Dose	Max daily dose	Peak effect	Monitoring	Notes
Diphenhydramine (antihistamine)	PO/IM: 12.5-50 mg 1 mg/kg/dose	Child: 50-100 mg Adolescent: 100-200 mg	PO: 2 hours	-Disinhibition or delirium in younger or developmentally delayed patients	Avoid in delirium. May be given with haloperidol or chlorpromazine.
Lorazepam (benzodiazepine)	PO/IM/IV/NGT: 0.5-2 mg 0.05-0.1 mg/kg/dose	Child: 4 mg Adolescent: 6-8 mg Depending on weight/prior medication exposure	IV: 10 minutes PO/IM: 1-2 hours	-Disinhibition or delirium in younger or developmentally delayed patients	May be given with haloperidol, chlorpromazine or risperidone. Do not give within 1 hour of olanzapine.
Clonidine (alpha2 agonist)	PO: 0.05-0.1 mg	27-40.5 kg: 0.2 mg/day 40.5-45 kg: 0.3 mg/day > 45 kg: 0.4 mg/day	PO: 30-60 minutes	-Hypotension -Bradycardia	Avoid giving with benzodiazepines or atypicals due to hypotension risk.
Chlorpromazine (antipsychotic)	PO/IM: 12.5-60 mg (IM should be half the PO dose) 0.55 mg/kg/dose	Child < 5 years: 40 mg/day Child > 5 years: 75 mg/day	PO: 30-60 minutes IM: 15 minutes	-Hypotension -QT prolongation	
Haloperidol (antipsychotic)	PO/IM: 0.5-5 mg (IM should be half a dose of PO) 0.55 mg/kg/dose	15-40 kg: 6 mg > 40 kg: 15 mg Depending on prior antipsychotic exposure	PO: 2 hours IM: 20 minutes	-Hypotension -QT prolongation, especially with IV administration.	Note EPS risk with doses of >3 mg/day. IV dosing with very high EPS risk.
Olanzapine (antipsychotic)	PO/ODT or IM: 2.5-10 mg (IM should be half or 1/4 dose of PO)	10-20 mg Depending on antipsychotic exposure	PO: 5 hours (range 1-8 hours) IM: 15-45 minutes		Do not give within 1 hour of any benzodiazepine, given risk for respiratory suppression.
Risperidone (antipsychotic)	PO/ODT: 0.25-1 mg 0.005-0.01 mg/kg/dose	Child: 1-2 mg Adolescent: 2-3 mg Depending on antipsychotic exposure	PO: 1 hour		Can cause akathisia (restlessness/agitation) in higher doses.
Quetiapine (antipsychotic)	PO: 25-50 mg 1-1.5 mg/kg/dose (or divided)	> 10 years: 600 mg Depending on prior antipsychotic exposure	PO: 30 minutes – 2 hours	-Hypotension	More sedating at lower doses.

Table 28-3 Comparison of Radiation Doses from Medical Imaging Tests and Background Radiation

Imaging		Radiation dose (mSv)[1]	Time to accumulate comparable natural background dose
Computed tomography	Multiphase abdomen and pelvis	31.0	10 years
	Abdomen and pelvis	10.0	3 years
	Chest (pulmonary embolism)	10.0	3 years
	Chest	7.0	2 years
	Head	2.0	8 months
	Sinuses	0.6	2 months
Fluoroscopy	Coronary angiography	5–15	20 months–5 years
	Barium swallow	1.5	6 months
Nuclear medicine	Cardiac perfusion (sestamibi)	12.5	4 years
	Bone scan	4.2	1 year 4 months
	Lung ventilation/ perfusion	2.0	8 months
Radiography	Abdomen	1.2	5 months
	Lumbar spine	0.7	3 months
	Chest	0.1	10 days
	Extremity	0.001	< 1 day
Other	Mammography	0.7	3 months
	Bone densitometry (DEXA[2])	0.001	< 1 day

[1]These doses are effective doses, which are theoretical quantities proposed by the International Commission on Radiation Protection to assess the health risks of low doses of ionizing radiation; millisievert (mSv). [2]DEXA: dual-energy X-ray absorptiometry.

Source: Lin EC. Radiation risk from medical imaging. Mayo Clin Proc. 2010;85(12):1142-1146. doi:10.4065 /mcp.2010.0260.

OVERVIEW

Drowning, or injury due to submersion or immersion in liquid, is the third leading cause of unintentional injury death worldwide and is in the top six causes of injury death in all childhood age groups.[1] Children are at an increased risk, but they also have better outcomes from resuscitation. Most drowning cases are nonfatal drownings and will be seen in the ED. Knowing which patients are at risk for morbidity and mortality is critical to identifying those who require observation and hospital-based care.

TERMINOLOGY

Drowning is defined by WHO as "the process of experiencing respiratory impairment from submersion/immersion in liquid; outcomes are classified as death, morbidity and no morbidity."[2] Historically used diagnoses, such as near-drowning, are discouraged. Terms such as "dry drowning," "wet drowning," "secondary drowning," "passive drowning," "silent drowning," and "delayed drowning" are not accepted medical terms or diagnoses.[3,4] Expert consensus now agrees on three outcomes possible after a submersion/immersion event: fatal drowning, nonfatal drowning with morbidity, and nonfatal drowning without morbidity.[1,5]

MANAGEMENT

Patients who present after submersion with no immediate symptoms have a 100% survival rate and can be dismissed from the scene or discharged from the ED without intervention. Patients presenting with cough and without auscultatory findings are also at a very low risk for mortality. These patients need to be observed in the ED and their vital signs, including pulse oximetry, monitored and can be considered for discharge if there is no worsening of symptoms. Those with severe symptoms, abnormal exam, and unstable hemodynamics should undergo resuscitation and stabilization with a focus on aggressive respiratory support, fluid resuscitation, management of hypothermia, and evaluation for traumatic injuries. The role of chest radiographs is unclear in minimally symptomatic patients and is more likely to be useful for the detection of pulmonary edema, aspiration pneumonia, or pneumonitis when used based on clinical indicators.

Figure 29-1 Drowning Grading and Mortality Risk

Grade	Dead	6	5	4	3	2	1	Rescue
Intervention	None	Start CPR (ABC sequence) After return of spontaneous ventilation, follow intervention for grade 4	Start artificial ventilation Respiratory arrest is usually reversed after a few imposed breaths After return of spontaneous ventilation, follow intervention for grade 4	Administer high-flow oxygen by face mask or orotracheal tube and mechanical ventilation Monitor breathing because respiratory arrest can still occur Start crystalloid infusion and evaluate for use of vasopressors	Administer high-flow oxygen by face mask or orotracheal tube and mechanical ventilation	Low-flow oxygen	Advanced medical attention and oxygen should not be required	None
Further Management	Forensic evaluation	Intensive care unit				Emergency department	If no coexisting conditions, evaluate further or release from the accident site	
Survival	0%	7–12%	56–69%	78–82%	95–96%	99%		

Figure 29-1 Drowning Grading and Mortality Risk (*Continued*)

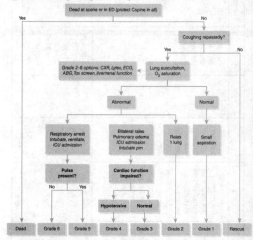

ABC—airway–breathing–circulation; CPR—cardiopulmonary resuscitation.
Szpilman D, Bierens JJ, Handley AJ, Orlowski JP. Drowning. *N Engl J Med.* 2012;366(22):2102-2110.

REFERENCES

1. Centers for Disease Control and Prevention. 10 leading causes of injury deaths by age group highlighting unintentional injury deaths, United States—2017. https://www.cdc.gov/injury/images/lc-charts/leading_causes_of_death_by_age_group_unintentional_2017_1100w850h.jpg.
2. World Health Organization. *Facts About Injuries: Drowning.* Geneva: World Health Organization; 2003.
3. Hawkins SC, Sempsrott J, Schmidt A. "Drowning" in a sea of misinformation. *Emerg Med News.* 2017;39(8):1.
4. Idris AH, Berg RA, Bierens J, et al. Recommended guidelines for uniform reporting of data from drowning: the "Utstein style." *Circulation.* 2003;108(20):2565-2574.
5. van Beeck E, Branche C. Definition of drowning: a progress report. In *Drowning* (pp. 85-89). Berlin: Springer; 2014.

OVERVIEW

Abdominal pain is a common reason children present to the pediatric emergency department (PED). The ED provider has the difficult task of differentiating the child with a surgical condition that requires acute intervention from the many children presenting with more benign causes. Table 30-1 outlines common etiologies of abdominal pain in children presenting to the PED.

Table 30-1 Common Causes of Abdominal Pain by Age

Age	Emergent	Urgent	Common (and more benign)
<3 months	Trauma NEC Omphalitis Adhesions Testicular torsion		Colic GERD Milk protein allergy
≥3 months to 1 year	Trauma Midgut volvulus Incarcerated hernia Pyloric stenosis Intussusception	Acute gastroenteritis	GERD Constipation
1–5 years	Trauma Appendicitis	Acute gastroenteritis HSP Pneumonia Meckel diverticulum	UTI Constipation
5–12 years	Trauma Appendicitis Testicular or ovarian torsion DKA	Acute gastroenteritis IBD Pneumonia	UTI Constipation FGID GAS
>12 years	Trauma Appendicitis Testicular or ovarian torsion Ectopic pregnancy DKA	Acute gastroenteritis IBD Pneumonia Hepatitis Pancreatitis Nephrolithiasis PID	UTI Constipation FGID GAS Ruptured ovarian cyst

NEC—necrotizing enterocolitis; GERD—gastroesophageal reflux disease; HSP—Henoch-Schönlein purpura; UTI—urinary tract infection; DKA—diabetic ketoacidosis; IBD—inflammatory bowel disease; FGID—functional gastrointestinal disorders; GAS—group A strep; PID—pelvic inflammatory disease.
Data from Smith J, Fox SM. Pediatric abdominal pain. *Emerg Med Clin of North Am.* 2016;34(2):341-361. doi:10.1016/j.emc.2015.12.010.

APPROACH

Initial approach to a child with abdominal pain should include assessment and stabilization as needed depending on vital signs, hydration, and mental status. Children with severe pain should receive analgesia. Following this, the history and physical examination should guide your evaluation.

Key history questions:

- Onset
- Provoking/Palliating factors
- Quality of pain
- Radiation of pain
- Time course
- Trauma
- Associated symptoms:
  - Fever
  - Oral intake (fluids and food)
  - Nausea
  - Vomiting (If yes, bloody? Coffee grounds? Bilious?)
  - Last bowel movement (Frequency? Consistency? Painful? Blood? Tarry?)
  - Urine output and urinary symptoms
  - Weight loss
  - Bloating
  - Testicular pain, swelling, or trauma
- Past medical history
- Past surgical history (specifically any prior abdominal surgeries)
- Physical examination:
- Vital signs: Fever? Tachycardic? Hypotensive?
- Constitutional: Is the child ill appearing? Sitting up playing? Running around the room?
- Abdominal examination: Inspection, palpation, percussion
- In boys: Testicular examination
- Be sure to complete remainder of exam to look for other sources of abdominal pain (pharyngitis, pneumonia)

The history and physical exam should help guide your next steps. The following is an overview of the more common and/or serious abdominal surgical conditions in children.

BILIOUS VOMITING

Bilious vomiting may be a sign of intestinal obstruction and should be evaluated expeditiously. Table 30-2 outlines the etiology by age. In neonates, bilious vomiting represents a surgical disorder in nearly half of all cases.[1] After initial stabilization, including IV placement and fluid resuscitation, neonates with bilious vomiting should be transferred to a facility with pediatric surgeons for further evaluation and definitive care; transfer is time-critical.[2,3] Evaluation will include an upper-gastrointestinal contrast study and consultation with a pediatric surgeon to identify surgical causes of bilious emesis. Older children presenting with bilious emesis should also receive initial stabilization as necessary. Evaluation should be based on history and a physical; considerations include abdominal X-rays (upright and lateral decubitus) to assess for bowel gas pattern, ultrasound to assess for appendicitis or intussusception, and/or laboratory studies to assess for pancreatitis.

Table 30-2 Causes of Bilious Vomiting in Infants and Children[1]

Age	Cause	% of cases
0–4 weeks[2]	**Surgical disorders:** Midgut volvulus, hernia, bowel atresia, meconium ileus/plug, Hirschsprung's	**20–51**
	Nonsurgical: Mostly idiopathic/unknown cause	**49–80**
1–12 months	**Surgical disorders:**	**14**
	Intussusception	(7)
	Bowel obstruction or hernia	(7)
	Nonsurgical disorders:	**86**
	Gastroenteritis	(64)
	Bronchiolitis	(18)
	Urinary infection	(4)
>12 months	**Surgical disorders:**	**11**
	Appendicitis	(5)
	Small bowel obstruction	(2)
	Pancreatitis (not all surgical) or cholecystitis	(2)
	Intussusception	(1)
	Ventricular shunt failure	(1)
	Nonsurgical disorders:	**89**
	Gastroenteritis or cyclic vomiting	(74)
	Respiratory infection, pharyngitis, otitis, asthma	(11)
	Other (pelvic infection, DKA, HSP, pregnancy)	(4)

[1]In neonates and older children, green emesis more likely to indicate surgical disorder than yellow emesis. [2]Consult surgeon at this age (0–4 weeks) for all bilious emesis.

Modified from Godbole P, Stringer MD. Bilious vomiting in the newborn: How often is it pathologic? *J Pediatr Surg.* 2002;37(6):909-911; Mohinuddin S, Sakhuja P, Bermundo B, et al. Outcomes of full-term infants with bilious vomiting: observational study of a retrieved cohort. *Arch Dis Child.* 2015;100(1):14-17.

APPENDICITIS

In children, appendicitis is most common between 10 and 19 years of age. Appendicitis in children typically presents with the gradual onset of abdominal pain that initially starts in the periumbilical region and then migrates to the right lower quadrant.[4] This pattern is not always presenting in children with appendicitis. Pain may be accompanied by nausea, vomiting, anorexia, and fever. Pain precedes vomiting (though in young children they may not be able to tell you which started first). The risk of perforation increases after 24 hours and is often present in patients with symptoms longer than 48 hours. When perforation occurs, the pain may decrease initially, but then the pain becomes more diffuse.[4] Table 30-3 reviews the presentation of appendicitis and Table 30-4 reviews evaluation of appendicitis.

Table 30-3 Appendicitis

Frequency of historical features at different ages					
0–2 years (rare)		**2–5 years (<5% all cases)**		**6–12 years**	
Vomiting	85–90%	Abdominal pain	89–100%	Pain	98%
Pain	35–77%			↑ with movement	41–75%
Fever	40–60%	Vomiting	66–100%		
Diarrhea	18–46%	*(unlike*		Vomiting	68–95%
Irritability	35–40%	*older children*		*before pain*	≤ 18%
Cough/Rhinitis	40%	*and adults,*		Anorexia	47–75%
Grunting	8–23%	*vomiting*		Diarrhea	9–16%
Hip pain/ stiffness	3–23%	*may precede*		Constipation	5–28%
		pain)		Dysuria	4–20%
		Fever	80–87%		
		Anorexia	53–60%		

Frequency of physical exam features at different ages					
0–2 years (rare)		**2–5 years (<5% all cases)**		**6–12 years**	
Temperature > 100°F	87–100%	Temperature > 100°F	82%	Temperature > 100.4°F	4%
Diffuse tender	55–92%	RLQ tender	58–85%	<24 hours pain	64%
RLQ tender	<50%	Diffuse tender	19–28%		
Distention	30–52%	Involuntary guarding	85%	>24 hours pain and RLQ tender	>80–95%
Lethargy	40%				
Mass	30%	Rebound tender	50%	Diffuse tenderness	15%
				Rebound	~50%

Risk of appendicitis[1,2]	Item	M	PAS
MANTRELS (M) score	**M**igration of pain to RLQ	1	1
Total > 6 candidates for surgery	**A**norexia or acetone in urine	1	1
4–6 serial exam or CT/US	**N**ausea with vomiting	1	1
< 4 very low risk of appendicitis	**T**ender right lower quadrant	2	2
	Rebound or equivalent	1	0

Table 30-3 Appendicitis (*Continued*)

Pediatric Appendicitis Score (PAS)	Pain with coughing, hopping, or percussion	0	2
In separate studies, a PAS ≥ 3 and ≥ 5 were each 98% sensitive at diagnosing appendicitis	Elevated temp. (> 38°C/100.4°F)	1	1
	Leukocytosis > 10,000–10,500	2	1
	Shift WBCs > 75% neutrophils	1	1

[1]PAS is more reliable in children, while M score is *unreliable* in children and primarily useful in adolescents and young adults. Calculate total points for M score or PAS by adding points from M or PAS column. [2]2008/(2009) studies recommended surgery for all PAS ≥ 6 (≥ *8*) and recheck, US, or CT if 3–6 (5–7).
Modified from Bhatt M, Joseph L, Ducharme FM, Dougherty G, McGillivray D. Prospective validation of the pediatric appendicitis score in a Canadian pediatric emergency department. *Acad Emerg Med.* 2009;16(7):591-596; Goldman RD, Carter S, Stephens D, Antoon R, Mounstephen W, Langer JC. Prospective validation of the pediatric appendicitis score. *J Pediatr.* 2008;153(2):278-282.

Table 30-4 Appendicitis Diagnosis and Management

Diagnosis	(1) Score—Table 30-3; (2) WBC count and CRP—poor utility (esp. < 24 hours of symptoms); (3) Serial WBC count useless; (4) US is 60–90% sensitive (diameter > 6 mm, target sign, wall > 2 mm)—some perform pre-CT and CT only if normal US; (5) CT is ≥ 95% sensitive (esp. if focused RLQ exam with 3–5 mm cuts/ reconstruction, using IV +/− colonic contrast).
Management	(1) Fluid resuscitation; (2) IV antibiotics if suspect perforation (page 143); (3) Surgical consultation; (4) Limited studies found that select children with symptoms <24 hours OR with >5 days (presumed perforation) treated nonoperatively with IV antibiotics may have superior or equivalent outcome to those treated operatively.

Modified from Henry MC, Gollin G, Islam S, et al. Matched analysis of nonoperative management vs immediate appendectomy for perforated appendicitis. *J Pediatr Surg.* 2007;42(1):19-23, discussion 23-24; Abeş M, Petik B, Kazil S. Nonoperative treatment of acute appendicitis in children. *J Pediatr Surg.* 2007;42(8):1439-1442; Rothrock SG, Pagane J. Acute appendicitis in children: emergency department diagnosis and management. *Ann Emerg Med.* 2000;36(1):39-51.

HIRSCHSPRUNG'S DISEASE

Hirschsprung's disease (congenital megacolon) is the congenital absence of parasympathetic ganglion cells in Auerbach's plexus (myenteric) and Meissner's plexus (submucosal) in the intestine, causing uncoordinated intestinal motility. In 80–90%, involvement is limited to the rectum and rectosigmoid colon including the internal anal sphincter. Hirschsprung's is noted in 1/5,000 births and is more common in males and Down syndrome. In newborns, it may present as complete obstruction or delayed passage of meconium with mild constipation. Most affected infants are full term. If left untreated, failure to thrive will be noted, with ill appearance, malnourishment, or chronic constipation. The most serious complication is the development of ulcerative enterocolitis, which may be lethal. In this complication, elevated luminal pressures in the proximal normal colon inhibit total colonic blood flow and shunt blood away from the mucosa. Bowel wall edema, mucosal necrosis, and sepsis occur. Diagnosis is made by barium enema (BE). If BE is nondiagnostic, consider rectal biopsy with acetylcholinesterase histochemistry on mucosa and submucosal biopsy specimens. Children with functional constipation are generally healthy appearing with bowel troubles beginning around the age of 2 years or the time of toilet training, have stool in rectal vault, and fecal soiling. In contrast, Hirschsprung's patients are generally younger, have empty rectal vault, and no fecal soiling.

INCARCERATED HERNIAS

Incarcerated hernias: Manual reduction may be useful regardless of time and may still work if the obstruction is present. Avoid manual reduction if peritonitis, unstable vitals, significant erythema, or other sign of strangulation. Bimanual abdominal/rectal exam may identify a mass between fingers, a finding absent in spermatic cord hydrocele. Palpation of the inguinal region may reveal a dilated external ring or a silk glove sign (smoothness felt as if two pieces of silk are being rubbed together when rolling the spermatic cord in a direction perpendicular to the inguinal canal).

PYLORIC STENOSIS

Pyloric stenosis (PS) is characterized by a hypertrophic pylorus. PS is rare in premature infants and more common in first-born males. Symptoms typically begin at 2 to 3 weeks but may present up to 5 months (though this late presentation is now rare with the increased availability of an ultrasound). Infants present with nonbilious vomit during/after feeding that progresses to projectile vomiting over the ensuing weeks. Patients are hungry with poor weight gain.

Physical examination: Abdomen—peristaltic waves or a palpable "olive" may be seen, but these findings are neither sensitive nor specific. Lab findings show a hypochloremic metabolic alkalosis.

Diagnosis/Management: Ultrasound is the gold standard for diagnosis. Ultrasonography (≥ 4 mm pyloric muscle thickness or ≥ 14 mm length) is $>95\%$ sensitive for diagnosing pyloric stenosis. Once the diagnosis is made, consult pediatric surgery for laparoscopic management.

INTUSSUSCEPTION

Intussusception is the telescoping of one intestinal segment into another and is the leading cause of obstruction from 3 months to 4 years. Mean age is 8 months, with 80% younger than 2 years. Origin is unknown in 90% unless younger than 1 month or older than 3 years where lead point (e.g., tumor) may be found.[5] This typically presents as a previously well infant who paroxysmally cries out, draws up legs, and may vomit. In some cases, the child may be lethargic, but in other cases the child initially appears well between episodes. An exam may reveal distention and/or a sausage-shaped mass in RUQ but an absence of this does not exclude this diagnosis.

DIAGNOSIS/TREATMENT

US is diagnostic with a classic bull's eye appearance in > 95%. BE, air-contrast enema, or saline enema reduces ~90%. Although an enema is usually therapeutic, it should be avoided in the presence of shock, peritoneal signs, perforation, or high-grade obstruction. After reduction, intussusception may recur in approximately 12% of patients; risk factors for recurrence include age older than 2 years, duration of symptoms > 48 hours, and rectal bleeding.[6,7]

REFERENCES

1. Mohinuddin S, Sakhuja P, Bermundo B, et al. Outcomes of full-term infants with bilious vomiting: observational study of a retrieved cohort. *Arch Dis Child.* 2015;100(1):14-17.
2. Burge DM. The management of bilious vomiting in the neonate. *Early Hum Dev.* 2016;02:41-45. doi:10.1016/j.earlhumdev.2016.09.002.
3. Godbole P, Stringer MD. Bilious vomiting in the newborn: how often is it pathologic? *J Pediatr Surg.* 2002;37(6):909-911. http://www.ncbi.nlm.nih.gov/pubmed/12037761.
4. Rentea RM, St. Peter SD. Pediatric appendicitis. *Surg Clin North Am.* 2017;97(1):93-112. doi:10.1016/j.suc.2016.08.009.
5. Gondek AS, Riaza L, Cuadras D, et al. Ileocolic intussusception: predicting the probability of success of ultrasound guided saline enema from clinical and sonographic data. *J Pediatr Surg.* 2018;53(4):599-604. doi:10.1016/j.jpedsurg.2017.10.050.
6. Gray MP, Li S-H, Hoffmann RG, et al. Recurrence rates after intussusception enema reduction: a meta-analysis. *Pediatrics.* 2014;134(1):110-119. doi:10.1542/peds.2013-3102.
7. Xie X, Wu Y, Wang Q, et al. Risk factors for recurrence of intussusception in pediatric patients: a retrospective study. *J Pediatr Surg.* 2018;53(11):2307-2311. doi:10.1016/j.jpedsurg.2018.03.023.

31 ■ TOXICOLOGY

Table 31-1 Toxins That Affect Vital Signs and Physical Examination

Hypotension			Hypertension
ACE inhibitors	Antidepressants	Nitroprusside	Amphetamines
α and β antagonists	Disulfiram	Opioids	Anticholinergics
Anticholinergics	Ethanol, methanol	Organophosphate	Cocaine
Arsenic (acutely)	Iron, isopropanol	Phenothiazines	Lead
Ca^{+2} channel block	Mercury, GHB	Sedatives	MAO inhibitors
Clonidine, cyanide	Nitrates	Theophylline	Phencyclidine
			Sympathomimetics

Tachycardia		Bradycardia	
Amphetamines	Ethylene glycol, iron	Antidysrhythmics	
Anticholinergics	Organophosphates	α agonists, β antagonists	
Arsenic (acutely)	Sympathomimetics	Ca^{+2} channel blockers	
Antidepressants	PCP, phenothiazines	Digitalis, opioids, GHB	
Digitalis, disulfiram	Theophylline	Organophosphates	

Tachypnea		Bradypnea	
Ethylene glycol	Salicylates	Barbiturates	Isopropanol
Methanol	Sympathomimetics	Botulism	Opioids
Nicotine	(cocaine)	Clonidine	Organophosphate
Organophosphate	Theophylline	Ethanol	Sedatives

Hyperthermia		Hypothermia
Amphetamines	Phencyclidine	Carbon monoxide
Anticholinergics	Phenothiazines	Ethanol
Arsenic (acute)	Salicylates	Hypoglycemic agents
Cocaine	Sedative-hypnotics	Opioids
Antidepressants	Theophylline	Phenothiazines
LSD	Thyroxine	Sedative-hypnotics

Mydriasis (pupillary dilation)		Miosis (pupillary constriction)	
Anticholinergics	Cyanide	Anticholinesterases	Nicotine
Antihistamines	Drug withdrawal	Insecticides	Opioids
Antidepressants	Sympathomimetics	Bromide	Phencyclidine
Anoxia—any cause	Select narcotics	Central α$_2$ agonists	Pilocarpine
Amphetamines	(meperidine, pen-	Clonidine,	Physostigmine
Camphor	tazocine, Lomotil,	guanefacine,	Yohimbine
Cocaine	propoxyphene)	Guanabenz,	
		imidazoline	
		Coma—any	
		sedative	

Table 31-2 Drugs and Toxins That Cause Seizures[1]

Amphetamines	Carbon monoxide, Cyanide	Lindane, Lithium	Withdrawal (etha-
Anticholinergics	Cocaine, Camphor	Nicotine,	nol, sedative)
Antidepressants	Diphenhydramine	Organophosphates	Theophylline
β blockers	GHB, Isoniazid	PCP, Propoxyphene	Tramadol
Bupropion	Lead, Lidocaine	Quinine, SSRIs	Venlafaxine

[1]All agents causing ↓ BP, fever, hypoglycemia and CNS depression can cause seizures.

Table 31-3 Drugs and Toxins That Cause Hypoglycemia

6-Mercaptopurine (6-MP)	Insecticides (carbamates/
Ackee fruit (unripe fruit Jamaican	organophosphates)
Ackee tree S. Florida/Caribbean)	Insulin (exogenous)
Alcohols (ethanol, methanol, isopropanol,	Isoniazid
ethylene glycol)	Lithium
Angiotensin-converting enzyme (ACE) inhibitors	Mamejava plant
β blockers	Methotrexate
Bishydroxycoumarin (rat poison)	Monoamine oxidase (MAO) inhibitors
Bitter melon gourds	Nonsteroidal anti-inflammatory agents
Chlorpromazine	P-aminobenzoic acid
Climbing ivory gourd	Pentamidine
Clofibrate	Phenylbutazone
Didanosine	Phenytoin
Disodium ethylenediaminetetraacetic acid	Pomegranate tree
(EDTA)	Probenecid
Disopyramide	Quinine
Fluoxetine	Ritodrine
Fenfluramine	Salicylates
Fenugreek herb	Sertraline
Ginseng plant (American, Asian, Siberian)	Steroids (anabolic: stanozolol)
Haloperidol	Sulfonamides
Hypoglycemic agents (sulfonylureas, bigu-	Thiazide diuretics
anides, α glucosidase inhibitor, thiazolidin-	Thioglycolate
ediones, benzoic acid derivatives)	Thyroid hormone
	Tremetol
	Tricyclic antidepressants (TCA)
	Trimethoprim

TOXICOLOGY

Phone numbers to ID hazardous chemical agents/spills and their management:
- CDC/Agency for Toxic Substances Disease Registry (ATSDR): (770) 488-7100
- Chemical Manufacturer's Association (CHEMTREC): (800) 424-9300

Table 31-4 Poisoning (Toxidromes)
See specific toxins within text for treatment.

Syndrome	Toxin	Manifestations
Anticholinergic	*Natural:* Belladonna alkaloids, atropine, homatropine, *Amanita muscuria. Synthetics:* Cyclopentolate, dicyclomine, tropicamide, antihistamines, phenothiazines, dextromethorphan, TCA	*Peripheral antimuscarinic:* Dry skin, thirst, blurred vision, mydriasis, ↑ pulse, ↑ BP, red rash, ↑ temperature, abdominal distention, urine retention. *Central symptoms:* Delirium, ataxia, cardiovascular collapse, seizures
Acetylcholinesterase inhibition	Insecticides (organophosphates, carbamates) Nerve gas agents (see page 36)	*Muscarinic effects (SLUDGE):* Salivation, lacrimation, urination, defecation, GI upset, emesis. Also ↓ or ↑ pulse and BP, miosis. *Nicotinic effects:* ↑ pulse, muscle fasciculations, weakness, paralysis, ↓ respirations, sympathetic stimulation. *Central effects:* Anxiety, ataxia, seizure, coma, ↓ respiration, cardiac collapse
Cholinergic	Acetylcholine, betel nut, bethanechol, clitocybe, methacholine, pilocarpine	See *muscarinic* and *nicotinic* effects mentioned previously
Hemoglobinopathy	Carbon monoxide, methemoglobin	Headache, nausea, vomiting, dizziness, coma, seizures, cyanosis, cutaneous bullae, "chocolate" blood with methemoglobinemia
Narcotic	Morphine, dextromethorphan, heroin, fentanyl, meperidine, propoxyphene, codeine, diphenoxylate, Dilaudid	CNS depression, miosis (except meperidine), ↓ respirations, ↓ BP, seizures (with propoxyphene and meperidine)
Sodium channel blockade	β-blockers *(not all),* Benadryl, calcium channel blockers, carbamazepine, citalopram, class I antiarrhythmic, cocaine, cyclic antidepressives, lamotrigine, loxapine, orphenadrine, phenothiazines, thioridazine, tetrodotoxin (TTX)	*SALT syndrome: S*hock, *A*ltered mental status, *L*ong QRS (wide complex), *T*erminal R in aVR. Other ECG features: wide QRS with bradycardia, wide complex tachycardia (ventricular or supraventricular)
Sympathomimetic	Aminophylline, amphetamines, cocaine, ephedrine, caffeine, methylphenidate	CNS excitation, seizures, ↑ pulse, ↑ BP (↓ BP with caffeine), hyperpyrexia, psychosis, sweating
Withdrawal syndrome	Alcohol, barbiturates, benzodiazepines, cocaine, narcotics	Diarrhea, mydriasis, piloerection, ↑ BP, ↑ pulse, insomnia, lacrimation, cramps, yawning, hallucinations

Table 31-5 Poisoning Antidotes and Treatments
See specific toxins within text for more detail.

Toxin	Antidote	Other considerations
Acetaminophen	N-acetyl cysteine see Table 31-13 for dose	Very effective if used within 8 hours, use Rumack-Matthew nomogram to guide management
β blockers	Glucagon 50–150 mcg/kg IV, SC, or IM may repeat	Glucagon may help reverse ↓ pulse and ↓ BP
Ca^{+2} channel blockers	CaCl$_2$ 45–90 mg/kg slow IV, glucagon—see β blocker dose	Glucagon may help reverse ↓ pulse and ↓ BP
Cyanide	Cyanide Kit and Cyanokit	See pages 35–36 for detail
Digoxin	Digoxin Fab fragments	See Table 31-23 for dose
Ethylene glycol	Fomepizole (Antizol) 15 mg/kg IV + 10 mg/kg IV every 12 hours × 4 doses	Ethanol if Antizol not available; ethanol dose see Table 31-33, dialysis
Hydrofluoric acid	IV, arterial, or SC or topical calcium gluconate	Acute or delayed deep tissue burn, systemic acidosis, dysrhythmias secondary to hypocalcemia, hypokalemia, and hypomagnesemia
Isoniazid	Pyridoxine—70–75 mg/kg IV up to 5 g	Reverses seizures
Methanol	Antizol, dialysis, ethanol	See pages 307–308 for detail
Methemoglobinemia	Methylene blue (0.2 ml/kg of 1% solution IV over 5 minutes)	Consider exchange transfusion if severe methemoglobinemia
Opiates	Naloxone 0.01–0.10 mg/kg up to 2 mg IV	Codeine, diphenoxylate, fentanyl, propoxyphene may require higher doses
Organophosphates	Atropine 0.05 mg/kg IV may double until effective + pralidoxime (2-PAM)	Exceptionally high atropine doses may be necessary; see Table 31-36
Salicylates	Dialysis Sodium bicarbonate 1 mEq/kg IV	Goal of alkaline diuresis is urine pH 7.50–7.55, see pages 309–311
Sodium channel block	Sodium bicarbonate 1 mEq/kg IV	Goal of narrowing QRS complex and reversing arrhythmias
TCA	Sodium bicarbonate 1 mEq/kg IV	Goal is serum pH 7.50–7.55 to alter protein binding, see pages 313–314

Table 31-6 Radio-Opaque Ingestions

Radio-opaque ingestions *(Mnemonic CHIPES)*
• **Ch**loral hydrate and chlorinated hydrocarbons
• **H**eavy metals (arsenic, Pb, mercury), health food (bone meal, vitamins)
• **I**odides, iron
• **P**otassium, psychotropics (e.g., phenothiazines, antidepressants)
• **E**nteric-coated tabs (KCl, salicylates)
• **S**olvents (chloroform, CCl$_4$)

Table 31-7 Drugs Cleared by Hemodialysis and by Hemoperfusion

Drugs cleared by hemodialysis[1]	
• Salicylates	• Isopropyl alcohol
• Ethylene glycol	• Chloral hydrate
• Methanol	• Lithium
• Bromide	• Iron
• Ethanol	• Isoniazid
• Theophylline	• Barbiturates
• Depakote	

Drugs cleared by hemoperfusion[1]
• Barbiturates (e.g., phenobarbital)
• Theophylline
• Phenytoin
• Possibly digoxin

[1]Consult local poison center for more detail concerning latest recommendations.

Table 31-8 General Approach to the Poisoned Child

• Treat airway, breathing, and BP.	• Dextrose 5–10 ml/kg of D$_{10}$W in neonate, 2–4 ml/kg D$_{25}$W ≤ 2 years, 1–2 ml/kg D$_{50}$W > 2 years
• Insert IV and apply cardiac monitor.	
• Apply pulse oximeter and administer O$_2$.	• Naloxone 0.01–0.10 mg/kg can be given as a therapeutic trial especially if opioid ingestion is suspected
	• Benzodiazepines (Ativan 0.05–0.10 mg/kg IV)

Table 31-9 Charcoal

Contraindications	Drugs cleared by multidose charcoal[1]
• Caustics (acids, alkalis) • Ileus, bowel obstruction • Risk of aspiration (if altered mental status) • Drugs bound poorly by charcoal (arsenic, bromide, K$^+$, toxic alcohols, heavy metals [iron, iodide, lithium], pesticides, solvents)	Carbamazepine, chlorpropamide, dapsone, diazepam, digoxin, nadolol, nonsteroidals, oleander, phenobarbital, phenytoin, propoxyphene, salicylates, theophylline, and TCA

[1]Administer repeat charcoal doses every 3–4 hours (use cathartic only for first dose).
Initial dose is 1 g/kg PO or per NG alone or with cathartic. American Academy of Clinical Toxicology does not recommend for most drugs ≥ 1 hour after ingestion.

Table 31-10 Cathartics

Cathartics theoretically help by ↑ fecal elimination of charcoal-bound toxins, and preventing concretions. Monitor electrolytes closely with their use.	Cathartic choices[1]
	• Sorbitol (35%)—1 g/kg PO or NG • Magnesium citrate 4 ml/kg PO or NG • Na$^+$ or MgSO$_4$—250 mg/kg PO or NG

[1]Only use cathartic one time (with first charcoal dose) or not at all.
Ipecac—Routine use of ipecac in the ED should be abandoned (AACT).

Table 31-11 Whole Bowel Irrigation

Administration	Indications
• Place NG tube • Administer polyethylene glycol (GoLYTELY) at 25–40 ml/kg/hour • Stop when objects recovered or when effluent is clear	• Iron, zinc, Li, sustained release meds • Ingested crack vials or drug packets
	Contraindications
	• CNS or respiratory depression • Ileus, bowel obstruction, perforation

Table 31-12 Acetaminophen Phases

Phase	Time after ingestion	Signs and symptoms
1	30 minutes to 24 hours	Asymptomatic, or minor GI irritant effects
2	24–72 hours	Relatively asymptomatic, GI symptoms resolve, possible mild elevation of LFTs or renal failure
3	72–96 hours	Hepatic necrosis with potential jaundice, hepatic encephalopathy, coagulopathy, and renal failure, sepsis
4	4 days–2 weeks	Resolution of symptoms or death

Toxicity Assessment: ≥ 150 mg/kg (200 mg/kg) is potentially toxic. Obtain level ≥ 4 hours after ingestion and plot on nomogram; 4-hour level ≥ 140 mcg/ml indicates need for N-acetyl cysteine. On nomogram, level above thick top line = probable risk. Levels above bottom thinner line = possible risk of toxicity. If unknown times, obtain level at 0 and 4 hours to calculate half-life. If half-life > 4 hours, give antidote.

Table 31-13 Management

Decontamination	• Charcoal is indicated only if toxic coingestants are present. • Some ↑ oral Mucomyst dose by 20% if charcoal given.
N-acetyl cysteine (NAC) Mucomyst (Acetadote—IV formulation)	• Assess toxicity based on nomogram. • If drug level will return in < 8 hours post-ingestion, treatment can be delayed until the level is known. NAC prevents 100% of toxicity if administered < 8 hours from ingestion. If level will return > 8 hours and ≥ 150 mg/kg ingested, administer first dose of Mucomyst. NAC is useful ≤ 24 hours after ingestion, possibly up to 72 hours. • *PO dose:* 140 mg/kg PO, then 70 mg/kg every 4 hours × 17 doses. Shorter course (20–36 hours) may be effective if normal liver function tests and undetectable serum acetaminophen level (<10 mcg/ml) at 20–36 hours. Contact poison center for short protocol specifics. Source: Betten DP, Cantrell FL, Thomas SC, Williams SR, Clark RF. A prospective evaluation of shortened course oral N-acetylcysteine for the treatment of acute acetaminophen poisoning. *Ann Emerg Med.* 2007;50(3):272–279. • *IV dose*—150 mg/kg IV (in D₅W) over 15 minutes, then 50 mg/kg (in D₅W) over 4 hours, then 100 mg/kg (in D₅W) over 16 hours. Up to 18% develop anaphylactoid reaction (especially if asthmatic or if they have had a prior NAC reaction). If this happens, discontinue and manage symptoms (e.g., antihistamines, epinephrine, inhaled β agonists, IV fluids). If symptoms stop and were mild, consider restarting NAC. Otherwise, do not restart. • Be aware that NAC can cause anaphylaxis.

Table 31-14 Acetaminophen Nomogram

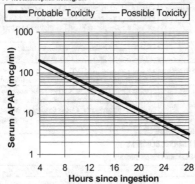

Winshall JS, Lederman RJ. *Tarascon Internal Medicine & Critical Care Pocketbook*, 4th ed. Jones and Bartlett Publishers, Inc; 2007.

β BLOCKERS

β1 stimulation—↑ contraction force + rate, AV node conduction, and renin secretion.

β2 stimulation—Blood vessel, bronchi, GI, and GU smooth muscle relaxation. Propranolol is nonselective, blocking β1 and β2 receptors. Other nonselective β blockers: nadolol, timolol, pindolol. Selective β1 blockers: metoprolol, atenolol, esmolol, + acebutolol. Pindolol + acebutolol have some β agonist properties.

Table 31-15 β Blockers

System	Clinical features
CNS	• Lethargy, slurring, confusion, coma, seizures, ↓ respirations
Cardiac	• ↓ HR, ↓ BP, AV block (1st, 2nd, or 3rd), sinus arrest, asystole
GI	• Nausea, vomiting, ileus, obstruction, bowel ischemia/infarction
Metabolic	• Hyperglycemia (esp. verapamil), lactic acidosis

Treatment of β blocker toxicity	
Option	Recommendations
Gastrointestinal decontamination	• Avoid ipecac. Aspiration and asystole are reported. Charcoal—Repeat doses (see page 295)
Glucagon	• Indications: ↓ HR or BP. Dose: 50–150 mcg/kg + 50 mcg/kg/hour IV

(Continued)

Table 31-15 β Blockers (*Continued*)

Glucose and insulin	• Insulin—1 unit/kg bolus, then 0.5 units/kg/hour • Glucose—0.5–1 g/kg bolus, then 0.5 g/hour. Monitor every 30–60 minutes glucose/K$^+$ until all infusions have been off for ≥ 6 hours.
Atropine	• No HR response is suggestive of β blocker toxicity. Administer 0.02 mg/kg IV prn (maximum of 0.5–1 mg).
Fluid/Vasopressors	• If ↓ BP does not respond to NS, administer α + β agonists (epinephrine/norepinephrine) or pure β agonist (dobutamine).
Other options	Consider NaHCO$_3$ 1–2 mEq/kg IV to reverse sodium channel blockade (SALT syndrome) if wide QRS, low BP, ± acidosis. Use pacemaker if no response to above. Consider dialysis if atenolol, nadolol, or acebutolol overdose. Inamrinone—Consult pharmacist, special dosing/monitoring.

CALCIUM CHANNEL BLOCKERS

Table 31-16 Calcium Channel Blockers

System	Clinical features
CNS	• Lethargy, slurring, confusion, coma, seizures, ↓ respirations
Cardiac	• ↓ HR, ↓ BP, AV block (1st, 2nd, or 3rd), sinus arrest, asystole
GI	• Nausea, vomiting ileus, obstruction, bowel ischemia/infarction
Metabolic	• Hyperglycemia (esp. verapamil), lactic acidosis

Option	Recommendations
Gastrointestinal decontamination	• Charcoal. Avoid ipecac. • Whole-bowel irrigation if sustained-release preparation
Calcium	• Usually ineffective at improving cardiac conduction defects • Primary indication is to reverse hypotension. • Administer Ca^{+2} gluconate 60–100 mg/kg IV over 5 minutes, repeat prn. Alternatively, CaCl$_2$ 20 mg/kg IV over ≥ 5 minutes.
Glucagon	• Indications: ↓ HR or BP • Dose: 50–150 mcg/kg IV bolus + 50 mcg/kg/hour IV
Glucose and insulin	• Insulin—1 unit/kg bolus, then 0.5 units/kg/hour • Glucose—0.5–1 g/kg bolus, then 0.5 g/hour. Monitor every 30–60 minutes glucose/K$^+$ until all infusions have been off for ≥ 6 hours.
Atropine	• Administer 0.02 mg/kg IV if symptomatic ↓ HR (repeat × 3).
Fluids/Pressors	• ↓ BP occurs from peripheral vasodilation. Give NS, then vasoconstrictor: norepinephrine, Neo-Synephrine, ↑ dose dopamine.
Other options	• Consider NaHCO$_3$ 1–2 mEq/kg IV to reverse sodium channel blockade (SALT syndrome) if wide QRS, low BP, ± acidosis • Pacemaker if no response to calcium, glucagon, atropine

CARBON MONOXIDE

Table 31-17 Carbon Monoxide Elimination

Carbon monoxide exposure can occur from fire, catabolism of heme compounds, cigarettes, pollution, ice-surfacing machines, and methylene chloride (dermally absorbed paint remover) degradation. Carbon monoxide displaces O_2 off Hb shifting O_2-Hb dissociation curve to left. Carbon monoxide also binds cytochrome-A cardiac and skeletal muscle myoglobin.	FIO_2	Carbon monoxide half-life
	Room air	4–6 hours
	100% rebreather	1–1.5 hours
	3 ATM hyperbaric O_2	15–30 minutes

Table 31-18 Clinical Features of Carbon Monoxide Poisoning

Clinical features[1]	
Carboxyhemoglobin level	Typical symptoms at given level of carbon monoxide toxicity
0–10%	Usually none, ± ↓ exercise tolerance, ↑ angina, and ↑ claudication
10–20%	Frontal headache, dyspnea with exertion
20–30%	Throbbing headache, dyspnea with exertion, ↓ concentration
30–40%	Severe headache, vomiting, visual changes
40–50%	Confusion, syncope on exertion, myocardial ischemia
50–60%	Collapse, seizures
> 60–70%	Coma and death
Variable	Cherry red skin, visual field defect, homonymous hemianopsia, papilledema, retinal bleed, hearing changes, pulmonary edema. GI upset with vomiting (esp. common < 8 years old)
Assessment of carbon monoxide intoxication	
Carboxyhemoglobin levels	Levels are unreliable and may be low in significant intoxication.
Anion gap	Cyanide and lactic acidosis may contribute to anion gap.
Saturation gap	Calculated—directly measured arterial O_2 saturation. This gap occurs with cyanide, methemoglobin, and sulfhemoglobin.

(Continued)

Table 31-18 Clinical Features of Carbon Monoxide Poisoning (*Continued*)

ECG	May show changes consistent with myocardial ischemia
Cardiac enzymes	May be elevated from direct myocardial damage

Treatment of carbon monoxide toxicity	
Criteria for admission	**Criteria for hyperbaric oxygen[2]**
• All with carboxyhemoglobin > 15–20% • Pregnancy and carboxyhemoglobin > 10% • Acidosis, ECG changes, myocardial ischemia, abnormal neurologic exam or history of unconsciousness • Symptoms after 100% $O_2 \times 3$ hours	• Cyanide toxicity, coma, unconscious > 20 minutes, abnormal neurological exam, ischemic changes on ECG, dysrhythmias, or neurologic symptoms after 100% $O_2 \times 3$ hours, also consider if pregnant with carboxyhemoglobin level > 15%, or at carboxyhemoglobinlevel > 20%.

[1]May cause fluilike symptoms (vomiting and diarrhea) in children (especially with use of combustion heaters in winter). [2]Per the American College of Emergency Physicians 2018 Clinical Policy, emergency physicians should use hyperbaric oxygen (HBO$_2$) therapy or high-flow normobaric therapy for acute carbon monoxide-poisoned patients. It remains unclear whether HBO$_2$ therapy is superior to normobaric oxygen therapy for improving long-term neurocognitive outcomes.

American College of Emergency Physicians Clinical Policies Subcommittee (Writing Committee) on Carbon Monoxide Poisoning; Wolf SJ, Maloney GE, Shih RD, et al. Clinical policy: critical issues in the evaluation and management of adult patients presenting to the emergency department with acute carbon monoxide poisoning. Ann Emerg Med. 2017;69(1):98.e6-107.e6.

CLONIDINE

Clonidine is an α-adrenergic agonist with BP-lowering and sedative properties with the ability to ameliorate opiate withdrawal symptoms. Serum half-life is 12 hours (6–24 hours).

Table 31-19 Clonidine

Clinical features	
General	• Up to 76% of children manifest symptoms by 1 hour and 100% by 4 hours (unless sustained release pill). Symptoms usually last < 24 hours. *Caution:* Ingestion of a clonidine patch may cause prolonged symptoms; therefore, admit for observation and consider whole bowel irrigation if this type of ingestion occurs.
CNS	• Lethargy, coma, recurrent apnea, miosis, hypotonia.
Cardiac	• Sinus bradycardia, hypertension (transient), later hypotension.
Other	• Hypothermia and pallor.
Treatment	
Monitor	• Cardiac monitor and pulse oximeter and observe closely for apnea. Apnea often responds to tactile stimulation.
Decontamination	• Charcoal—only consider if < 1 hour from ingestion. Avoid ipecac.
Atropine	• Indication: bradycardia. Dose: 0.02 mg/kg IV.

Table 31-19 Clonidine (*Continued*)

Treatment	
Antihypertensives	• Hypertension is usually transient. If needed, use short-acting titratable agent (e.g., nitroprusside).
Fluids/Pressors	• Treat hypotension with fluids and dopamine prn.
Naloxone	• 0.02 mg/kg IV may reverse CNS but not cardiac/BP effects. Up to 10 mg may be required. *Caution*: Naloxone may also precipitate hypertension.

COCAINE

Table 31-20 Cocaine Pharmacokinetics

Cocaine is the HCl salt of the alkaloid extract of the *Erythroxylum coca* plant. It can be absorbed across all mucous membranes. It is a local anesthetic (ester-type) that blocks the reuptake of norepinephrine, dopamine, and serotonin.	Route	Peak effect	Duration
	Nasal	30 minutes	1–3 hours
	GI	90 minutes	3 hours
	IV/Inhaled	1–2 minutes	≤ 30 minutes

Data from Cave G, Harvey MG. Should we consider the infusion of lipid emulsion in the resuscitation of poisoned patients? *Crit Care.* 2014;18(5):457; *Ann Emerg Med.* 2008;51:117-134.

Table 31-21 Clinical Features of Cocaine Toxicity

General	• Agitation, hyperthermia, sweat, rhabdomyolysis, GI perf/ischemia.
Cardiac	• A direct myocardial depressant prolongs QT with sympathetic hyperactivity, myocardial ischemia (often with atypical clinical features and ECG findings—acutely or during withdrawal), ↑ BP, ↑ HR, LVH, arrhythmias, ↑ platelet aggregation, accelerated atherosclerosis.
CNS	• Seizures, CNS infarct or bleed, CNS abscess, vasculitis, dystonia.
Lung	• Pneumothorax/Mediastinum, hemorrhage, pneumonitis, ARDS.
Psychiatric	• Paranoia, psychosis.
Management	
General	• Apply cardiac monitor, oxygen, pulse oximeter and observe for arrhythmia, seizures, and hyperthermia. Benzodiazepines are drug of choice for agitation, while haloperidol is also effective (without ↑ cocaine seizure threshold).
Hyperthermia and Rhabdomyolysis	• Benzodiazepines to reduce agitation and muscle activity; cool with mist and fan; continuous rectal probe temperature; check serum CK/CO₂; administer IV fluids and bicarbonate to prevent renal failure (page 78).

(Continued)

Table 31-21 Clinical Features of Cocaine Toxicity (Continued)

GI decontaminate	• *Body stuffers*—Charcoal and monitor for perf/ischemia. • *Body packer*—X-ray and whole bowel irrigation; if rupture, consider laparotomy to remove cocaine.
Cardiovascular (arrhythmias and hypertension)	• Administer benzodiazepines for ↑ BP, ↑ HR. Treat according to standard ALS protocols: Use nitroprusside or phentolamine if severe HTN. Use caution with labetalol: β > α block ± ↑ seizures. In the past, experts recommended avoiding β blockade (due to unopposed alpha effects). Limited studies suggest there may be a beneficial, protective effect of β blockade. Currently, clear recommendations cannot be given regarding their use or avoidance. • *Wide-complex tachycardia* due to quinidine like effect. Give $NaHCO_3$ 1 mEq/kg IV and cardiovert.
Cardiovascular (chest pain)	• Administer benzodiazepines, aspirin, and IV nitroglycerin if myocardial infarction. Phentolamine IV may reverse coronary vasoconstriction.
Neurologic	• Treat status epilepticus with benzodiazepines. Barbiturates are second line while phenytoin is not useful. Exclude coexisting disease (CT, glucose, electrolytes, R/O infection).

Data from Grant Cave & Martyn G Harvey, Should we consider the infusion of lipid emulsion in the resuscitation of poisoned patients?, *Ann Emerg Med.* 2008;51:117-134. Dattilo PB, Hailpern SM, Fearon K, Sohal D, Nordin C. Beta-blockers are associated with reduced risk of myocardial infarction after cocaine use. *Ann Emerg Med.* 2008; 51(2):117-25. DOI: 10.1016/j.annemergmed.2007.04.015; Hoffman RS. Cocaine and beta-blockers: should the controversy continue?. *Ann Emerg Med. 2008;* 51(2):127-9. DOI: 10.1016/j.annemergmed .2007.08.011; Freeman K, Feldman JA. Cocaine, myocardial infarction, and beta-blockers: time to rethink the equation?. *Ann Emerg Med.* 2008; 51(2):130-4. DOI: 10.1016/j.annemergmed.2007.08.020

DIGOXIN

Natural sources: foxglove, oleander, lily of the valley, and the skin of toads. Therapeutic range—0.5–2.0 ng/ml. Severe poisoning may not demonstrate ↑ levels.

Table 31-22 Digoxin Clinical Features—Acute Toxicity

Clinical features—acute toxicity	
Digoxin level	Usually markedly elevated (obtain > 6 hours after ingestion)
GI and CNS	Nausea, vomiting, diarrhea, headache, confusion, coma
Cardiac	Paroxysmal atrial tachycardia, AV blocks, bradyarrhythmias
Metabolic	Hyperkalemia from inhibition of the Na^+/K^+ ATP pump
Clinical features—chronic toxicity	
Digoxin level	May be normal[1]
History	URI symptoms, on diuretics, renal insufficiency, yellow-green halos

Table 31-22 Digoxin Clinical Features—Acute Toxicity (*Continued*)

Cardiac	Ventricular arrhythmias (PVCs) are more common than with acute toxicity
Metabolic	Potassium low or normal, magnesium is often low

Treatment of digoxin toxicity	
• Multidose charcoal • Atropine 0.02 mg/kg for ↓ HR • Ventricular arrhythmia: lidocaine 1 mg/kg IV ± MgSO₄ 25 mg/kg slow IV	• Treat ↑ K⁺: (page 91); avoid calcium. • Avoid cardioversion if possible (predisposes to ventricular fibrillation) • Digoxin Fab fragments (Digibind)

Indications for Digibind	Total body load digoxin—TBLD estimates
• Ventricular arrhythmias • Bradyarrhythmias unresponsive to therapy • Ingestion of > 0.1 mg/kg • Digoxin level > 5 ng/ml • Consider if K⁺ > 5.5 mEq/l	• First assess total body load of digoxin (TBLD) = [digoxin level (ng/ml) × weight (kg)] ÷ 100 • Acute ingestion—the total mg ingested if digoxin capsules or elixir is ingested • Acute ingestion—the total mg ingested × 0.8 if another form of digoxin is ingested • Or estimate Digibind dose based on serum levels

¹*Chronic ingestions* may have normal to mildly elevated digoxin levels.

Table 31-23 Dosing Digibind

• Dose (# vials) = [serum digoxin concentration (ng/ml) × weight (kg)]/100.
• If ingested quantity unknown, consider empiric administration of 2–10 vials.
• One 38 mg Digibind vial can bind 0.5 mg of digoxin if amount ingested known.
• Dilute Digibind to 10 mg/ml and administer IV over 30 minutes. Consider using 0.22-micron filter for infusion. Serum digoxin levels are useless after Digibind, as lab assay measures bound + unbound digoxin. These misleading levels may be exceptionally high, as Digibind draws digoxin back into the serum. Once bound, digoxin-Fab complex is renally excreted.

ETHYLENE GLYCOL

Ethylene glycol is found in coolants (e.g., automobile antifreeze), preservatives, lacquers, cosmetics, polishes, and detergents.

Table 31-24 Ethylene Glycol

Timing	Clinical features
1–12 hours	• *Early:* Inebriation, ataxia, slurring without ethanol on breath • *Later:* Coma, seizures, and death
12–24 hours	• *Cardiac:* Deterioration occurs during this phase • *Early:* Tachycardia, hypertension, tachypnea • *Later:* Congestive heart failure, ARDS, and cardiovascular collapse • Myositis occasionally occurs during this phase
24–72 hours	• Nephrotoxicity with calcium oxalate crystal precipitation leading to flank pain, renal failure, and hypocalcemia

Diagnosis	Treatment
• Anion gap acidosis. • Osmol gap[1] (measured—calculated osmol) > 10 mOsm/l (page 85). • Hypocalcemia (ECG—↑ QT interval). • Calcium oxalate crystals in urine (urine may fluoresce with UV light—e.g., Wood's lamp). • ↑ BUN and creatinine. • Serum ethylene glycol level > 20 mg/dl is toxic. • Serious toxicity has been reported in the *absence* of an elevated anion gap and crystalluria.	• Charcoal ineffective. • NaHCO₃ 1 mEq/kg IV—keep pH ~7.40. • Ca⁺² gluconate 10%, 100 mg/kg IV if low calcium. • Pyridoxine and thiamine IV. • Fomepizole[2] (Antizol)—15 mg/kg IV, + 10 mg/kg every 12 hours × 4 doses, then ↑ to 15 mg/kg IV every 12 hours until level < 20 mg/dl. • Ethanol if Antizol unavailable. • Dialysis if (1) oliguria/anuria, (2) severe acidosis, or (3) level > 50 mg/dl (> 20 mg/dl if fomepizole not used).

[1]Osmol gap may be normal in significant toxicity. [2]Consult poison center. Administer slow IV over 15 minutes. If unavailable, load IV ethanol (see "Methanol," page 307, Table 31-33).

FLUNITRAZEPAM—ROHYPNOL "ROOFIES"

Rohypnol is a benzodiazepine marketed outside the United States for insomnia, sedation, and pre-anesthesia. It is 10 times as potent as diazepam. It potentiates and prolongs the effects of heroin, methadone, and alcohol and attenuates the withdrawal of cocaine. It produces disinhibition and amnesia and has been used as a "date rape" drug.

Table 31-25 Flunitrazepam—Rohypnol "Roofies"

Onset/Duration	• Maximal absorption is 0.5–1.5 hours with $t_{1/2}$ of nearly 12 hours.
Major clinical effects	• *CNS*—Sedation, incoordination, hallucinations. Paradoxical excitement, especially with alcohol use. ↓ DTRs, mid to small pupils. • *CV-Pulm*—Respiratory depression, hypotension, aspiration.
Management	• NOT routinely detected in urine benzodiazepine screen. • Charcoal if < 1 hour from ingestion. • Protect airway and apply cardiac monitor, pulse oximeter. • Flumazenil (see dose, page 23) may reverse CNS effects. • Admit if lethargic or unstable after 2–4 hours of observation.

GAMMA HYDROXYBUTYRIC ACID (GHB)

Gamma hydroxybutyric acid (GHB) has been promoted as a steroid alternative, a weight control agent, and as a narcolepsy treatment.

Table 31-26 Gamma Hydroxybutyric Acid

Features	Details
Onset/Duration	• Onset of symptoms is ~15 minutes, with spontaneous resolution from 2 to > 48 hours (depending on dose and coingestant).
Major clinical effects	• *CNS*: Acts with ethanol to produce CNS/respiratory depression. At ↑ levels patients are unresponsive to noxious stimuli and lose pharyngeal reflexes. Seizures, clonic arm/leg/face movements, vomit, amnesia, ↓ DTRs, vertigo, nystagmus, and ataxia occur. • *CV-Pulm*: ↓ HR, irregular or ↓ respirations, ↓ BP.
Management	• Protect airway and apply cardiac monitor, pulse oximeter. • Treat symptomatically (e.g., atropine for persistent ↓ HR). • Exclude coingestant or other diagnosis (e.g., CNS trauma). • Admit if symptoms do not resolve after 6 hours of observation.

IRON

Iron is a chemical element that naturally exists in the body. It plays an active role in various metabolic processes and is found mainly in hemoglobin and myoglobin. These two proteins allow for oxygen transport and storage via the hematopoietic system. There are several formulations of iron that can be taken as dietary supplements and a severe overdose can be lethal.

Table 31-27 Iron

Iron formulations	Elemental iron	Mechanisms of iron toxicity
Ferrous gluconate	12%	• Direct GI mucosal damage with hemorrhagic gastritis, bleeding
Ferrous sulfate	20%	
Ferrous fumarate	33%	• Hepatic necrosis
Ferrous phosphate	37%	• Mitochondrial damage
Ferrous or ferric pyrophosphate	12%	• Venodilation and hypotension • Third-spacing of fluids
Ferrocholinate	12%	• Thrombin inhibition-coagulopathy

Table 31-28 Clinical Features—Staging of Iron Poisoning

Stage	Time post ingestion	Findings
I	1–6 hours	Local toxicity: GI bleeding, perforation, diarrhea, and shock due to direct corrosion and vasodilation
II	2–12 hours	Relative stability and resolution: Stage I symptoms resolve
III	12–36 hours	Metabolic disruption: Metabolic acidosis, circulatory collapse, neurologic deterioration, hepatic failure, renal failure, coagulation defects, and third-spacing of fluids
IV	2–4 days	Liver failure: Hepatic necrosis
V	2–6 weeks	Late sequelae: GI tract scarring

Table 31-29 Clinical Features—Suggestive of Iron Toxicity

Vomiting and diarrhea (esp. ≤ 6 hours)	Hypotension	
Mental status changes	Coagulopathy, acidosis	
Estimate of quantity elemental iron ingested and toxicity potential	Elemental iron (Table 31-27)	Toxicity
	< 20 mg/kg	None
	20–60 mg/kg	Mild to moderate
	> 60 mg/kg	Severe

Table 31-30 Serum Iron and TIBC levels

Obtain serum iron and total iron-binding capacity (TIBC) at least 4 hours post-ingestion. Absorption may be delayed for slow-release forms, if so obtain second level at 8 hours. Iron levels ≥ 350 mcg/dl (normal 50–150) are serious, as the TIBC (350–500 mcg/dl) is exceeded. High iron falsely lowers TIBC level, rendering test unreliable.	Serum iron (mcg/dl)	Toxicity
	< 100	None
	100–300	Mild
	300–500	Moderate
	500–1,000	Severe
	> 1,000	Possibly lethal

Table 31-31 Adjunctive Diagnostic Tests

WBC count	> 15,000 cells/mm^3 is associated with a serum iron > 300 mcg/dl.
Glucose	> 150 g/dl is associated with a serum iron > 300 mcg/dl.
KUB	Radio-opaque tablets on plain films indicate potential for further absorption/toxicity; 50% with iron > 300 mcg/dl = negative X-ray.

Table 31-32 Treatment of Iron Poisoning

Fluid/Blood	• Use NS ± blood prn. Consult surgeon if suspect perforation.
Decontaminate	• Charcoal is ineffective.
Whole bowel irrigation	• Administer polyethylene glycol (GoLYTELY; Table 31-11). This option is especially useful if X-ray shows tablets beyond pylorus.
Deferoxamine	• Do not rely on deferoxamine challenge to make decisions. • 15 mg/kg/hour IV infusion. Do not wait for iron levels to return if the patient is symptomatic. Deferoxamine given IV or IM causes ↓ BP, which is usually the limiting factor in infusion rate. Seizures can occur following deferoxamine. If improving, discontinue deferoxamine when urine clears and iron level < 100 mcg/dl.
Dialysis	• If renal failure prevents excretion of ferrioxamine.
Indications for chelation with deferoxamine	• Multisystem toxicity (e.g., vomiting, diarrhea, GI bleeding, ↓ BP, acidosis, altered mental status, coagulopathy). • Tablets seen on plain abdominal radiograph. • Serum iron > 350 mcg/dl or serum iron > TIBC (TIBC can be unreliable when serum iron levels are high).

METHANOL

Methyl alcohol sources are wood alcohol, solvents, paint removers, shellacs, windshield washing fluids, and antifreeze. Toxicity is from formaldehyde/formic acid. Death has been reported after ingestion of 15 ml of 40% solution.

Table 31-33 Methanol Toxicity

Clinical features		Treatment
0–12 hours	• Inebriation, drowsiness • Asymptomatic period	• Charcoal • $NaHCO_3$ 1 mEq/kg IV—keep pH > 7.35
12–36 hours	• Vomiting, hyperventilation • Abdominal pain, pancreatitis • Visual blurring, blindness with mydriasis and papilledema • CNS depression	• Folate • Consult poison center • Fomepizole (Antizol)—(see ethylene glycol dosing, Table 31-24).
Diagnostic studies		
• Osmol gap[1] may occur before anion gap acidosis (see page 85). • Anion gap and lactic acidosis.		• Ethanol (10%) in D_5W (if no Antizol)—(1) IV loading dose 10 ml/kg over 1–2 hours, (2) then 1.6 ml/kg/hour (3) Ethanol goal: = 100–150 mg/dl.

(Continued)

Table 31-33 Methanol Toxicity (*Continued*)

Diagnostic studies	Treatment

• Hemoconcentration, hyperglycemia.
 • Methanol levels > 20 mg/dl are toxic.
   (1) CNS symptoms occur > 20 mg/dl
   (2) Visual symptoms occur > 50 mg/dl
	• Dialyze if (1) visual symptoms, (2) CNS depression, (3) level > 50 mg/dl, (4) severe metabolic acidosis, or (5) history of ingestion of > 30 ml.
	 • Stop dialysis and ethanol when methanol levels fall to < 20 mg/dl.v

[1]Osmol gap may be normal in significant toxicity.

ORGANOPHOSPHATES AND CARBAMATES

Organophosphates irreversibly bind and inhibit cholinesterases at CNS receptors, postganglionic parasympathetic nerves (muscarinic effects), and autonomic ganglia and skeletal myoneural junctions (nicotinic effects). Carbamates irreversibly bind cholinesterases and are less toxic.

Table 31-34 Clinical Features of Insecticide Toxicity

Onset of symptoms	• Usually begin < 24 hours after exposure. Lipid-soluble organophosphates (e.g., fenthion) may take days to produce symptoms with persistence for weeks to months and periodic relapses.
CNS	• Cholinergic excess: delirium, confusion, seizures, respiratory depression. Carbamates have less central effects.
Muscarinic	• SLUDGE: Salivation, lacrimation, urination, defecation, GI upset, emesis; miosis, bronchoconstriction, bradycardia.
Nicotinic	• Fasciculations, muscle weakness, sympathetic ganglia stimulation (hypertension, tachycardia, pallor, rarely mydriasis).

Table 31-35 Diagnostic Studies in Insecticide Poisoning

Labs	• ↑ Glucose, ↑ K⁺, ↑ WBC, ↑ amylase, glycosuria, proteinuria
ECG	• Early—↑ in sympathetic tone (tachycardia) • Later—Extreme parasympathetic tone (sinus bradycardia, AV block, and ↑ QT)
Serum (*pseudo*) RBC (*plasma*) Cholinesterase	• Serum levels are more sensitive but less specific than RBC • Plasma levels return to normal before RBC levels • Mild cases: Levels are < 50% of normal • Severe cases: Levels are < 10% of normal

Table 31-36 Treatment for Insecticide Poisoning

General	• First take off all clothing that may contain the toxin. • Wash toxin off patient if dermal exposure. • Support airway, breathing, and blood pressure. Respiratory depression is the most common cause of death. • Medical personnel should gown and glove if dermal exposure. • Administer charcoal if oral ingestion.
Atropine *Extremely large doses often needed*	• Competitively blocks acetylcholine (ACh) at muscarinic (not nicotinic) receptors. Atropine may reverse CNS effects. • *Dose:* ≥ 0.05 mg/kg every 5 minutes. Mix 50 mg in 500 ml NS and titrate. • *Goal:* Titrate to mild anticholinergic signs (dry mouth, secretions) and not to pupil size or heart rate. • Treatment failure most often due to not using enough atropine.
Pralidoxime (2-PAM)	• PAM has endogenous anticholinergic effects, while reversing nicotinic and central effects. It does not reverse carbamate toxicity. • *Dose:* 20–50 mg/kg IV over 15 minutes. May repeat in 1–2 hours, then may repeat every 10–12 hours. Onset of effect is 10–40 minutes after administration.
Atrovent	• Ipratropium bromide 0.5 mg nebulized every 4–6 hours may dry secretions.

SALICYLATES

Methyl salicylate (oil of wintergreen) is the most toxic form. Absorption generally is within 1 hour of ingestion (delays ≥ 6 hours occur with enteric-coated and viscous preparations). At toxic levels, salicylates are renally metabolized. Alkaline urine promotes excretion. At different acidosis/alkalosis states, measurable salicylate levels change, therefore, measure arterial pH at the same time as the drug level.

Table 31-37 Salicylate Toxicity—Levels

Ingestion	Severity	Signs and symptoms
< 150 mg/kg	Mild	Vomiting, tinnitus, and hyperpnea
150–300 mg/kg	Moderate	Vomiting, hyperpnea, diaphoresis, and tinnitus
>300 mg/kg	Severe	Acidosis, altered mental status, seizures, and shock

Table 31-38 Clinical Features of Salicylate Toxicity

Direct	• Irritation of GI tract with reports of perforation
Metabolic	• *Early:* Respiratory alkalosis from respiratory center stimulation • *Later:* Anion gap acidosis—uncoupled oxidative phosphorylation • Hypokalemia, ↑ or ↓ glucose, ketonuria, and either ↑ or ↓ Na+
CNS	• *Early:* Tinnitus, deafness, agitation, hyperactivity • *Later:* Confusion, coma, seizure, CNS edema (esp. < 4 years old)
GI	• Vomiting, gastritis, pylorospasm, ↑ liver enzymes, perforation
Pulmonary	• Noncardiac pulmonary edema (esp. with chronic toxicity)

Table 31-39 Indicators of Salicylate Toxicity

Clinical	• See Table 31-38 for features associated with toxicity.
Ingestion	• Ingestion of ≥ 150 mg/kg is associated with toxicity.
Ferric chloride	• Mix 2 drops $FeCl_3$ + 1 ml urine. Purple = salicylate ingestion.
Phenistix	• Dipstick test for urine. Brown indicates salicylate or phenothiazine ingestion (not toxicity). Adding 1 drop 20N H_2SO_4 bleaches out color for phenothiazines but not salicylates.
Salicylate levels	• A level > 30 mg/dl drawn ≥ 6 hours after ingestion is toxic. Clinical picture more important than levels (esp. if chronic component to overdose). Do not wait for 6 hours to treat ill patients. • Follow serial levels (every 2–3 hours) until downward trend established. • In patients with a low pH, CNS penetration increases and toxicity can occur at lower levels. • *Done nomogram* is unreliable indicator of toxicity.
Nontoxic ingestion	• If each of the following are present, acute toxicity is unlikely (1) < 150 mg/kg ingested, (2) absent clinical features, (3) level < 30 mg/dl obtained ≥ 6 hours after ingestion (unless enteric-coated preparation, viscous preparation, or chronic ingestion).

Table 31-40 Treatment of Salicylate Poisoning

General	• Treat dehydration, electrolyte abnormalities. CSF hypoglycemia occurs with normal serum glucose—add D_5W or $D_{10}W$ to all fluids.
Decontaminate	• Multidose charcoal. Whole bowel irrigation (if enteric coated).
Alkalinization	• Add 100 mEq $NaHCO_3$ to 1 l D_5W 1/2NS (± 20–40 mEq/l K+ if no renal failure). *Goal*—urine pH > 7.5.
Hemodialysis	• *Indications:* Renal failure, noncardiogenic pulmonary edema, congestive heart failure, persistent CNS disturbances, deterioration of vital signs, unable to correct acid–base or electrolyte imbalance, salicylate level > 100 mg/dl (acutely).

Table 31-41 Chronic Salicylate Toxicity

Presentation	• Patients are older, on chronic salicylates. Neuro changes and non-cardiogenic pulmonary edema are more common. Many are treated for infectious/neuro disease prior to correct dx.
Toxicity	• Salicylate levels are often normal to therapeutic.
Treatment	• Supportive measures and urinary alkalinization are recommended. Dialyze if acidosis, confusion, or pulmonary edema.

SELECTIVE SEROTONIN REUPTAKE INHIBITORS AND NON-TRICYCLIC ANTIDEPRESSANTS

Table 31-42 Selective Serotonin Reuptake Inhibitors and Non-tricyclic Antidepressants

Selective serotonin reuptake inhibitors (SSRIs)	SSRIs
Overdose is relatively benign. Most common symptoms: ↑ HR, tremor, vomiting, and drowsy. ECG: ↑ HR, nonspecific ST-T changes. Seizures, cardiotoxicity (wide QRS/QTc) can occur at high levels (esp. fluvoxamine). ↓ HR is seen with fluvoxamine at high or low doses. *Treatment:* (1) exclude coingestants, (2) observe for 6 hours, (3) Charcoal 1 g/kg (< 1 hour post-ingest.), (4) NaHCO₃ IV if wide QRS tachycardia, (5) observe for potentially lethal *serotonin syndrome.*	Citalopram (Celexa)
	Escitalopram (Lexapro)
	Fluoxetine (Prozac)
	Fluvoxamine (Luvox)
	Paroxetine (Paxil)
	Sertraline (Zoloft)

Monoamine oxidase inhibitors (isocarboxazid/Marplan, phenelzine/Nardil, selegiline/Eldepryl, tranylcypromine/Parnate). Overdose may have onset up to 12 hours later. Excess α+β adrenergic symptoms: Headache, tremor, ↑ BP, ↑ DTR rigidity, chest pain, ↑ temp. Later ↓ BP, ↓ HR, seizures. *Treatment:* (1) Nipride or phentolamine for ↑ BP (No β blockers), (2) NS + Norepi. for ↓ BP, (3) charcoal, (4) benzodiazepines, (5) treat hyperthermia (see malignant hyperthermia/rhabdomyolysis page 78).

Serotonin, norepinephrine reuptake inhibitors—Venlafaxine (Effexor), duloxetine (Cymbalta)—Overdose causes ↑ HR and ↓ level of consciousness, brief and limited seizures, mild hypotension. Treat with supportive care.

Norepinephrine and dopamine reuptake inhibitor—Bupropion (Wellbutrin). Overdose causes lethargy (41%), tremors (24%), and seizures (21%). Mean seizure onset is 3.7 hours. Treat with benzodiazepines, phenytoin. One case prolonged QRS/QTc.

Noradrenergic and serotoninergic antidepressants—Mirtazapine (Remeron) inhibits presynaptic α₂ receptors increasing serotonin and norepinephrine transmission. Serotonin-2 and -3 receptors are blocked diminishing anxiety and GI side effects. Overdose is rare—with sedation and drowsiness requiring rare intubation. No cardiac conduction effects or seizures have been noted to date.

Serotonin-2 receptor antagonists—Nefazodone (Serzone), trazodone (Desyrel) (esp. trazodone) cause sedation, lightheadedness, GI upset, headaches. Trazodone has been associated with nonsustained ventricular tachycardia and other dysrhythmias. Treatment for overdose of either agent is supportive.

Table 31-43 Serotonin Syndrome

	Mild	Moderate	Severe
CNS	Confused, restless	Agitated, sleepy	Coma, seizures
Autonomic	Temp. (T) < 38°C, mydriasis, diarrhea, ↑ HR	T < 39.5°C, BP low or high, mydriasis	T > 39.5°C, dyspnea, diaphoresis, ↑ HR
Neuromuscular	Clonus, ataxia, akathisia, ↑ DTRs	Myoclonus, clonus, ataxia	Muscle rigidity (rhabdomyolysis)

Causes: Coingestion SSRIs, TCA, MAOI, meperidine, codeine, dextromethorphan
Treatment: Stop drug, manage complications (hyperthermia/rhabdomyolysis), administer benzodiazepines. Some experts recommend cyproheptadine.

Data from Reilly TH, Kirk MA. Atypical antipsychotics and newer antidepressants. *Emerg Med Clin North Am.* 2007;25:477.

SULFONYLUREAS

Examples: Chlorpropamide, tolbutamide, glipizide, gliclazide, glimepiride, glyburide. Clinical: 50% of children develop symptoms of hypoglycemia in 2 hours, while 96% develop symptoms by 8 hours unless long-acting pill ingested (XL preps). Neurologic (lethargy, seizure, headache, focal deficits) and autonomic symptoms (sweat, hypertension, tachycardia, pallor) occur.

Table 31-44 Sulfonylureas Treatment/Disposition

Treatment: If hypoglycemia, IV glucose (age < 1 month: 10 ml/kg D_{10}W, 1–24 months: 4 ml/kg D_{25}W; > 2 years: 2 ml/kg of D_{50}W). Drip: D_{10-20}W/ D_{10-20}NS. If no IV, glucagon 0.02–0.03 mg/kg SC (if < 20 kg) or 1 mg if > 20 kg. If recurrent: octreotide (2 mcg/kg IV/SC every 6–12 hours) OR if unavailable, diazoxide (1–3 mg/kg) IV over 30 minutes every 4 hours. Charcoal does not absorb all sulfonylureas and may be aspirated. Consider risks/benefits of whole bowel irrigation if XL prep.

Disposition: Admit for 24 hours if first-generation overdose, symptomatic, or XL ingestions since delayed onset 16–24 hours after ingestion can occur. If second or third generation (gliclazide, glimepiride, glipizide, glyburide), asymptomatic, normal glucose and unintentional overdose, some experts observe ≥ 8–12 hours post-ingestion, then discharge.

SYMPATHOMIMETICS

Table 31-45 Sympathomimetics (Amphetamines and Derivatives)

Effects of amphetamines are (1) *sympathomimetic*—α and β adrenergic—mydriasis, $\uparrow$ HR, $\uparrow$ BP, $\uparrow$ temp., arrhythmias, myocardial infarction, rhabdomyolysis, psychosis, CNS bleed, $\uparrow$ sweat, seizures; (2) *dopaminergic*—restlessness, anorexia, hyperactive, movement disorders, parania; (3) *serotonergic*—mood, impulse control, serotonin syndrome.

Ice/Crank (crystal methamphetamine) is one of most commonly synthesized illicit drugs. Onset is minutes, lasts 2–24 hours. **MDMA (Ecstasy)**—popular at "raves" and consumed orally. Low dose—euphoria, mild sympathomimetic symptoms last ~4–6 hours. Potent serotonin releaser (no impulse control). High dose—effects (1–3) above.

Treatment: (1) supportive care, cardiopulmonary and neuro monitoring; (2) benzodiazepines for agitation; (3) labetalol or Nipride or phentolamine for $\uparrow$ BP; (4) if $\downarrow$ BP, dopamine or norepinephrine; (5) consider charcoal; (6) treat complications.

TRICYCLIC ANTIDEPRESSANTS

Table 31-46 Tricyclic Antidepressants (TCA)

Clinical features are due to α adrenergic block ($\downarrow$ BP), anticholinergic effects (altered mentation, seizures, $\uparrow$ HR, mydriasis, inhabitation of norepinephrine uptake ($\uparrow$ catecholamines), Na^+ channel block (quinidine-like cardiac depression).

ECG findings in TCA overdose	
Sinus tachycardia • $\uparrow$ QRS > 100 ms, $\uparrow$ PR interval, $\uparrow$ QT interval, BBB (esp. right BBB) • Right axis deviation of the terminal 40 ms of the QRS > 120° (prominent terminal R in AVR—see figure) • AV conduction blocks (all degrees) • Ventricular fibrillation or tachycardia	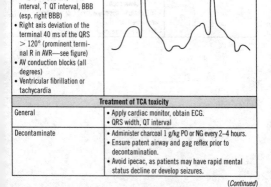

Treatment of TCA toxicity	
General	• Apply cardiac monitor, obtain ECG. • QRS width, QT interval
Decontaminate	• Administer charcoal 1 g/kg PO or NG every 2–4 hours. • Ensure patent airway and gag reflex prior to decontamination. • Avoid ipecac, as patients may have rapid mental status decline or develop seizures.

(Continued)

Table 31-46 Tricyclic Antidepressants (TCA) (*Continued*)

$NaHCO_3$	• *Indications:* (1) acidosis, (2) QRS width > 100 ms, (3) ventricular arrhythmias, or (4) hypotension. • Alkalinization enhances TCA protein binding and reverses Na^+ channel blockade and toxic cardiac manifestations. • *Dose:* 1–2 mEq/kg IV. May repeat or initiate drip. • *Goal:* Arterial pH of 7.50–7.55 or normal QRS. • $NaHCO_3$ is ineffective for CNS manifestations (e.g., seizures).
Fluids/Pressors	• Administer 10–20 ml/kg NS for hypotension. Repeat 1–2×. • If fluids are ineffective administer phenylephrine or norepinephrine (not dopamine) due to prominent α effects.
Antiseizure medications	• Use lorazepam followed by phenobarbital. • Phenytoin may be ineffective in TCA-induced seizures.
$MgSO_4$	• 25 mg/kg administered slow IV (over 15 minutes) may be useful for ↓ BP, and arrhythmias.
Disposition	*May transfer to psychiatric facility if all of following are present:* • No major evidence of toxicity during 6 hours ED observation. • Active bowel sounds. • ≥ 2 charcoal doses are given (not all experts recommend this). • There is no evidence of toxic coingestant.

32 ■ TRAUMA

- Leading cause of death/disability for people under the age of 19 in the United States.
- Major causes of death are airway compromise and inadequate fluid resuscitation.
- Blunt trauma > penetrating trauma.
- Fatal injuries involve those to the head, chest, and abdomen.
- Injury characteristics vary by age.
- Earliest sign of shock = tachycardia.
- Firearms cause the highest percentage of fatality/incidence, though overall incidence is low.

Sources: Tisherman SA, Forsythe, RM, Kellum, JA. *Trauma Intensive Care.* New York, NY: Oxford University Press; 2013:251-271; Schneeweiss S, Leilani A. *The Hospital for Sick Children Handbook of Pediatric Emergency Medicine.* Sudbury, MA: Jones and Bartlett; 2008:37-42.

Table 32-1 Guidelines for Field Triage of Injured Patients[1]

Step 1: Are any of following present?: GCS < 14, SBP < 90 mm Hg [*while 70 + age × 2 numerically estimates hypotension in children, the expert panel used higher cutoff (< 90 mm Hg) to ensure appropriate overtriage of children*], or RR < 10 or > 29 breath/minute (< 20 if < 1 year old)	NO →	Go to Step 2

↓ YES

Take to Highest-Level Trauma Center

Step 2: Are any of following present?: Penetration to head, neck, torso, extremity proximal to elbow, or knee, amputation proximal to wrist/ankle, flail chest, 2 or more proximal long bone fractures, mangled/crushed or degloved extremity, pelvic fracture, open or depressed skull fracture or paralysis	NO →	Go to Step 3

↓ YES

Take to Highest-Level Trauma Center

Step 3: Are any of following present?: Fall > 10 feet or > 2–3 × child's height, high-risk auto crash (intrusion > 12 inches occupant side, or > 18 inches any side), ejection, death in same passenger compartment, high-risk car telemetry data, auto vs. pedestrian/bicyclist with one of following: thrown, run over, > 20 mph impact; or motorcycle crash > 20 mph, or EMS provider judgment	NO →	Go to Step 4

↓ YES

Take to Closest Appropriate Trauma Center, Which Need Not Be the Highest-Level Trauma Center

Step 4: Children (esp. those < 5 years old) are triaged preferentially to closest pediatric-capable trauma center. Patients with bleeding disorder (e.g., blood thinner) with burns, time-sensitive injury (fracture that is open or neurovascular compromise), on dialysis, or pregnancy > 20 weeks	NO →	Go to Step 5

↓ YES

Step 5: Contact medical control and consider transport to a trauma center or specific resource hospital (e.g., isolated burns without trauma to burn center), if significant trauma, still transport to resource hospital.	NO →	Follow local transport protocols

[1]GCS—Glasgow coma scale (see Pediatric GCS); SBP—systolic blood pressure; RR—respiratory rate. Modified from Sasser SM, Hunt RC, Sullivent EE, et al. Guidelines for field triage of injured patients. Recommendations of the National Expert Panel on Field Triage. *MMWR Recomm Rep.* 2009;58(RR-1):1-35.

TRAUMA SCORING AND ASSESSMENT

Table 32-2 Pediatric Trauma Score[1]

		Patient Features				
		Weight (kg)	Airway	Systolic BP (mm Hg)	Mental status	Open wounds	Extremity fractures
Score	−1	<10	Nonmaintainable	<50	Comatose	Major	Open or multiple
	+1	10–20	Maintainable	50–90	Obtunded	Minor	Closed
	+2	>20	Normal	>90	Awake	None	None

[1]A total score of ≤8 suggests possible serious injury, <1 predicts mortality rate of >98%, 4 = 50% mortality, > 8 predicts < 1% mortality.
Data from Ramenofsky, M. L., Ramenofsky, M. B., Jurkovich, G. J., Threadgill, D., Dierking, B. H., & Powell, R. W. The Predictive Validity of the Pediatric Trauma Score. The Journal of Trauma: Injury, Infection, and Critical Care; 1998:28(7),1038-1042. doi:10.1097/00005373-198807000-00021

Table 32-3 Pediatric Glasgow Coma Scale[1]

Eye opening	Best motor	Best verbal
0–1 year	0–1 year	0–2 years
4 Spontaneous	6 Spontaneous movement	5 Normal cry, smile, coo
3 To shout	5 Localizes pain	4 Cries
2 To pain	4 Flexion withdrawal	3 Inappropriate cry, scream
1 No response	3 Flexion/Decorticate	2 Grunts
	2 Extension/Decerebrate	1 No response
	1 No response	
> 1 year	> 1 year	2–5 years
4 Spontaneous	6 Obeys	5 Appropriate words
3 To verbal	5 Localizes pain	4 Inappropriate words
2 To pain	4 Flexion withdrawal	3 Cries or screams
1 No response	3 Flexion/Decorticate	2 Grunts
	2 Extension/Decerebrate	1 No response
	1 No response	
		> 5 years
		5 Oriented
		4 Disoriented but converses
		3 Inappropriate words
		2 Incomprehensible
		1 No response

[1]Total score indicates that injury is mild (13–15), moderate (9–12), or severe (≤8).

Table 32-4 Revised Trauma Score (RTS)[1]

RTS—add each category	GCS	Systolic BP (mm Hg)	Respiratory rate
4	13–15	> 89	10–29
3	9–12	76–89	> 29
2	6–8	50–75	6–9
1	4–5	1–49	1–5
0	3	0	0

[1]RTSC—modified for children. RR > 29 is normal (4) if aged 0–3 years, RTS < 12 indicates possibility of significant trauma, RTS < 7 = 79% probability of emergent surgery.

Table 32-5 Initial Approach to Pediatric Trauma

Primary survey (0–5 minutes)			
Assessment	**Action**		
Airway—Assess air movement, while immobilizing cervical spine.	Endotracheal intubate if (1) unable to ventilate, (2) altered mentation/aspiration risk, (3) need for hyperventilation in head injury, (4) flail chest, (5) severe shock. See pages 15–17 for ET tube size and rapid sequence technique.		
Breathing—Assess ventilation effectiveness and oxygenation.	Apply pulse oximeter (± end-tidal CO_2 monitor), O_2, perform needle thoracostomy for tension pneumothorax, occlusive dressing for sucking chest wound, and ET tube if needed.		
Circulation—Assess strength, rate, quality of peripheral pulses, while stopping external bleed.	Attach cardiac monitor, apply pressure to external bleed. Insert two large peripheral venous lines, and draw blood for type and cross-match, and basic labs.		
See pages 5–6 for a complete list of normal vitals by length, weight, and age. See pages 10–11, 14 for central venous catheter sizes, and IO technique.	*Age*	*IV catheter size*	*Intraosseous size*
	0–1 year	20–22 gauge	17F
	> 1–6 years	18–20 gauge	15F
	8–12 years	16–20 gauge	—
	> 15 years	14–18 gauge	—
Disability—Assess pupils and alertness (AVPU)	Assess pupils + Pediatric GCS (page 317), **A**lert, responds to **V**oice, **P**ain, **U**nresponsive (AVPU)		
Exposure	Completely undress patient (begin radiant warming)		
Resuscitation (simultaneously performed during primary survey)			
Airway/Breathing	Reassess, see airway and breathing boxes above in this table		
Circulation	Note: Do not spend > 2–3 minutes attempting peripheral IV. If hypotensive, obtain IO or central venous access. Administer NS 20 ml/kg IV for hypotension/shock. Reassess, and repeat NS 20 ml/kg IV if needed. Administer O negative whole blood or packed RBCs 10–20 ml/kg.		

Table 32-5 Initial Approach to Pediatric Trauma (*Continued*)

Primary survey (0–5 minutes)	
Assessment	**Action**
	Insert NG tube, Foley catheter (see page 5 for size). A base deficit (BD) ≤ −8 mEq/L predicts a 15 × increased risk of transfusion requirement compared to a normal BD.
Secondary survey and definitive care	
Reassess ABCDE	Address any deterioration or new abnormalities. Insert chest tube prn (e.g., if prior needle thoracostomy).
Head-to-toe examination	Complete vital signs (do not forget back and rectal exams).
Address extremity injuries	Reduce dislocations compromising circulation.
Initial X-rays	Cervical spine, chest, pelvis, extremities, and CT scans as indicated by the physical exam.
Pain control, infection risk	Administer analgesics, antibiotics, tetanus.
Begin disposition	Call surgeon and consultants as need is identified. Initiate transfer, admission, or prepare for operating room. Splint fractures and dress wounds.
Documentation	Document all abnormalities (including X-ray, lab abnormalities), consults, and times. Talk with family.

ABDOMINAL TRAUMA

Table 32-6 Abdomen CT Criteria if Significant Pediatric Blunt Torso Trauma

Predictor panel[1]	Predictive values of predictor panel (95% confidence interval)	
• Low systolic BP	Sensitivity	95% (90–98%)[2]
• Abdomen tender	Specificity	49% (34–40%)
• Femur fracture	Negative predictive value	98% (96–99%)
• ALT > 125 U/L	Positive predictive value	20% (17–23%)
• AST > 200 U/L		
• Hematocrit < 30%		
• UA with > 5 RBC/hpf		
• Seat belt sign		

[1]Listed panel + GCS < 14 = author's prior cited indicators for abdominal CT. [2]Sensitivity for surgical intervention was 100% (1 nontherapeutic laparotomy performed).

Data from Holmes JF, Mao A, Awasthi S, McGahan JP, Wisner DH, Kuppermann N. Validation of a prediction rule for the identification of children with intra-abdominal injuries after blunt torso trauma. *Ann Emerg Med.* 2009;54(4):528-533; Borgialli DA, Ellison AM, Ehrlich P, et al. Association between the seat belt sign and intra-abdominal injuries in children with blunt torso trauma in motor vehicle collisions. *Acad Emerg Med.* 2014;21(11):1240-1248.

320 Trauma

Table 32-7 Predictors of Abdominal, GU Injury, and Death Based on Pelvic Fracture Class

Torode class[1]	Mortality	GU injury	Other fracture[2]	Neuro. injury	Abd. surgery
II	0%	6%	39%	61%	11%
III	3%	26%	49%	57%	13%
IV	13%	38%	56%	56%	40%

[1]See Table 26-10 for Torode and Zieg Class. [2]Others found that multiple pelvic fracture sites (80% associated injury) + RTS < 11 (see Table 32-4) predicted abdominal/GU injuries. If only single fracture site and RTS of 11 or 12, only 0.5% had intra-abdominal injury.
Data from Torode I, Zieg D, Pelvic fractures in children. *J Pediatr Orthop.* 1985;5:76; Silber JS, Flynn JM. Changing patterns of pediatric pelvic fractures with skeletal maturation: implications for classification and management. *J Pediatr Orthop.* 2002;22:22; Bond SJ, Gotschall CS, Eichelberger MR. Predictors of abdominal injury in children with pelvic fracture. *J Trauma.* 1991;31:1169-1173.

Table 32-8 Management of Blunt Abdominal and Flank Trauma

• 10% of trauma-related deaths
• Spleen > liver
• Main complications: bleeding; solid organ or vascular injury; peritonitis—hollow viscus perforation
• Validity of single pediatric FAST exam controversial—negative FAST cannot rule out intra-abdominal injury
• + FAST = immediate abdominal CT if stable
• Hemodynamically unstable patient needs OR

Modified from Tisherman SA, Forsythe, RM, Kellum, JA. *Trauma Intensive Care.* New York, NY: Oxford University Press; 2013:251-271; Schacherer N, Miller J, Petronis K. Pediatric blunt abdominal trauma in the emergency department: evidence-based management techniques. *Pediatr Emerg Med Pract.* 2014;11(10):1-23. Eric Brader, and Christina Halldorson. "Updates in Pediatric Trauma, Part I." *Pediatric Emergency Medicine Reports,* vol. 20, no. 4, AHC Media LLC, 3/24/2015. "Blunt Pelvic Trauma." *Trauma Reports,* vol. 15, no. 6, AHC Media, LLC, 11/1/2014.

HEAD AND NECK TRAUMA

Table 32-9 High Yield Criteria for Cranial Computed Tomography in Children < 2 Years Old After Trauma[1]

Predictors	Predictive values[4,5]	
• Altered mental status[2]	Sensitivity	100% (86–100%)
• Scalp hematoma[2]	Specificity	54% (52–56%)
• Loss of consciousness ≥ 5 seconds	Negative predictive value	100% (99.7–100%)
• Severe mechanism[3]	Positive predictive value	2% (1–2%)
• Palpable fracture		
• Not acting normal per parents		

[1]*Study inclusion criteria*—Head trauma within prior 24 hours with GCS 14–15 (page 317). *Exclusion criteria*—Penetrating trauma, known brain tumor, preexisting neurological disorder, prior CT pretransfer, ventricular shunt, bleeding disorder, or GCS < 14. [2]*Altered mental status*—GCS < 15, agitation, sleepy, slow response, repetitive questioning. *Scalp hematoma*—Frontal hematoma allowed. [3]*Severe mechanism*—Ejection from vehicle, death of another passenger, rollover, pedestrian or bicyclist without helmet struck by motor vehicle, fall > 3 feet, head struck by high-impact object. [4]*Predictive value* in detecting clinically important traumatic brain injury (ciTBI) if any one of predictors present with (95% confidence intervals). [5]*ciTBI detected by criteria*—Death from TBI, intubation > 24 hours for TBI, hospital admit ≥ 2 nights for abnormal CT.
Data from Kuppermann N, Holmes JF, Dayan PS, et al. Identification of children at very low risk of clinically-important brain injuries after head trauma: a prospective cohort study. *Lancet.* 2009;374(9696):1160-1170.

Table 32-10 PECARN Head Injury Criteria for Imaging (with Risk of ciTBI)[1]

	CT recommended	Dependent on clinical factors	CT not recommended
Age < 2 years old	GCS = 14 or other signs of altered mental status, or palpable skull fracture (4.4%)	Occipital/parietal/temporal scalp hematoma, history of loss of consciousness more than 5 seconds, severe mechanism of injury, or not acting normally per parent Observation vs. CT dependent on: Physician experience Multiple or isolated findings Worsening symptoms or signs after ED observation Age < 3 months old Parental preference (0.9%)	Previously mentioned features not present (<0.02%)
Age < 2 years old	GCS = 14 or other signs of altered mental status, or signs of basilar skull fracture (4.3%)	History of loss of consciousness, history of vomiting, severe mechanism of injury, or severe headache Observation vs. CT dependent on: Physician experience Multiple or isolated findings Worsening symptoms or signs after ED observation Parental preference (0.8%)	Previously mentioned features not present (<0.05%)

[1]For use in patients with GCS (Glasgow Coma Scale) scores of 14–15 following head trauma; ciTBI—clinically important traumatic brain injury.

Data from Kuppermann N, Holmes JF, Dayan PS, Hoyle JD Jr, Atabaki SM, Holubkov R, Nadel FM, Monroe D, Stanley RM, Borgialli DA, Badawy MK, Schunk JE, Quayle KS, Mahajan P, Lichenstein R, Lillis KA, Tunik MG, Jacobs ES, Callahan JM, Gorelick MH, Glass TF, Lee LK, Bachman MC, Cooper A, Powell EC, Gerardi MJ, Melville KA, Muizelaar JP, Wisner DH, Zuspan SJ, Dean JM, Wootton-Gorges SL; Pediatric Emergency Care Applied Research Network (PECARN). Identification of children at very low risk of clinically-important brain injuries after head trauma: a prospective cohort study. *Lancet*. 2009;374(9696):1160-70. doi: 10.1016/S0140-6736(09)61558-0.

Recognize signs and symptoms of Increased ICP:

- Vital sign changes: bradycardia, hypertension, abnormal respirations
- Pupillary dilation
- Extensor posturing
- Temporary treatment
- Hyperventilation titrated to reversal of pupillary dilation;
- Mannitol (0.5–1 g/kg) over 10 minutes, or hypertonic saline 3%; 1–3 mL/kg, up to a maximum dose of 250 mL
- Avoid hypoxia
- Ensure hemodynamic stability

source: Kochanek PM et al. Management of Pediatric Severe Traumatic Brain Injury: 2019 Consensus and Guidelines-Based Algorithm for First and Second Tier Therapies. Pediatr Crit Care Med. 2019;20(3):269.

Table 32-11 Consensus Statement on Concussion in Sports—Fifth International Conference, Berlin 2016

Suspected diagnosis of sports-related concussion (SRC) can include one or more of the following clinical domains: (a) Symptoms: somatic (e.g., headache), cognitive (e.g., feeling like in a fog), and/or emotional symptoms (e.g., lability) (b) Physical signs (e.g., loss of consciousness, amnesia, neurological deficit) (c) Balance impairment (e.g., gait unsteadiness) (d) Behavioral changes (e.g., irritability) (e) Cognitive impairment (e.g., slowed reaction times) (f) Sleep/Wake disturbance (e.g., somnolence, drowsiness)	
Step 1	**Immediately** remove from play.
Step 2	**Neuroimaging** only if concerned regarding bleed or increased ICP Concussion is clinical diagnosis. Consider possibility of C-spine injury. *Advanced neuroimaging, fluid biomarkers, and genetic testing are important research tools, but require further validation to determine their ultimate clinical utility in evaluation of SRC.*
Step 3	**Neurocognitive testing**—Prior *grading* systems have been abandoned in favor of individualized evaluation of each athlete. Standardized Sports Concussion Assessment Tool (SCAT5) or other sideline assessment tool. This evaluation tool includes a symptom score, physical sign score, GCS, balance assessment, coordination exam, and a cognitive assessment that are followed over time.
Step 4	**Observation**—The player should not be left alone after the injury, and serial monitoring for deterioration is essential over the initial few hours after injury. The patient should go to the hospital immediately if he or she experiences a new headache, drowsiness, the inability to recognize people or places, repeated vomiting, abnormal behavior (e.g., irritability), seizures, weakness, or sensory changes in arms or legs, unsteady gait, or speech changes. If concern regarding brain bleed, avoid NSAIDs and aspirin.
Step 5	**Return to play (RTP)**—See Table 32-13. Recommended that all athletes should have a clinical neurological assessment (including an evaluation of mental status/cognition, oculomotor function, gross sensorimotor, coordination, gait, vestibular function, and balance) as part of their overall management. Patients should spend at least 24 hours without any concussive symptoms or neurocognitive abnormalities at each RTP stage before progressing to the next step.

Modified from McCrory P, Meeuwisse W, Dvořák J, et al. Consensus statement on concussion in sport—the 5th international conference on concussion in sport held in Berlin, October 2016. *Br J Sports Med.* 2017;51(11):838-847.

Concussion is defined as a disturbance in brain function from trauma with or without loss of consciousness (LOC). Suspect if any: symptoms (headache, feel like in fog, emotion labile), LOC, amnesia, behavior change, impaired cognition, or sleep problem.

Table 32-12 Return to Play (RTP) Guidelines for Sports Concussions[1]

Stages of graduated return-to-sport (RTS) strategy

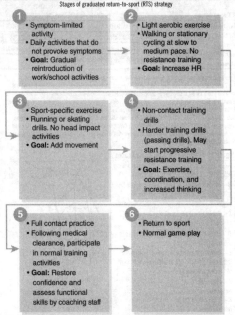

1.
- Symptom-limited activity
- Daily activities that do not provoke symptoms
- **Goal:** Gradual reintroduction of work/school activities

2.
- Light aerobic exercise
- Walking or stationary cycling at slow to medium pace. No resistance training
- **Goal:** Increase HR

3.
- Sport-specific exercise
- Running or skating drills. No head impact activities
- **Goal:** Add movement

4.
- Non-contact training drills
- Harder training drills (passing drills). May start progressive resistance training
- **Goal:** Exercise, coordination, and increased thinking

5.
- Full contact practice
- Following medical clearance, participate in normal training activities
- **Goal:** Restore confidence and assess functional skills by coaching staff

6.
- Return to sport
- Normal game play

[1]An initial period of 24–48 hours of both relative physical rest and cognitive rest is recommended before beginning the RTS progression.

There should be at least 24 hours for each step of the progression. If any symptoms worsen during exercise, the athlete should go back to the previous step. Resistance training should be added only in the later stages (stage 3 or 4 at the earliest). If symptoms are more than 10–14 days in adults or more than 1 month in children, the athlete should be referred to a healthcare professional who is an expert in the management of concussion.

McCrory P, Meeuwisse W, Dvořák J3, Aubry M, Bailes J, Broglio S, Cantu RC, Cassidy D, Echemendia RJ, Castellani RJ, Davis GA, Ellenbogen R, Emery C, Engebretsen L, Feddermann-Demont N, Giza CC, Guskiewicz KM, Herring S, Iverson GL, Johnston KM, Kissick J, Kutcher J, Leddy JJ, Maddocks D, Makdissi M, Manley GT, McCrea M, Meehan WP, Nagahiro S, Patricios J, Putukian M, Schneider KJ, Sills A, Tator CH, Turner M, Vos PE. Consensus statement on concussion in sport-the 5th international conference on concussion in sport held in Berlin, October 2016. *Br J Sports Med.* 2017;51(11):838-847. doi: 10.1136/bjsports-2017-097699.

Table 32-13 NEXUS Criteria for Cervical Spine Imaging in Pediatric Blunt Trauma[1]

NEXUS criteria	Operator characteristics (95% confidence interval)	
Midline tenderness	Sensitivity[1]	100% (89–100%)
Impaired consciousness, poor history	Specificity	20% (19–21%)
Neurologic deficit	Negative predictive value	100% (99–100%)
Distracting/Painful injury Intoxication	Positive predictive value	1% (1–2%)

[1]CT preferred if high risk, NEXUS C-spine (prospective) study included 3,065 children <18 years old (88 ≤2 years, 817 = 2–8 years, and 2,160 = 8–17 years). Other retrospective studies found that NEXUS criteria were only 43–94% sensitive in detecting significant pediatric C-spine injury with 100% sensitivity if >8 years old. NEXUS may not apply if ≤2–8 years old, or if underlying congenital/acquired spine instability. Data from Viccellio P, Simon H, Pressman BD. A prospective multicenter study of cervical spine injury in children. *Pediatrics.* 2001;108:e20; Garton HJ, Hammer MR. Detection of pediatric cervical spine injury. *Neurosurgery.* 2008;62:700–708; Ehrlich PF, Wee C, Drongowski R, Rana AR. Canadian C-spine rule and the national emergency X-radiography utilization low-risk criteria for C-spine radiography in young trauma patients. *J Pediatr Surg.* 2009;44:987.

Figure 32-1 Normal Cervical Spine Spaces

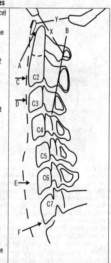

A—Atlantal dens interval—(*Predental space*) <5mm if <8 years, >8 years <3 mm.

B—Posterior cervical line, spino-laminar line of C2 should be within 2 mm anterior or posterior to line.

C—Prevertebral space ≤7 mm in front of C2 or < 1/3 width of C2 vert. body.

D—Limit of overriding of vertebral bodies is 2.5 mm.

E—Retrotracheal space should be <14 mm in front of C6 or < 5/4 of width of C5 in front of C5 (# are inexact)

F—Prevertebral fat stripe—should not bulge out.

X ÷ Y = Power's ratio

Normal value is 0.7–1.0

Value < 0.7 suggests anterior subluxation atlantooccipital (AA) joint.

Also, a line from the anterior margin of the foramen magnum to the tip of the odontoid should be <10–12 mm. If greater, atlanto-occipital dislocation may be present.

Wackenheim line—a line drawn along posterior clivus usually intersects tip of odontoid tangentially. If displaced, suspect atlantooccipital joint laxity. May be unreliable in young children.

Table 32-14 Cervical Spine Anatomy in Children < 8 Years Old

Normal lordosis to cervical spine is absent in 14% of children.
Normal posterior angulation of odontoid seen in up to 4% of children.
Majority of injuries occur at C1–C2 ≤ 8 years old and lower cervical spine > 8 years.
Os odontoideum—Congenital anomaly where odontoid does not fuse with C2.[1]
Ossiculum terminale—A secondary center of ossification for odontoid tip, appears by age 3 (in 26% of children) and fuses with odontoid by 12 (may never fuse).
Prevertebral space at C3 is ≤ 1/3–2/3 of C3 vertebral body width or ≤ 5–7 mm.[2]
Prevertebral space at C5 is ≤ 5/4 of (C5 or C6) vertebral body width or ≤ 14 mm.[2]
Predental space up to 5 mm ≤ 8 years (up to 3 mm > 8 years).
Pseudo-Jeffersonian fracture-C1 lateral masses grow faster than C2 so C1 overlaps C2 (usually <6 mm). Present in 90% age 1–2, 18% aged 7 years.
Pseudosubluxation of C2/C3 or C3/C4 in 40% (normal variant where anterior aspect of C2 spinolaminar line is ≤ 2 mm anterior or posterior to posterior cervical line; see page 324).

[1]Spine injury with minor trauma occurs. [2]These norms can be unreliable in children.

Table 32-15 Development of Cervical Spine

Age	Feature
<6 months	C1 ring invisible and all synchondroses are open, vertebrate are normally wedged anteriorly, and there is often no lordosis to the uninjured spine.
1 year	Body of C1 becomes visible radiographically.
3 years	Posteriorly located spinous process synchondroses fuse. Dens becomes ossified (visible radiographically).
3–6 years	Neurocentral (body) and C2-odontoid synchondroses fuse. Summit ossification center appears at the apex (top) of the odontoid. Anterior wedging of the vertebral bodies resolve (now is not normal if seen).
8 years	Pseudosubluxation and predental widening resolve, lordosis is normal now.
12–14 years	Secondary ossification centers appear at spinous process tips (mistaken for fractures), summit ossification center of odontoid fuses (if it does not, *os odontoideum* occurs), superior/inferior epiphyseal rings appear on the body.
25 years	Secondary ossification centers at tips of spinous processes fuse, superior/inferior epiphyseal rings fuse to the vertebral body.

SPINAL CORD INJURY WITHOUT RADIOLOGIC ABNORMALITY (SCIWORA)

SCIWORA accounts for 1/5 of all pediatric spinal cord injuries. Immediate plain films, CT are always normal, immediate MRI is normal in up to 50% with atrophy of spinal cord evident on MRI performed 1–3 months after the accident. Those with initial normal MRI almost always have 100% recovery. Delayed onset of neurologic deficit occurs in 54% (mean 1.2 days), with half of the delayed subset complaining of paresthesias at the time of the accident; 83% of cases involve the cervical cord, and 2/3 are 8 years old or younger; 44% have isolated sensory, 31% isolated motor, and 25% motor plus sensory deficits. For children with delayed paralysis, progression of weakness is rapid and usually causes complete cord lesion.

Sources: Kriss VM, Kriss TC. SCIWORA (spinal cord injury without radiographic abnormality) in infants and children. *Clin Pediatr (Phila).* 1996;35:119; Baker C, Kadish H, Schunk JE. Evaluation of pediatric cervical spine injuries. *Am J Emerg Med.* 1999;17:230; Grabb PA, Pang D. Magnetic resonance imaging in the evaluation of spinal cord injury without radiographic abnormality in children. *Neurosurgery.* 1994;35:406.

Table 32-16 Spinal Cord Injury Syndromes[1]

Anterior cord syndrome	Central cord syndrome
• Flexion or vertical compression injury to anterior cord or spinal artery	• Hyperextension injury
• Complete motor paralysis	• Motor weakness in hands > arms
• Hyperalgesia with preserved touch and proprioception (position sense)	• Legs are unaffected or less affected
• Loss of pain and temperature sense	• Variable bladder/sensory deficit
• Most likely cord injury to require surgery	• Prognosis is generally good and most do not require surgery

Complete cord injury	Brown-Séquard syndrome
• Flaccid below injury level	• Hemisection of cord
• Absent deep tendon reflexes	• Ipsilateral weakness
• Decreased sympathetics	• Ipsilateral loss of proprioception
• Warm skin, low BP, and slow HR	• Contralateral loss of pain and temperature sensation
• Sensation may be preserved	

	Posterior cord syndrome
• Priapism may be present	• Pain, tingling of neck and hands
• If lasts > 24 hours, will be complete	• 1/3 have upper extremity weakness
	• Mild form of central cord syndrome

[1] Diffuse flexion withdrawal can occur in children with paralyzed limbs if stimulated.

STEROID PROTOCOL FOR TREATMENT OF ACUTE SPINAL CORD INJURY

According to the American Association of Neurological Surgeons and Congress of Neurological Surgeons and American Academy of Emergency Medicine, the use of steroids in acute spinal cord injury is not recommended.

Source: Hurlbert RJ, Hadley MN, Walters BC, et al. Pharmacological therapy for acute spinal cord injury. *Neurosurgery.* 2013;72 (Suppl 2):93-105.

Table 32-17 Management of the Penetrating Neck Injury

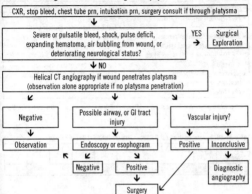

Modified from Múnera F, Cohn S, Rivas LA. Penetrating Injuries of the neck: use of helical computed tomographic angiography. J Trauma. 2005;58(2):413–418; Hogan AR, Lineen EB, Perez EA, Neville HL, Thompson WR, Sola JE. Value of computed tomographic angiography in neck and extremity pediatric vascular trauma. J Pediatr Surg. 2009;44(6):1236–1241.

Table 32-18 Evaluation of Suspected Urethral Trauma

Retrograde urethrogram indications	Retrograde urethrogram technique
• Penile, perineal, vaginal, or scrotal trauma • Blood at urethral meatus or cannot void • Extravasation of blood/urine to scrotum, perineum, abdominal wall, or penile shaft • Abnormal prostate examination • Significant pelvic fracture • Inability to easily pass Foley catheter	• Obtain preinjection KUB film • Place Cooke adapter or Christmas tree adapter on end of 30–60 ml syringe (may substitute Foley) • Inject 0.2 ml/kg of contrast dye over 60 seconds • Take X-ray during last 10 seconds

Table 32-19 Evaluation of Suspected Bladder Trauma

Cystogram indications	Cystogram technique
• Penetrating injury to low abdomen or pelvis • Blunt lower abdominal-perineal trauma with significant microscopic hematuria (> 20 RBC/hpf), gross blood, blood at meatus • Significant pelvic fracture • Unable to void or minimal urine after Foley	• After urethrogram, empty bladder • Instill contrast into bladder until 5 ml/kg or discomfort or bladder is full (see formula below for normal bladder volumes[1]) • Obtain oblique, and AP films of bladder, empty bladder then repeat films

[1]*Bladder volume* if [< 1 year = weight (kg) × 10 ml]; if [≥ 1 year = (age in years + 2) × 30 ml].

Table 32-20 Estimated Urethral Catheter Size (French/Fr) Based on Age

Age (years)	1 day	3 months	1	3	6	8	10	12	Teen
Size (Fr)	5	8	8–10	10	10	10–12	12	12–14	16+

Table 32-21 Independent Predictors of Intrathoracic Injury if Significant Pediatric Blunt Torso Trauma

Predictors	Predictive values[1] (95% confidence interval)	
• ↓ BP or ↑ resp rate • Chest wall tender • Abraded/Contused • Specificity • ↓ Breath sounds, or rales or rhonchi • Femur fracture • GCS < 15	Sensitivity	98% (91–100%)[2]
	Specificity	37% (34–40%)
	Negative predictive value	99% (98–100%)
	Positive predictive value	12% (10–15%)

[1]Predictive value if any one of the identified predictors is present. [2]100% sensitive in predicting abnormality requiring therapy in this single study.

Data from Holmes JF, Sokolove PE, Brant WE, Kuppermann N. A clinical decision rule for identifying children with thoracic injuries after blunt torso trauma. *Ann Emerg Med.* 2002;39(5):492-499.

Table 32-22 Rib Fracture Etiology in Infants < 1 Year

Abuse	82%	Fragile bones[1]	8%
Nonintentional	8%	Birth trauma	3%

[1]Includes osteogenesis imperfecta, rickets, prematurity.

Table 32-23 Chest Tube Sizes (French/Fr) for Hemothorax/Pneumothorax Based on Age

Age (years)	1 month	0.5	1	3	5–6	8	12	16
Size (Fr)	12–18	14–20	14–24	16–28	20–32	24–32	28–36	28–40

Modified from Schafermeyer R. Pediatric trauma. *Emerg Med Clin North Am.* 1993;11:187-205.

33 ■ UROLOGY

GENITAL DISORDERS—MALE

Table 33-1 Clinical Features of Common Conditions Associated with Scrotal Pain in Children and Adolescents[1]

	Acute epididymitis	Testicular torsion	Torsion of appendage
History			
Duration of pain	> 24 hours	< 12 hours	> 12 hours
Dysuria/Pyuria	Common	Rare	
Nausea/Vomiting	Uncommon	Common	Uncommon
onset of pain	Gradual	Acute/Sudden	
Peak incidence	< 2 years old and postpubertal	Perinatal and puberty	Prepubertal
Previous episode	Unusual	Typical	Unusual
Trauma	Unusual	Occasional	Unusual
Imaging			
Blood flow on color Doppler ultrasound	Normal or increased	Decreased	Normal or increased
Physical examination			
Cremasteric reflex	Usually present	Usual absent	Usually present
Scrotal edema/ erythema	Common > 12 hours		
Suggestive findings	None	High-riding testicle in horizontal plane	Palpable nodule "blue-dot"
Tenderness	Epididymis, then diffuse	Testis, then diffuse	Appendage, then testis

[1]Adapted from Brenner J, Ojo A. Causes of scrotal pain in children and adolescents. UpToDate. https://www.uptodate.com/contents/causes-of-scrotal-pain-in-children-and-adolescents. Accessed June 2018.

1. Testicular torsion
   * Testicular torsion results from inadequate fixation of the testis to the tunica vaginalis through the gubernaculum testis, leading to "bell clapper" deformity (testis resting in horizontal plane).
   * Testicular torsion is a clinical diagnosis and immediate urology consultation is imperative when suspected for surgical detorsion and fixation. Do not wait for the ultrasound to confirm the diagnosis.
   * Color Doppler ultrasound of the scrotum is the first-line imaging modality given its timely accessibility compared to the nuclear scan. It is generally indicated for cases with equivocal clinical findings. The reported sensitivity and specificity range from 69 to 100% and 77–100%, respectively.[1–7]
   * Consider manual detorsion prior to surgery if emergency operative care is not available in a timely manner. Use the "open book maneuver"—the external rotation of the testicle 360 degrees one to two times under appropriate sedation and analgesia.
2. Torsion of appendage
   * Torsion of appendix testis or appendix epididymis. The physical examination typically reveals a nontender testicle and a tender localized mass at the superior or inferior pole. A "blue dot" represents a gangrenous appendage seen through the scrotum.
   * Torsion of appendage is a clinical diagnosis. Color Doppler ultrasound is indicated for cases where testicular torsion cannot be excluded.
   * Supportive management with analgesics and scrotal support.
3. Acute epididymitis
   * Commonly occurs in sexually active late adolescents but also seen in prepubertal boys with anatomical/functional abnormalities in the urinary tract.
   * Perform urinalysis and urine culture. Consider further testing for sexually transmitted infections such as nucleic acid amplification for *Chlamydia trachomatis* and *Neisseria gonorrhea*.
   * Antibiotic treatment options vary depending on the etiology, if indicated. Refer to "epididymitis antibiotic recommendations" on page 148.
4. Other common conditions associated with scrotal pain in children and adolescents include:
   * Trauma
   * Incarcerated inguinal hernia
   * Orchitis (mumps, coxsackie, and parvovirus)
   * IgA vasculitis (Henoch-Schönlein purpura)

REFERENCES

1. Kadish HA, Bolte RG. A retrospective review of pediatric patients with epididymitis, testicular torsion, and torsion of testicular appendages. *Pediatrics.* 1998;102:73.
2. Lam WW, Yap TL, Jacobsen AS, Teo HJ. Colour Doppler ultrasonography replacing surgical exploration for acute scrotum: myth or reality? *Pediatr Radiol.* 2005;35:597.
3. Paltiel HJ, Connolly LP, Atala A, et al. Acute scrotal symptoms in boys with an indeterminate clinical presentation: comparison of color Doppler sonography and scintigraphy. *Radiology.* 1998;207:223.
4. Baker LA, Sigman D, Mathews RI, et al. An analysis of clinical outcomes using color Doppler testicular ultrasound for testicular torsion. *Pediatrics.* 2000;105:604.
5. Yazbeck S, Patriquin HB. Accuracy of Doppler sonography in the evaluation of acute condition of the scrotum in children. *J Pediatr Surg.* 1994;29:1270.
6. Kass EJ, Stone KT, Cacciarelli AA, Mitchell B. Do all children with an acute scrotum require exploration? *J Urol.* 1993;150:667.
7. Nussbaum-Blask AR, Bulas D, Shalaby-Rana E, et al. Color Doppler sonography and scintigraphy of the testis: a prospective, comparative analysis in children with acute scrotal pain. *Pediatr Emerg Care.* 2002;18:67.

APPENDIX

Table A-1 Commonly Used Oral Medications

Medication	Strength (mg/5 ml)	mg/kg/dose	Age:	2 months	4 months	6 months	9 months	12 months	15 months	2 years	3 years	5 years
			Weight (kg):	5	6.5	8	10	10	11	13	15	19
			Frequency	ml per dose								
acetaminophen	160 mg/5 ml	15	every 6 hours	2.3	3	3.8	4.2	4.7	5.2	6.1	7	8.9
ibuprofen	100 mg/5 ml	10	every 6 hours	–	–	4	4.5	5	5.5	6.5	7.5	9.5
amoxicillin	125 mg/5 ml	25	bid	5	6.5	8	9	10	11	13	15	19
amoxicillin	250 mg/5 ml	25	bid	2.5	3.3	4	4.5	5	5.5	6.5	7.5	9.5
amoxicillin	400 mg/5 ml	45[1]	bid	2.8	3.7	4.5	5.1	5.6	6.2	7.3	8.4	10.7
amoxicillin/ clavulanic acid	200 mg/28.5 mg/5 ml	20 (amox)	bid	2.5	3.3	4	4.5	5	5.5	6.5	7.5	9.5
azithromycin[3,4]	100 mg/5 ml	5	daily	1.3[2]	1.6[2]	2	2.3	2.5	2.8	3.3	3.8	4.8
azithromycin[3,4]	200 mg/5 ml	5	daily	0.6[2]	0.8[2]	1	1.1	1.3	1.4	1.6	1.9	2.4
cefaclor[3]	125 mg/5 ml	20	bid	4	5.2	6.4	7.2	8	8.8	10.4	12	15.2
cefaclor[3]	250 mg/5 ml	20	bid	2	2.6	3.2	3.6	4	4.4	5.2	6	7.6
cefadroxil	125 mg/5 ml	15	bid	3	3.9	4.8	5.4	6	6.6	7.8	9	11.4
cefadroxil	250 mg/5 ml	15	bid	1.5	2	2.4	2.7	3	3.3	3.9	4.5	5.7
cefdinir	125 mg/5 ml	14	daily	2.8[2]	3.6[2]	4.5	5	5.6	6.2	7.3	8.4	10.6
cefixime[4]	100 mg/5 ml	8	daily	2	2.6	3.2	3.6	4	4.4	5.2	6	7.6

cefprozil	125 mg/5 ml	15	bid	3[2]	3.9[2]	4.8	5.4	6	6.6	7.8	9	11.4
cefprozil	250 mg/5 ml	15	bid	1.5[2]	2[2]	2.4	2.7	3	3.3	3.9	4.5	5.7
cephalexin	125 mg/5 ml	12.5	four times per day	2.5	3.3	4	4.5	5	5.5	6.5	7.5	9.5
cephalexin	250 mg/5 ml	12.5	four times per day	1.3	1.6	2	2.3	2.5	2.8	3.3	3.8	4.8
clindamycin	75 mg/5 ml	10	three times per day	3.3	4.3	5.3	6	6.7	7.3	8.7	10	12.7
penicillin V[5]	250 mg/5 ml	250 mg/dose	bid/three times per day	—	5	5	5	5	5	5	5	5
SMX/TMP(Bactrim)	200 mg SMX: 40 mg TMP/5 ml	5 (TMP)	bid	3.1	4.1	5	5.6	6.3	6.9	8.1	9.4	11.9
diphenhydramine	12.5 mg/5 ml	1.25	every 6 hours	2.5	3.3	4	4.5	5	5.5	6.5	7.5	9.5
cetirizine	5 mg/5 ml	2.5 mg/dose	daily	—	—	2.5	2.5	2.5	2.5	2.5	2.5	2.5
prednisolone	15 mg/5 ml	1	daily	1.7	2.2	2.7	3	3.3	3.7	4.3	5	6.3
prednisone	5 mg/5 ml	1	daily	5	6.5	8	9	10	11	13	15	19

[1]AAP recommends 80–90 mg/kg/day for otitis media in children. Augmentin used as ES only. [2]Dosing at this age/weight is NOT recommended by the manufacturer. [3]Dose shown is for otitis media only; see dose in text for alternative indications. [4]Give a double dose of drug (azithromycin) for the first day. [5]AHA dosing for streptococcal pharyngitis. Treat for 10 days.

Table A-2 Critical Drugs and IV Infusions[1]

adenosine	• 0.1 mg/kg IV *rapid* push (max dose 6 mg), second dose 0.2 mg/kg IV *rapid* push (max dose 12 mg).
amiodarone	• 5 mg/kg IV bolus if pulseless VT/VF (max dose 300 mg). Administer over 20–60 minutes if perfusing rhythm. May repeat to daily max of 15 mg/kg.
atropine	• 0.02 mg/kg IV (max dose 0.5 mg)[2].
diazepam	• 0.1–0.3 mg/kg IV (max dose 10 mg). 0.5 mg/kg PR (2–5 years old); 0.3 mg/kg PR (6–11 years old); 0.2 mg/kg (≥ 12 years old). Max PR dose 20 mg.
dobutamine	• 0.5–20 mcg/kg/minute IV infusion. Titrate to desired effect.
dopamine	• 2–20 mcg/kg/minute IV infusion. Titrate to desired effect.
enalaprilat	• 0.005–0.01 mg/kg IV (max dose 1.25 mg).
epinephrine	• Pulseless arrest: 0.01 mg/kg IV every 3–5 minutes (max single dose 1 mg). • Infusion: 0.1–1 mcg/kg/minute. • Anaphylaxis: 0.01 mg/kg IM every 15 minutes prn (max single dose 0.3 mg).
esmolol	• 100–500 mcg/kg IV bolus (optional), followed by infusion of 25–100 mcg/kg/minute. Titrate infusion by 25–50 mcg/kg/minute every 5–10 minutes up to 500 mcg/kg/minute.
fosphenytoin[3]	• 15–20 mg PE/kg IV (preferred) or IM. Max infusion rate for loading dose: 150 mg PE/minute.
isoproterenol	• 0.05–1 mcg/kg/minute IV infusion. Titrate to desired effect.
labetalol	• 0.2–1 mg/kg IV bolus (max 40 mg). Infusion: 0.25–3 mg/kg/hour (initiate infusion at low end of dosing range & titrate slowly).
levetiracetam	• 20–60 mg/kg IV bolus (max 3,000–4,500 mg/dose).
lidocaine	• 1 mg/kg IV; infusion: 20–50 mcg/kg/minute.
lorazepam	• 0.05–0.1 mg/kg IV (max single dose 4 mg).
midazolam	• 0.05–0.2 mg/kg IV/IM (max 10 mg); 0.2 mg/kg intranasal (max 10 mg). Infusion: 0.03–0.12 mg/kg/hour. Titrate to desired effect.
milrinone	• 50 mcg/kg IV over 10–60 minutes (optional), followed by infusion of 0.25–0.75 mcg/kg/minute IV infusion.
nicardipine	• 0.5–5 mcg/kg/minute IV infusion.
nitroprusside	• 0.3–10 mcg/kg/minute IV infusion.
norepinephrine	• 0.05–2 mcg/kg/minute IV infusion.

Table A-2 Critical Drugs and IV Infusions[1] (*Continued*)

pentobarbital	• 1–2 mg/kg IV bolus, followed by infusion of 0.5–1 mg/kg/hour[4]. Titrate slowly to desired effect.
phenobarbital	• 15–20 mg/kg IV (max dose 1,000 mg). Max infusion rate for loading dose: 1 mg/kg/minute, not to exceed 30 mg/minute.
phenylephrine	• 5–20 mcg/kg IV q 10–15 minutes. Infusion: 0.1–2 mcg/kg/minute.
procainamide	• 10–15 mg/kg (max 1,500 mg) IV over 30–60 minutes. Infusion: 20–80 mcg/kg/minute. Stop for hypotension or QRS widens by 50% of original width.
prostaglandin E₁ (alprostadil)	• 0.05–0.1 mcg/kg/minute IV infusion initially. Once therapeutic response is achieved, decrease rate to lowest effective dose. Usual dosing range: 0.01–0.4 mcg/kg/minute.

[1]Details regarding indications, dosing, side effects, and contraindications are listed for resuscitation (Table 2-11), cardiovascular (pages 48–49), HTN (Table 16-2), seizures (Table 22-5). [2]Minimum dose of 0.1 mg is controversial and not recommended in patients < 5 kg due to reports of toxicity. [3]PE—phenytoin equivalents. [4]Higher loading dose (10–15 mg/kg) may be used to induce pentobarbital coma.

INDEX

A

AARS. *See* atlantoaxial rotary subluxation
abbreviated cross-match blood test, 131
abdominal complications of sickle cell anemia, 119
abdominal pain, causes of, 283
abdominal trauma, 319–320
abscess
  antibiotics, 143
  brain, 144
  epidural, 244, 260
  retropharyngeal, 261
abuse (nonaccidental trauma), 1–4
acetabulum/femur, 256
acetaminophen
  dose, 20
  overdose, 296–297
acidosis, inborn errors, 197
acrodermatitis enteropathica, 59
ACS. *See* acute chest syndrome
activated factor VIIa, 121
acute asthma exacerbation, 263
acute cerebellar ataxia, 208
acute chest syndrome (ACS), 117–118
acute gastroenteritis (AGE), 106
acute leukemia, 65
acute otitis media (AOM), 186
acute radiation syndrome, 36–37
acyanotic heart disease, 52
AD. *See* atopic dermatitis
adenosine, 48
adrenal crisis therapy, 69–70
adrenal insufficiency, 69–70

advanced life support. *See* life support, advanced
aerosolized racemic epinephrine, 273
AGE. *See* acute gastroenteritis
agitated patient
  evaluation and management of, 276
  medication management for, 277–278
airway and anesthesia, 15–24
  airway management, 15–20
  analgesia, 20–24
airway management, 15–20
albumin, 131
albuterol, 26
allergic dermatitis, 62
alpha viruses, 35
ALTE. *See* apparent life-threatening event
altered level of consciousness, assessment of, 202
altered mental status, infant/child with, 202–203
amicar, 121
amiodarone, 48
ampicillin, 32
analgesia, 20–24
anaphylaxis, 25–27, 131
  hereditary angioedema, 27
  management of, 25–26
anemia, 115–116
angioedema, hereditary, 27
ankle, 255, 257–258
anterior cord syndrome, 326
anthrax, 30–32
anthrax vaccine adsorbed (AVA) BioThrax, 31
antiarrhythmic agents, 48–49

AOM. *See* acute otitis media
aortic coarctation (CoA), 134
Apgar scoring, 9
aplastic anemia, 65
aplastic crisis in sickle cell anemia, 118
apophysitis, 248, 250, 257, 258
apparent life-threatening event (ALTE), 28
appendicitis, 285–287
Apt-Downey test, 112
arrhythmias, 45
arrhythmogenic right ventricular cardiomyopathy, 41
arthritis, 237–245
  bacterial. *See* bacterial arthritis
  septic. *See* septic arthritis
Ask Suicide-Screening Questions (ASQ), 275
asthma, 263–267
  guidelines for ED management of, 265
  inhaled medications, 266–267
  oral medications, 267
  parenteral agents, 266
  peak expiratory flow rate, 263
  pediatric asthma severity score, 264
  -related death, risk factors for, 264
  severity of acute asthma exacerbation, 263
ataxia, 207–208
atlantoaxial rotary subluxation (AARS), 260
atopic dermatitis (AD), 61–62
atrial fibrillation, 46–47